BIOCHEMICAL CHARACTERIZATION OF LYMPHOKINES

PROCEEDINGS OF THE SECOND INTERNATIONAL LYMPHOKINE WORKSHOP

ACADEMIC PRESS RAPID MANUSCRIPT REPRODUCTION

PROCEEDINGS OF THE SECOND INTERNATIONAL LYMPHOKINE WORKSHOP HELD IN ERMATINGEN, SWITZERLAND, MAY 27–31, 1979

BIOCHEMICAL CHARACTERIZATION OF LYMPHOKINES

PROCEEDINGS OF THE SECOND INTERNATIONAL LYMPHOKINE WORKSHOP

edited by

ALAIN L. DE WECK
FLEMMING KRISTENSEN
Institute for Clinical Immunology
University of Bern, Switzerland

MAURICE LANDY
Schweizerisches Forschungsinstitut
Davos, Switzerland

ACADEMIC PRESS
A Subsidiary of Harcourt Brace Jovanovich, Publishers
New York London Sydney Toronto San Francisco 1980

ACADEMIC PRESS, INC.
111 Fifth Avenue, New York, New York 10003

United Kingdom Edition published by
ACADEMIC PRESS, INC. (LONDON) LTD.
24/28 Oval Road, London NW1 7DX

Library of Congress Cataloging in Publication Data

International Lymphokine Workshop, 2d, Ermatingen,
Switzerland, 1979.
Biochemical characterization of lymphokines.

1. Lymphokines—Congresses. I. de Weck,
Alain L. II. Kristensen, Flemming. III. Landy,
Maurice. IV. Title. [DNLM: 1. Lymphokines—
Congresses. W3 IN729 2d 1979b / QW568 I595 1979b]
QR185.8.L93I57 1979 616.07′9 80-289
ISBN 0-12-213950-X

PRINTED IN THE UNITED STATES OF AMERICA

80 81 82 83 9 8 7 6 5 4 3 2 1

CONTENTS

SESSION VI: NONANTIGEN SPECIFIC MONOKINES AND LYMPHOKINES INFLUENCING T AND B CELL FUNCTIONS

Chairmen: J. J. Oppenheim and B. Waksman

SESSION VII: ANTIGEN-SPECIFIC HELPER AND SUPPRESSOR FACTORS

Chairmen: M. Feldmann and E. Diener

SESSION VIII: EFFECTS OF LYMPHOKINES *IN VIVO*

Chairmen: S. Cohen

CONTRIBUTORS

Numbers in parentheses indicate the pages on which the authors' contribution begin.

N. ADELMAN (47), Department of Pathology, University of Connecticut Health Center, Farmington, Connecticut

M. ALTIN (489), Department of Molecular Biology, Vanderbilt University, Nashville, Tennessee 37235

A. ALTMAN (519), Department of Cellular and Developmental Immunology, Scripps Clinic and Research Foundation, La Jolla, California 92037

R. N. APTE (227), Department of Life Sciences, Bar-Ilan University, Ramat-Gan, Israel

H. ARNHEITER (393), Division of Experimental Microbiology Institute for Medical Microbiology, University of Zürich, Zürich 8028, Switzerland

T. BABA (593), Department of Pathology, University of Connecticut Health Center, Farmington, Connecticut 06032

P. E. BAKER (253), Department of Medicine, Dartmouth Medical School, Hanover, New Hampshire 03755

G. D. BALL (343), Department of Virology, Wellcome Research Laboratories, Beckenham, Kent, England

T. E. BECHTOLD (519), Department of Cellular and Developmental Immunology, Scripps Clinic and Research Foundation, La Jolla, California 92037

D. I. BELLER (427), Harvard Medical School, Boston, Massachusetts 02115

B. BENACERRAF (551), Department of Pathology, Harvard Medical School, Boston, Massachusetts 02115

K. BENDTZEN (99), TUFTS—New England Medical Center, Boston, Massachusetts

H. A. BERNHEIM (79), Department of Internal Medicine, Yale University, New Haven, Connecticut 06510

N. BERSCH (221), Department of Medicine, UCLA School of Medicine, Los Angeles, California 90024

L. H. BLOCK (79), Department of Internal Medicine, Yale University, New Haven, Connecticut 06510

B. BÖDEKER (133), Gesellschaft für Biotechnologische Forshung mbH, Braunschweig, BRG

D. L. BOROS (599), Department of Immunology and Microbiology, Wayne State University School of Medicine, Detroit, Michigan 48201

D. BOUT (75), Harvard Medical School, Boston, Massachusetts 02115

J. A. BRAATZ (87), Laboratory of Immunodiagnosis, National Cancer Institute, Bethesda, Maryland

I. A. BRAUDE (331), Interferon Laboratories, Memorial Sloan–Kettering Cancer Center, New York, New York 10021

A. P. BROWN (93), Department of Medicine, Harvard Medical School, Robert B. Brigham Hospital, Boston, Massachusetts 02115

M. J. BRUNDA (369), Laboratory of Immunodiagnosic National Cancer Institute, Bethesda, Maryland 20014

K. T. BRUNNER (513), Department of Immunology, Swiss Institute for Experimental Cancer Research, Epalinges s/Lausanne, Switzerland

S. J. BUCHOK (193), Cancer Research Center, Columbia, Missouri 65201

C. J. BURMAN (343), Department of Virology, Wellcome Research Laboratories, Veckenham, Kent, England

D. CAMERON (137), Department of Medicine, Harvard Medical School, Boston, Massachusetts 02115

K. CANTELL (375), Central Public Health Laboratory, Helsinki, Finland

J. M. CARDENAS (519), Department of Cellular and Developmental Immunology, Scripps Clinic and Research Foundation, La Jolla, California 92037

L. CARRICK, JR. (599), Department of Immunology and Microbiology, Wayne State University School of Medicine, Detroit, Michigan 48201

A. C. CARVALHO (531), Departments of Pathology and Medicine, Harvard Medical School, Boston, Massachusetts 02114

J-Ch. CEROTTINI (513), Unit of Human Cancer Immunology, Ludwig Institute for Cancer Research, Epalinges s/Lausanne, Switzerland

C. M. CHANG (199), Virginia Mason Research Center, Seattle Washington

M. CHUN (473), Department of Immunology, Memorial Sloan–Kettering Cancer Center, New York, New York 10021

W. H. CHURCHILL (137, 531), Department of Medicine, Harvard Medical School, Boston, Massachusetts 02115

M. C. COHEN (7), Department of Pathology, University of Connecticut Health Center, Farmington, Connecticut 06032

S. COHEN (7, 47, 593), Department of Pathology, University of Connecticut Health Center, Farmington, Connecticut 06032

J. R. F. CORVALAN (571), Lilly Research Center, Erl Wood Manor, Windlesham, Surrey, England

S. CROME (249), Immunology Unit, The Rayne Institute,St. Thomas' Hospital, London, England

H. DALÜGGE (365), Medical School of Hanover, Hanover FRG

J. R. DAVID (1, 75), Harvard Medical School,Boston, Massachusetts 02115

J-M. DAYER (439), Harvard Medical School, Massachusetts General Hospital, Boston, Massachusetts 02114

J. H. DEAN (353), Department of Immunology, Litton Bionetics, Kensington, Maryland

E. DE MAEYER (383), Institut Curie-Biologie Université de Paris–Sud, Orsay, France

J. DEMAEYER-GUIGNARD (383), Institut Curie-Biologie Université de Paris–Sud, Orsay, France

F. C. DEN HOLLANDER (109), Organon Scientific Development Group, Oss, the Netherlands

J.-P. DESSAINT (435), Department of Pathology and Biology, Yale University, New Haven, Connecticut 06510

A. L. DE WECK (15, 67), Institute for Clinical Immunology, Instelspital, Bern, Switzerland

E. DIENER (557), Department of Immunology and MRC Group on Immunoregulation, University of Alberta, Edmonton, Alberta, Canada

G. Di SABATO (489), Department of Molecular Biology, Vanderbilt University, Nashville, Tennessee 37235

J. Y. DJEU (369), Division of Virology, Bureau of Biologics, Bethesda, Maryland

W. DOMZIG (169), Max-Planck-Institut für Immunbiologie, Freiburg, FRG

M. E. DORF (551), Department of Pathology, Harvard Medical School, Boston, Massachusetts 02115

D. C. DUMONDE (249), Immunology Unit, The Rayne Institute, St. Thomas' Hospital, London, England

A. M. DVORAK (205, 531), Departments of Pathology and Medicine, Harvard Medical School, Boston, Massachusetts 02114

H. F. DVORAK (205, 531), Departments of Pathology and Medicine, Harvard Medical School, Boston, Massachusetts 02114

J. S. ECONOMOU (419), Department of Microbiology, Johns Hopkins University, School of Medicine, Baltimore, Maryland

P. EGGENA (105), Department of Medicine, UCLA San Fernando Valley Program, Los Angeles, California 91343

B. A. ELLIS (249), Immunology Unit, The Rayne Institute, St. Thomas' Hospital, London

A. ENGLARD (235), Laboratory of Immunopharmacology, Memorial Sloan–Kettering Cancer Center, New York, New York 10021

L. B. EPSTEIN (353), Cancer Research Institute, University of California, San Francisco, California 94143

P. ERB (541), Institute for Microbiology, University of Basel, Basel, Switzerland

M. ERNST (175), Max-Planck-Institut für Immunbiologie, Freiburg, FRG

M. EVINGER (315), Roche Institute of Molecular Biology, Nutley, New Jersey 07110

P. FAMILLETTI (315), Roche Institute of Molecular Biology, Nutley, New Jersey 07110

K. H. FANTES (343), Department of Virology, Wellcome Research Laboratories, Beckenham, Kent, England

J. J. FARRAR (303, 455), National Institute of Dental Research, NIH, Bethesda, Maryland 20014

J. FEDER (531), Monsanto Company, St. Louis, Missouri

M. FELDMANN (541, 563), ICRF Tumour Immunology Unit, Department of Zoology, University College, London, England

W. B. FINTER (343), Department of Virology, Wellcome Research Laboratories, Beckenham, Kent, England

H. FISCHER (149, 175), Max-Planck-Institut Immunbiologie, Freiburg, FRG

W. H. FRIDMAN (503), Laboratorie d'Immunologie Cellulaire, Institute de Recherches Scientifiques sur le Cancer, Villejuif, France

J. FULLER-BONAR (455), National Institutes of Health, Bethesda, Maryland 20014

A. GALLI (205), Department of Pathology, Massachusetts General Hospital, Boston, Massachusetts 02114

S. J. GALLI (205, 531), Departments of Pathology and Medicine, Harvard Medical School, Boston, Massachusetts 02114

W.-D. GASSEL (209, 215), Medizinische Poliklinik und Klinik, Universität Marburg, Marburg, West Germany

C. L. GECZY (243), Kolling Institute of Medical Research, Royal North Shore Hospital, St. Leonards, N.S.W. Australia

R. N. GERMAIN (551), Department of Pathology, Harvard Medical School, Boston, Massachusetts 02115

G. E. GIFFORD (307), Department of Immunology and Medical Microbiology, University of Florida, J. Hillis Miller Health Center, College of Medicine, Gainesville, Florida 32610

K. GILBERT (473), Department of Immunology, Memorial Sloan–Kettering Cancer Center, New York, New York 10021

C. D. GILLILAND (193), Cancer Research Center, Columbia, Missouri 65201

S. GILLIS (253, 399, 463), Department of Medicine,Dartmouth Medical School, Hanover, New Hampshire, 03755

H. P. GODFREY (43), Department of Pathology, Health Science Center, S.U.N.Y. at Stony Brook, Stony Brook, New York 11794

D. GOLDBLATT (353), Cancer Research Institute, University of California, San Francisco, California 94143

D. W. GOLDE (105, 221), School of Medicine, Center for the Health Sci ences, University of California, Los Angeles, California 90024

I. GOLDMAN (261), Department of Life Sciences and Medical Laboratories, Bar-Ilan University and Meir Hospital, Ramat-Gan and Kfar Saba, Israel

A. L. GOLDSTEIN (273), The George Washington University Medical Center, Washington D.C. 20037

J. W. GOODMAN (483), Department of Microbiology and Immunology, University of California, San Francisco, California

G. A. GRANGER (279, 285, 291), Department of Molecular Biology and Biochemistry, University of California, Irvine, California 92717

A. GREENHILL (399), National Institute for Dental Research/NIAID, Bethesda, Maryland 20014

D. K. GREINEDER (1), Department of Medicine, Robert B. Brigham Hospital, Harvard Medical School, Boston, Massachusetts 02115

I. GRESSER (393), Institut de Recherches Scientifiques sur le Cancer, Villejuif 94800, France

M. GROSS (315), Roche Institute of Molecular Biology, Nutley, New Jersey 07110

J. W. HADDEN (235), Memorial Sloan-Kettering Cancer Center, New York, New York 10021

E. M. HADDEN (235), Laboratory of Immunopharmacology, Memorial Sloan-Kettering Cancer Center, New York, New York 10021

O. HALLER (393), Division of Experimental Microbiology, Institute for Medical Microbiology, University of Zürich, Zürich 8028, Switzerland

M. E. HAMMOND (205), Department of Pathology, Massachusetts General Hospital, Boston, Massachusetts 02114

K. HAVEMANN (209, 215), Medizinische Poliklinik und Klinik Universität Marburg, Marburg, West Germany

C. S. HENNEY (507), Basic Immunology Program, Huchinson Cancer Research Center, Seattle, Washington 98104

R. B. HERBERMAN (353, 369), National Cancer Institute, National Institues of Health, Bethesda, Maryland 20014

Ch. F. HERTOGS (227), Department of Life Sciences, Bar-Ilan University, Ramat-Gan, Israel

M. L. HILFIKER (455), National Institute of Health, Bethesda, Maryland 20014

K. HIRAMATSU (577), Laboratories for Immunology, School of Medicine, Chiba University, Chiba, Japan

J. C. HISERODT (279), Department of Molecular Biology and Biochemistry, University of California, Irvine, California 92717

M. K. HOFFMANN (473), Memorial Sloan-Kettering Cancer Center, New York, New York 10021

H. T. HOLDEN (87,369), Laboratory of Immunodiagnosis, National Cancer Institute, Bethesda, Maryland 20014

A. HOLLIMAN (571), Department of Immunology, ARC Institute of Animal Physiology, Barbraham, Cambridge, England

J. C. HOUCK (199), Virginia Mason Research Center, 1000 Seneca Street, Seattle, Washington 98101

L. HÜBNER (447), Institut für Virologie und Immunbiology, Universität Würzburg, FRG

H. JAKSCHE (79), Sandoz Forschungsinstitut GES. mbH, Vienna, Austria

M. D. JOHNSTON (343), Department of Virology, Wellcome Research Laboratories, Beckenham, Kent, England

M. JOSKOWICZ (503), Laboratorie d'Immunologie Cellulaire, Institut de Recherches Scientifique sur de Cancer, Villejuif, France

S.-T. JU (551), Department of Pathology, Harvard Medical School, Boston, Massachusetts 02115

D. H. KATZ (519), Department of Cellular and Developmental Immunology, Scripps Clinic and Research Foundation, La Jolla, California 92037

S. P. KATZ (435), Department of Pathology and Biology, Yale University, New Haven, Connecticut

Y. KEISARI (113), Department of Human Microbiology, Sackler School of Medicine, Tel-Aviv University, Tel-Aviv, Israel

B. KICKHÖFEN (149), Max-Planck-Institut für Immunbiologie, Freiburg, FRG

H. KIRCHNER (365), German Cancer Research Center, Heidelberg, FRG

V. KLIMETZEK (75), Harvard Medical School, Boston, Massachusetts 02115

W. KLINKERT (31), Department of Experimental Dermatology, University of Münster, Münster, Germany

E. M. KNIEP (149, 175), Max-Planck-Institut für Immunbiologie, Freiburg, FRG

S. KONTIANEN (563), Department of Microbiology, University of Helsinki, Helsinki, Finland

S. M. KRANE (439), Massachusetts General Hospital, Boston, Massachusetts 02114

A. L. KÜHNER (75), Harvard Medical School, Boston, Massachusetts 02115

T.-H. KUO (479), Department of Immunology and Microbiology, Wayne State Univeristy Medical School,Detroit, Michigan 48201

L. B. LACHMAN (405), Division of Immunology, Duke University Medical Center, Durham, North Carolina 27710

H. LANG (169), Max-Planck-Institut für Immunbiologie, Freiburg, FRG

H. LAUKEL (209, 215), Medizinische Poliklinik und Klinik, Universität Marburg, Marburg, West Germany

S. LAZARY (15, 67), Institute for Clinical Immunology, Inselspital, Bern, Switzerland

J. LEHMANN (133), Geseltschaft für Biotechnologische Forschung mbH, Braunschweig, FRG

R. LENZ (227), Department of Life Sciences, Bar-Ilan University, Ramat-Gan, Israel

M. A. LEON (479), Department of Immunology and Microbiology, Wayne State University Medical School,Detroit, Michigan 48201

E. J. LEONARD (161), National Institutes of Health,Bethesda, Maryland 20014

G. K. LEWIS (483), Department of Microbiology and Immunology, University of California, San Francisco, California

L. S. LIN (331), Interferon Laboratories, Memorial Sloan–Kettering Cancer Center, New York, New York 10021

J. LINDENMANN (393), Division of Experimental Microbiology, Institute for Medical Microbiology, University of Zürich, Zürich 8028, Switzerland

B. H. LITTMAN (185), Division of Immunology and Connective Tissue Diseases, Medical College of Virginia, Richmond, Virginia 23298

M.-L. LOHMANN-MATTHES (169), Max-Planck-Institut für Immunbiologie, Freiburg, FRG

T. L. K. LOW (273), Department of Biochemistry, The George Washington University, School of Medicine and Health Science, Washington D.C.

R. A. LUBEN (55), Division of Biomedical Sciences, University of California, Riverside, California 92521

A. J. LUSIS (221), Department of Medicine, UCLA School of Medicine, Los Angeles, California 90024

R. MCCANDLISS (315), Roche Institute of Molecular Biology, Nutley, New Jersey 07110

P. L. MCCARTHY (23), Department of Medicine, Robert B. Brigham Hospital, Harvard Medical School, Boston, Massachusetts

M. C. MCDANIEL (145), College of Medicine, East Tennessee State University, Johnson City, Tennessee 37601

A. B. MACDONALD (493), Department of Microbiology, University of Texas, Austin, Texas

J. E. McENTIRE (193), Cancer Research Center, P. O. Box 1268, Colombia, Missouri 65201

S. MAEDA (315), Roche Institute of Molecular Biology, Nutley, New Jersey 07110

D. N. MÄNNEL (303), National Institutes of Health, Bethesda, Maryland 20014

G. D. MARSHALL, JR. (273), Department of Biochemistry, The George Washington University, School of Medicine and Health Sciences, Washington D.C.

B. J. MATHIESON (399), National Institute for Dental Research and NIAID, Bethesda, Maryland 20014

M. M. MAYER (297), Johns Hopkins University School of Medicine, Department of Microbiology, Baltimore, Maryland 21205

M. S. MELTZER (161), National Institutes of Health, Bethesda, Maryland 20014

S. E. MERGENHAGEN (267, 303), National Institutes of Health, and NIDR, Bethesda, Maryland 20014

R. S. METZGAR (405), Department of Immunology and Microbiology, Duke University Medical Center, Durham, North Carolina

JUN MINOWADA (67), Roswell Park Memorial Institute, Buffalo, New York

S. B. MIZEL (441, 455), National Institutes of Health, Bethesda, Maryland 20014

M. A. MOHLER (55), Division of Biomedical Sciences, University of California, Riverside, California 92521

E. MOZES (545), Department of Chemical Immunology, The Weizmann Institute of Science, Rehovot, Israel

P. F. MÜHLRADT (133), Gesellschaft für Biotechnologische Forschung mbH, Braunschweig, BRG

H. L. MULCAHY (493), Department of Microbiology, University of Texas, Austin, Texas

G. MÜLLER (447), Institut für Virologie und Immunbiologie Universität Würzburg, FRG

G. R. MUNDY (123), Department University of Connecticut Health Center, Farmington, Connecticut 06032

C. A. NACY (161), Walter Reed Army Institute of Research, Washington D.C.

C. NEAUPORT-SAUTÈS (503), Laboratoire d'Immunologie le Cellulaire, Institut de Recherches Scientifiques sur le Cancer, Villejuif, France

R. NETA (587), Department of Microbiology, University of Pittsburgh School of Medicine, Pittsburgh, Pennsylvania 15261

C. NEUMANN (359), Department of Experimental Dermatology, University of Münster, Münster, Germany

H. NORTHOFF (399), National Institute for Dental Research and NIAID, Bethesda, Maryland

I. NOWOWIEJSKI (499), Roche Institute of Molecular Biology, Nutley, New Jersey 07110

C. A. OGBURN (339), Medical College of Pennsylvania, Graduate School of Medical Sciences, Philadelphia, Pennsylvania 19129

M. OKADA (507), Program in Basic Immunology, Fred Hutchinson Cancer Research Center, Seattle, Washington

J. J. OPPENHEIM (353, 397, 399), National Institute of Dental Research and NIH, Bethesda, Maryland 20014

N. S. ORENSTEIN (531), Departments of Pathology and Medicine, Harvard Medical School, Boston, Massachusetts 02114

J. OSTROVE (307), Department of Immunology and Medical Microbiology, University of Florida College of Medicine, Gainesville, Florida 32610

U. OTZ (15, 67), Institute for Clinical Immunology, Inselspital, Bern, Switzerland

B. W. PAPERMASTER (193), Cancer Research Center, Columbia, Missouri 65201

K. PAUCKER (339), Department of Microbiology, Medical College of Pennsylvania, Philadelphia, Pennsylvania 19129

B. PESKAR (175), Pharmakologisches Institut, Freiburg, FRG

S. PESTKA (315), Roche Institute of Molecular Biology, Nutley, New Jersey 07110

H.-H. PETER (365), Medical School of Hannover, Hannover, FRG

K. PFIZENMAIER (527), Institute of Medical Microbiology, University of Mainz, Mainz, West Germany

E. PICK (113), Department of Human Microbiology, Sackler School of Medicine, Tel-Aviv University, Tel-Aviv, Israel

M. PIERRES (551), Department of Pathology, Harvard Medical School, Boston, Massachusetts 02115

D. H. PLUZNIK (227), Department of Life Sciences, Bar-Ilan University, Ramat-Gan, Israel

G. POSSANZA (7), Department of Pathology, University of Connecticut Health Center, Farmington, Connecticut

D. PRIMI (483), Department of Microbiology and Immunology, University of California, San Francisco, California 94143

S. G. QUAN (221), Department of Medicine, UCLA School of Medicine, Los Angeles, California 90024

C. RABOURDIN-COMBE (503), Laboratorie d'Immunologie Cellulaire, Institut de Recherches Scientifiques sur le Cancer, Villejuif, France

A. REES (563), Department of Zoology, University College, London, England

L. W. REDMON (87), Laboratory of Immunodiagnosis, National Cancer Institute, Bethesda, Maryland

T. H. REIDARSON (291), Department of Molecular Biology and Biochemistry, University of California, Irvine, California 92717

H. G. REMOLD (1, 23, 75), Harvard Medical School, Boston, Massachusetts 02115

E. REMOLD-O'DONNELL (23), Center for Blood Research, Boston, Massachusetts

G. E. RESTRICK (249), Immunology Unit, The Rayne Institute, St. Thomas' Hospital, London, England

H. RINDERKNECHT (105), Department of Medicine, UCLA San Fernando Valley Program, Los Angeles, California 91343

R. E. ROCKLIN (93, 353), Department of Medicine, TUFT–NEMC, Boston, Massachusetts 02111

T. J. ROGERS (499), Roche Institute of Molecular Biology, Nutley, New Jersey 07110

M. RÖLLINGHOFF (527), Institute of Medical Microbiology, University of Mainz, Mainz, West Germany

M. W. ROSS (279), Department of Molecular Biology and Biochemistry, University of California, Irvine, California 92717

L. A. ROZENSZAJN (261), Department of Life Sciences and Medical Laboratories, Bar-Ilan University and Meir Hospital, Ramat-Gan and Kfar Saka, Israel

A. S. RUBIN (493), Department of Microbiology, University of Texas, Austin, Texas 78712

M. RUBINSTEIN (315), Roche Institute of Molecular Biology, Nutley, New Jersey 07110

S. RUBINSTEIN (315), Roche Institute of Molecular Biology, Nutley, New Jersey 07110

M. RUFF (307), Department of Immunology and Medical Microbiology, University of Florida College of Medicine, Gainesville, Florida 32610

J.-E. RYSER (513), Department of Immunology, Swiss Institute for Experimental Cancer Research, Epalinges s/Lausanne, Switzerland

J. R. SADLIK (235), Laboratory of Immunopharmacology, Memorial Sloan-Kettering Cancer Center, New York, New York 10021

T. SAITO (577), Laboratories for Immunology, School of Medicine, Chiba University, Chiba, Japan

E. SAKSELA (375), Departments of Obstetrics and Gynaecology, University Central Hospital, Helsinki, Finland

M. G. SALIT (339), Department of Microbiology, Medical College of Pennsylvania, Philadelphia, Pennsylvania 19129

S. B. SALVIN (587), Department of Microbiology, University of Pittsburgh School of Medicine, Pittsburgh, Pennsylvania 15261

A. SCHIMPL (447), Institut für Virologie und Immunbiologie, Universität Würzburg, Federal Republic of Germany

L.B. SCHOOK (15, 67), Institute for Clinical Immunology, Inselspital, Bern, Switzerland

M. H. SCHREIER (535), Basel Institute for Immunology, Basel, Switzerland

A. H. W. M. SCHUURS (109), Organon Scientific Development Group, OSS, The Netherlands

U. SCHWULÉRA (129), Biotest-Serum-Institute GmbH, Flughafenstrasse 4, D-6000 Frankfurt, BRD

H. S. SHIN (419), Department of Microbiology, Johns Hopkins University School of Medicine, Baltimore, Maryland 21205

M. L. SHIN (297), Department of Microbiology, Johns Hopkins University School of Medicine, Baltimore, Maryland 21205

C. SHIOZAWA (557), Department of Immunology and MRC Group on Immunoregulation, University of Alberta, Edmonton, Alberta, Canada

B. SINGH (557), Department of Immunology and MRC Group on Immunoregulation, University of Alberta, Edmonton, Alberta, Canada

A. SLOMA (315), Roche Institute of Molecular Biology, Nutley, New Jersey 07110

K. A. SMITH (253, 399, 463), Hematology Research, Dartmouth Medical School Hanover, New Hampshire 03755

M. E. SMITH (193), National Institutes of Health, Bethesda, Maryland 20014

S. SONIK (557), Department of Immunology and MRC Group on Immunoregulation, University of Alberta, Edmonton, Alberta, Canada

H. H. SONNEBORN (129), BIOTEST-Serum-Institut GmbH, Flughafenstrasse 4, D-6000 Frankfurt, BRD

C. SORG (31, 37, 359), Department of Experimental Dermatology, University of Münster, Münster, Germany

L. SPOLTER (105), Department of Medicine, UCLA San Fernando Valley Program, Los Angeles, California 91343

B. SREDNI (261), Department of Life Sciences and Medical Laboratories, Bar-Ilan University and Meir Hospital, Ramat-Gan and Kfar Saka, Israel

M.-J. STARUCH (423), Department of Immunology, Merck Institute for Therapeutic Research, Rahway, New Jersey

W. E. STEWART II (331), Interferon Laboratories, Memorial Sloan–Kettering Cancer Center, New York, New York 10021

M. SUGIYAMA (353), Department of Otorhinolaryngology, Osaka City Medical School, Osaka, Japan

M. SUKO (593), Department of Pathology, University of Connecticut Health Center, Farmington, Connecticut 06032

I. T. SULEA (323), Department of Microbiology, New York University School of Medicine, New York, New York 10016

J. TABOR (315), Roche Institute of Molecular Biology, Nutley, New Jersey 07110

T. TADA (577), Department of Immunology, Faculty of Medicine, Tokyo University,Tokyo, Japan

I. TAKEI (577), Laboratories for Immunology, School of Medicine, Chiba University, Chiba, Japan

H. TAKESHIMA (315), Roche Institute of Molecular Biology, Nutley, New Jersey 07110

M. TANIGUCHI (577), Laboratories for Immunology, School of Medicine Chiba University, Chiba, Japan

M. J. TAUSSIG (571), Department of Immunology, ARC Institute of Animal Physiology, Babraham, Cambridge, England

G. B. THURMAN (273), Department of Biochemistry, The George Washington University, School of Medicine and Health Science, Washington, D.C.

T. TIMONEN (375), Department of Obstetrics and Gynaecology, University Center Hospital, Helsinki, Finland

R. P. TRIGLIA (483), Department of Microbiology and Immunology, University of California, San Francisco, California

E. R. UNANUE (427), Department of Pathology, Harvard Medical School, Boston, Massachusetts 02115

J. I. VAN LIESHOUT (109), Organon Scientific Development Group, OSS, The Netherlands

J. VILČEK (323), Department of Microbiology, New York University School of Medicine, New York, New York 10016

F. VOLVOVITZ (323), Department of Microbiology, New York University School of Medicine, New York, New York 10016

H. WAGNER (527), Institute of Medical Microbiology, University of Mainz, Mainz, West Germany

L. M. WAHL (161, 267), National Institute of Health, NIDR, Bethesda, Maryland 20014

S. M. WAHL (267), National Institute of Health, NIDR, Bethesda, Maryland 20014

B. H. WAKSMAN (435), Department of Pathology, Yale University School of Medicine, New Haven, Connecticut 06510

C. F. WARE (285, 291), Department of Molecular Biology and Biochemistry, University of California, Irvine, California 92717

A. H. WARFEL (235), Laboratory of Immuno-Pharmacology, Memorial Sloan–Kettering Cancer Center, New York, New York 10021

J. D. WATSON (463), Department of Medical Microbiology, University of California, Irvine, California 92717

D. R. WEBB (499), Department of Cell Biology, Nutley, New Jersey 07110

E. WECKER (447), Institut für Virologie und Immunbiologie, Universität Würzburg, Federal Republic of Germany

R. H. WEISBART (105), UCLA San Fernando Valley Program School of Medicine, Veterans Administration Hospital, Sepulveda, California 91343

Y. WEISER (1), Department of Medicine, Robert B. Brigham Hospital, Harvard Medical School, Boston, Massachusetts 02115

K. WENC (79), Department of Internal Medicine, Yale University, New Haven, Connecticut

K. WIEDER (499), Department of Cell Biology, Roche Institute of Molecular Biology, Nutley, New Jersey 07110

J. B. WILLOUGHBY (297), Department of Microbiology, Johns Hopkins University School of Medicine, Baltimore, Maryland 21205

M. WIRANOWSKA-STEWART (331), Interferon Laboratories, Memorial Sloan–Kettering Cancer Center, New York, New York 10021

R. A. WOLSTENCROFT (249), Immunology Unit, The Rayne Institute, St. Thomas' Hospital, London, England

V. WOLSTENCROFT (249), Immunology Unit, The Rayne Institute, St. Thomas' Hospital, London, England

D. D. WOOD (423), Department of Immunology, Merck Institute for Therapeutic Research, Rahway, New Jersey 20014

J. N. WOODY (563), Department of Pediatrics and The Lombardi Cancer Center, Georgetown University School of Medicine, Washington D.C.

R. S. YAMAMOTO (279), Department of Molecular Biology and Biochemistry, University of California, Irvine, California 92717

Y. K. YIP (323), Department of Microbiology, New York University School of Medicine, New York, New York 10016

T. YONEDA (123), Department of Medicine, University of Connecticut Health Center, Farmington, Connecticut 06032

T. YOSHIDA (7, 47, 593), Department of Pathology, University of Connecticut Health Center, Farmington, Connecticut 06032

K. YU (353), Cancer Research Institute, University of California, San Francisco, California 94143

R. ZAWATZKY (365), German Cancer Research Center, Heidelberg, FRG

A. ZEEVI (261), Department of Life Sciences and Medical Laboratories, Bar-Ilan University and Meir Hospital, Ramat-Gan and Kfar Saka, Israel

N. J. ZVAIFLER (563), Department of Internal Medicine, University of California at San Diego,San Diego, California

PREFACE

For more than half a century antibody has been the focus of immunologic thinking and investigation. Even during the past 25 years or so, the era of "modern" immunology, antibody continued to dominate concepts and mechanisms that sought to explain the functioning of the immune system. Only in the 1970s is there emerging an awareness and a still modest appreciation that lymphocytic products other than immunoglobulins are largely responsible for a complex array of cell cooperative activities. It is these activities, including in particular helper and suppressor functions, that we now know to have essential roles in the operation of the immune system, especially in its regulation. Moreover, it is these lymphokines and monokines that constitute the molecular "messengers" by which immunocompetent and accessory cells "communicate."

At this still rather early stage of development of the lymphokine field, it is not possible to state with any certainty the number, types, array of functions and the sequence of activities in biochemical or enzymatic cascades by which this growing spectrum of glycoprotein molecules fit precisely into the multicellular network that constitutes the immune system. Until recently, most lymphokines and monokines had been only scantily characterized at the molecular level. Consequently, the field had a distinctly phenomenological character not at all attractive to biochemists and molecular biologists. The establishment of lymphoid and hybrid cell lines capable of producing the desired lymphokines and monokines in large amounts, the improvement in techniques for purification and analysis of small amounts of glycoproteins, as well as the development of the technology for production of monoclonal antibodies have widened the horizons of lymphokine studies.

As this field now matures and advances, it appears more certain that the two broad categories of lymphokines, the nonspecific and the antigen-specific (such as T-cell-derived helpers and suppressors), together with the monokines, will point the way to the immunology of the 1980s, in which the potential of the immune system, i.e., its information library, heretofore ascribed solely to classical Ig, will be amplified to encompass these new kinds of immunologic or paraimmunologic information. This assemblage of lymphocyte and macrophage glycoproteins may yet rival Ig in the critical and diverse ways in which they make for the versatility, plasticity, and remarkable adaptability of the immune system to fulfill its essential functions. Moreover, their significance appears to extend beyond the confines of the lymphoid sytem, since some of these molecules are also produced by rapidly growing cells such as tumor cells and fibroblasts. These "cytokines" may in fact serve as biochemical messengers among populations of nonlymphoid cells.

Until rather recently, no serious attempt had been made to assemble and assess the data base for the lymphokine field. Several years ago a number of the leading lymphokine investigators in the United States decided that the time had come to organize a workshop–conference to report new findings and to provide a forum for ideas and points of view. The First International Workshop on Mechanism of Action and Characterization of Lymphocyte Mediators was held in Bethesda, Maryland, November 8–10, 1976. No proceedings volume was prepared to report the scientific record of that meeting. However, the abstracts of presented papers were published in Cellular Immunology ***27,*** 332–358 (1976) and, subsequently, a group of the key participants drafted a progress report "Current State of Studies of Mediators of Cellular Immunology," which appeared in Cellular Immunology ***33,*** 233–244 (1977), providing an interpretive account of the highlights of that workshop–conference. The informally constituted steering committee decided that, in view of the productivity and effectiveness of that meeting, others would be scheduled regularly at three-year intervals.

In planning the second workshop, the organizers felt that this time, and for the future, a permanent record of scientific progress was an important and essential consideration. Accordingly, a special effort was made to develop a proceedings volume that would reflect the accomplishments of this second international lymphokine workshop and in which a pattern would be established for the meetings to take place in the 1980s.

Much of the organization of this volume reflects the distinctive programming developed for this workshop. Sessions devoted to individual major topics were each given a separate, different structure suited to the issue being dealt with; some consisted solely of major reports with accompanying free discussion, others of a larger number of brief reports, still others of summaries reflecting poster presentations. Opportunity was afforded for open, uninhibited discussions and comments in all sessions, only a few being limited by the time available. Essentially, complete retrieval of the discussions was effected by arranging for participants to write out their queries or comments on standard numbered forms. These were collected during each session to assure completeness and sequential continuity. Additionally, all discussions were tape recorded as a fail-safe procedure and to permit rechecking of any written comment that seemed inconsistent or ambiguous. Cooperation was excellent and most of the 400 or so written statements were exemplary in their conciseness and relevance. Their editing was limited largely to improvement in clarity, directness of expression, and revised sequencing for continuity of topics or issues.

The research reports and accompanying technical comments, queries, discussion of issues, and individual interpretations altogether indicate the ways in which this field has progressed since the 1976 workshop. This volume also mirrors the present state of our information on such elements as advantageous source materials for lymphokine production, bioassay technology, characterization, mode of action, and the beginning of integrating these findings into the present knowledge of immune function and regulation. In bringing together the work of the principal investigators in this growing field, their critical comments and analyses, and a goodly number of notable, landmark advances, the reader—be he immunologist, cell biologist, geneticist, or biochemist—is offered a kind of comprehensive cross section, as it were, of the state of this endeavor in 1979. Perhaps as important and even more provocative, there is also provided a glimpse of new directions, new possibilities, and the swiftly mounting potential of this speciality to resolve issues that for so long have been out of the mainstream of traditional immunology research.

HETEROGENEITY OF HUMAN MIF[1]

Weishui Y. Weiser
Dirk K. Greineder[2]
Heinz G. Remold[3]
John R. David

Department of Medicine
Robert B. Brigham Hospital
Harvard Medical School
Boston, Massachusetts

Previous reports on human migration inhibitory factor (MIF) by Rocklin *et al.* (Rocklin *et al.*, 1972) and Block *et al.* (Block *et al.*, 1978) have shown that this lymphocyte mediator has an apparent molecular weight of approximately 25,000 as determined by Sephadex G-100 chromatography. In contrast, guinea pig MIF is more heterogeneous (Yoshida and Reisfeld, 1970; Remold and Mednis, 1977; Remold and Mednis, 1979; Sorg and Klinkert, 1978). For instance, Remold and Mednis have demonstrated two distinct molecular species with different isoelectric points, buoyant densities, and differential susceptibility to proteases. In light of these findings, we have reexamined the properties of human MIF produced by blood mononuclear cell preparations stimulated by concanavalin A (Con A) and now demonstrate that this human MIF, like guinea pig MIF, is also heterogeneous (Weiser *et al.*, 1979).

Blood mononuclear cells, purified on Ficoll-Hypaque gradients were cultured at 10×10^6 cells/ml of serum-free minimal essential medium with penicillin, streptomycin, and L-glutamine. To one aliquot, 10 μg Con A/ml was added, and the cells were cultured at 37°C. The supernatants from the cultures were collected after 24 hr, and these are referred to as the 1st day supernatants. Fresh media were then added and the cultures incubated for a second 24 hr. The resultant supernatants are referred to as the 2nd day supernatants.

[1]*Supported in part by USPHS grants AI-07685, AI-10921, and AM-05577.*
[2]*Recipient of Junior Faculty Research Award from the American Cancer Society.*
[3]*Recipient of an Established Investigatorship from the American Heart Association.*

ISBN 0-12-213950-X

Control supernatants were processed in exactly the same way, except that Con A was added only at the end of each incubation period. The supernatants were dialyzed against distilled water for 24 hr, lyophilized and then fractionated on Sephadex G-100 (Remold *et al.*, 1972). MIF activity was assayed using guinea pig peritoneal exudate cells as indicator cells.

CHROMATOGRAPHY ON SEPHADEX G-100

The peak of MIF activity obtained from day 1 supernatants was consistently recovered in fractions eluting around the chymotrypsinogen marker, thus having an apparent molecular weight of approximately 23,000. This is in agreement with the previous findings (Rocklin *et al.*, 1972; Block *et al.*, 1978). We were quite surprised by the results of the fractionation of the 2nd day supernatants. They contained more MIF activity and the activity was spread out over a broad range from albumin to RNase markers. This elution pattern indicates molecular heterogeneity and is different from previous findings on human MIF. It resembles, however, the patterns found for Con A-induced MIF from guinea pig lymph node cells (Remold *et al.*, 1972).

ISOELECTROFOCUSSING

The enriched MIF fractions and their control counterparts obtained from Sephadex G-100 gel filtration were subjected to isoelectrofocussing (IEF) in 0-47% sucrose density gradient using pH 2.5-6.0 ampholines (Remold and Mednis, 1977). The capacity of the isoelectrofocussing column was 440 ml. Fractions were extensively dialyzed against physiological saline to remove the ampholines before concentration and assay for MIF activity.

The MIF activity from the 1st day IEF fractions clustered between pH 4.1 to 5.2. In contrast, MIF activity from the 2nd day IEF fractions showed two peaks. One clustered in the same area as the 1st day MIF, around pH 4.3-5.3. An additional peak of activity was found between pH 2.9-3.6. For convenience, these will be referred to as pH5- and pH3-MIF.

The active IEF fractions were subjected to further chromatography on Sephadex G-75. pH5-MIF eluted with an apparent molecular weight between 23,000 and 43,000 whereas pH3-MIF eluted with an apparent molecular weight of 65,000.

The results indicate that human MIF, obtained by stimulating blood mononuclear cell preparations with Con A is heterogeneous; the properties are summarized in Table I.

TABLE I. Heterogeneity of Human MIF[a]

	pH3-MIF	*pH5-MIF*
Molecular weight (Sephadex G-75)	*65,000*	*23,000-43,000*
pI (Isoelectrofocussing)	*2.9-3.6*	*4.1-5.3*

[a]*Human blood mononuclear cells stimulated by Concanavalin A. Two MIFs found in 2nd 24 hr supernatants.*

These results are similar to the findings of distinct MIFs using Con A stimulated guinea pig and mice lymphocytes. Studies by several other laboratories have also documented heterogeneity of other lymphocyte mediators including lymphotoxin (Hiseredt *et al.*, 1976; Walker *et al.*, 1976) and leukocyte inhibitory factor (Brown and Rocklin, 1979).

Further studies will be required to show whether lymphocytes stimulated by other antigens or whether lymphocyte cell lines produce MIFs with similar properties, and to determine the interrelationship between these two MIFs and their other physical properties.

It is of note that Churchill and Remold have shown that guinea pig macrophages incubated with either pH5- or pH3-MIF become activated and exhibit an enhanced ability to kill tumor cells. Recently, in collaboration with Cameron and Churchill, we have obtained preliminary evidence that fractions containing human MIF also enhance the cytotoxicity of human monocytes for human tumor cells but not for normal cells. These studies further suggest that MIF and macrophage activating factor (MAF) are the same mediator. Formal proof of identity or nonidentity will only come when they are better characterized, or if their activities can be separated on further purification.

REFERENCES

Block, L.H., Jaksche, J., Bamberger, J., and Ruhenstroth-Bauer, G. (1978). *J. Exp. Med. 146*, 541.

Brown, A.P., and Rocklin, R.E. (1979). *J. Immunol. 122*, 1059.

Hiserodt, J.C., Prieur, A.M., and Granger, G.A. (1976). *Cell. Immunol. 24*, 277.
Remold, H.G., David, R.A., and David, J.R. (1972). *J. Immunol. 109*, 578.
Remold, H.G., and Mednis, A.D. (1977). *J. Immunol. 118*, 2015.
Remold, H.G., and Mednis, A.D. (1979). *J. Immunol. 122*, 1920.
Rocklin, R.E., Remold, H.G., and David, J.R. (1972). *Cell. Immunol. 1*, 436.
Sorg, C., and Klinkert, W. (1978). *Fed. Proc. 37*, 2748.
Walker, S.M., Lee, S.C., and Lucas, Z.L. (1976). *J. Immunol. 116*, 807.
Weiser, W.Y., Greineder, D.K., and David, J.R. (1979). *Fed. Proc. Abstr. 38*, 1215.
Yoshida, T., and Reisfeld, R.A. (1970). *Nature 226*, 856.

DISCUSSION

YOSHIDA: Since MIF heterogeneity is not evident in supernatants from cultures continued for 48 hr, does David think there is a possibility that products (perhaps inhibitors or suppressors) in 24 hr supernatants could interfere with those in 48 hr supernatants? Is there any difference between the first 24 hr of culture and the second 24 hr of culture as regards cell viability? Has David considered the possibility that the cell populations producing MIF may be different between the first and the second 24 hr of culture?

DAVID: It is quite possible that inhibitors are produced, that prevent further MIF production in the 48 hr uninterrupted assay. We have often noticed the production of more MIF when the medium is changed after 48 hr, suggesting feedback inhibition. It is also possible that a second subpopulation of cells is turned on during the second 24 hr.

MAYER: What is the shape of the dose-response curve of the MIF assay? Does it depart from linearity? If so, conversion of %-migration inhibition to "relative concentration" would yield a more meaningful distribution curve in fractionation experiments. This would be important in assessing the degree of heterogeneity.

DAVID: The dose-response curve departs from linearity. More detailed dose-response curves need to be carried out, particularly with each of the two MIF species. Mayer's suggestion of conversion to "relative concentration" compared to a standard is a good one.

PAPERMASTER: With regard to David's larger molecular weight fraction, has he determined whether MIF activity is bound to albumin, and whether this serum protein in the culture medium maybe acting as a carrier? Smith and McEntire in our laboratory, have obtained evidence that ^{3}H-amino acid biosynthetically labelled human and mouse cultured lymphoid cell line lymphotoxin, MIF and other factors bind to ^{125}I-labelled serum albumin and α-2 macroglobulin, acting as carriers in the culture medium. These biologic activities remain bound to the carrier proteins during gel filtration and electrophoresis and appear to be the result of hydrophobic binding. Dissociation of ^{3}H counts from ^{125}I-labelled carrier proteins occurs only in the presence of SDS.

DAVID: Although Rocklin showed that LIF with MW 68'000 does not bind to an anti-albumin affinity column, we have not done this yet with pH 3 human MIF.

SALVIN: Do LIF, lymphotoxin or similar toxic or inhibitory lymphokines follow this 1st day and 2nd day pattern?

DAVID: We have not looked into 1st day and 2nd day patterns for other human mediators.

LITTMAN: pH 3.5 MIF can be obtained by isoelectric focusing of a Sephadex G 100 fraction corresponding to a MW of 25'000. This differs from the monocyte-complement stimulator (MCS) which has a neutral isoelectric point. David's data indicate that pH 3.5 MIF has a MW of 68'000. This may be due to binding to another protein or to self-aggregation.

DAVID: I believe Littman's MIF of MW 25'000 is induced by antigenic stimulation. The possibility that the MW of 68'000 is due to aggregation of binding to another protein needs to be investigated.

EVIDENCE FOR THE EXISTENCE OF A COFACTOR NECESSARY FOR HUMAN MIF ACTIVITY[1]

Marion C. Cohen
Genus Possanza[2]
Takeshi Yoshida
Stanley Cohen

Department of Pathology
University of Connecticut Health Center
Farmington, Connecticut

There is great variation in the observed molecular weight of Migration Inhibition Factor (MIF) obtained from various species, and even within species (1-4). In the guinea pig, it ranges from approximately 45,000 to 67,000 daltons (4-6), whereas in man, the lower limit is usually given as 22,000 to 25,000 daltons (4-7). However, Yoshida and Reisfeld reported the existence of a guinea pig MIF with molecular weight of 12,000 (8) and similar findings have been recently obtained for human MIF (9,10). It is possible that MIF as well as other lymphokines may exist in various degrees of polymerization. Since the only presently available assays for MIF are bioassays, no information has been available as to the existence of functionally inactive subunits. In this report, we present evidence that human MIF can be dissociated into two components, each of which is devoid of activity, and which can be reassociated to restore activity. For these studies, human long-term lymphoid cell culture lines (RPMI 8392, RAJI, RPMI 8402, and Molt 4F) were used as sources of MIF. The cells were maintained in suspension culture. They were resuspended in RPMI 1640 medium containing antibiotics but no serum for 24 hours prior to harvest of the supernatants. Such culture fluids, which we have previously characterized, are known to contain lymphokines that are indistinguishable from those obtained from antigen or mitogen-stimulated normal human lymphocytes (10). MIF activity was assayed against guinea pig macrophages by the standard capillary tube technique and Migration Indices (MI) were calculated as previously described (11,12). In accordance with standard criteria,

[1] *Supported by NIH Research Grant CA-19286*
[2] *Present address: Boehringer Ingelheim Ltd, Ridgefield, CT*

ISBN 0-12-213950-X

MI $\leq$ 80.0 represent significant MIF activity. The usual controls for lack of cytotoxicity and reversibility of effect on prolonged incubation of macrophages with mediator were performed in all experiments.

The first indication that human MIF in these preparations might be capable of dissociation into inactive fragments came from routine dialysis experiments. The MIF-containing supernatants were dialyzed against RPMI 1640 medium for 18 hours at 4°C at a ratio of 1 part supernatant to 15 parts medium (dialysis tubing: Fischer Scientific Co., Pittsburgh, PA, cat. no. 8-667). In a total of 12 out of 15 separate experiments, MIF activity was completely lost on dialysis. In one experiment, activity fell to a borderline value, and in the other two experiments, there was significant but incomplete loss of activity.

These findings were surprising since the sizing data as well as previous reports in the literature (4,5) suggest that human MIF should be non-dialyzable. We therefore attempted to determine whether the loss of activity was an artifact, and simply due to adsorption on the dialysis tubing. For this purpose, supernatants were placed in dialysis tubing and held, in the absence of external fluid for dialysis, in a sealed test tube to prevent dehydration. After 18 hours of incubation at 4°C full MIF activity was retained. Similarly, when samples of MIF-containing supernatants were mixed with pieces of dialysis tubing and incubated in Petri dishes for 18 hours at 4°C in order to increase the contact area between mediator and tubing no loss of activity was observed. These results demonstrate not only that adsorption could not explain our findings but also that inactivation by degradation or denaturation does not occur under the conditions utilized.

These results suggested that we were losing a low molecular weight subunit necessary for the expression of MIF activity. If this were the case, then dialyzing repeatedly samples of MIF against the same dialysis medium should ultimately saturate the dialysate and prevent further loss of activity. In three such experiments, by the 4th sample, a point was reached at which MIF activity was fully retained in the retentate. Such a preparation, dialyzed against fresh medium showed total loss of activity, as expected. It should be noted that at no point in these experiments could MIF activity be found in the dialysate.

We next demonstrated that the two putative subunits could reassociate to restore activity. For this purpose, we utilized as inactive retentate a sample dialyzed against RPMI 1640 as described above. To obtain the smaller component, lost on dialysis, we utilized the dialysate from the final run of the saturation experiment, concentrated back to 2X that of the

TABLE I. Reconstitution of MIF Activity on Mixing Inactive Retentate and Inactive Dialysate

Material	*Migration Index*		
	Expt. 1	*Expt. 2*	*Expt. 3*
Untreated, intact MIF	*44.5 ± 1.1*	*32.8 ± 1.3*	*33.7 ± 1.4*
Retentate	*91.3 ± 2.9*	*90.0 ± 2.3*	*95.1 ± 2.6*
Dialysate	*94.7 ± 2.6*	*87.7 ± 2.0*	*85.7 ± 2.5*
Mixture (Retentate & Dialysate)	*58.6 ± 1.3*	*62.5 ± 1.5*	*62.3 ± 1.1*

original preparation by Amicon ultrafiltration on a DM5 membrane, which retains substances of molecular weight greater than 5,000 daltons. Retentate and dialysate were combined in equal quantities and assayed in capillary tube preparations without preincubation. The results are given in Table I. In each case, although retentate and dialysate are each devoid of MIF activity, mixtures of both have significant activity.

In a final set of experiments, we sought to determine if either the large MIF fragment in the retentate or the small fragment in the dialysate could competitively inhibit the activity of intact MIF. Equal volumes of either retentate, concentrated dialysate, or RPMI 1640 medium as control were mixed with fresh MIF and the mixtures assayed. In three separate experiments, we found that the presence of the retentate abolished detectable MIF activity. The dialysate, under these conditions, had no effect. These results suggest that reassociation of subunits cannot occur in the environment of the cell surface. Otherwise, one might expect that the smaller subunit from intact MIF could associate with the added large subunit to create functional units. Another possibility is that the molar ratios of these components are critical for interaction with the target cell. This could come about, for example, if cooperative effects between adjacent MIF molecules are important for the activity, in analogy to the situation for complement activation by membrane-bound IgG.

The initial observation that led to the above experiments was that, in our hands, human MIF loses activity upon dialysis. As stated above, it is widely held that human MIF is nondialyzable (reviewed in 6). Nevertheless, in those cases where dialysis results are reported, substantial amounts of MIF activity may, in fact, disappear (9,13). Non-dialyzability of human MIF is also inferred from the fact that chromatographic separation procedures often involve a step of dialysis. This, however, is usually done under conditions of high salt and mediator concentration since fractions are first concentrated by lyophilization. Under these conditions, we find that we can partially prevent loss of human MIF activity by dialysis. It may be that the stability of subunit association is critically dependent upon the ionic composition of the medium. Preliminary experiments suggest that calcium gradients across the dialysis membrane may be of critical importance in this regard.

Although the experiments described all utilized MIF from cultured lymphoid cell lines, we obtained identical results in two experiments utilizing MIF prepared by antigen stimulation of human peripheral blood lymphocytes. This, in conjunction with the data on the correspondences between lymphokines from these sources, suggest the general validity of these observations for materials derived from human sources. In contrast to these, and in agreement with all reports in the literature, we find that guinea pig MIF does not lose activity on dialysis.

The model of human MIF structure that emerges from these studies appears to be one in which two non-covalently linked fragments are involved in the expression of activity; one interacts with membrane receptors to facilitate the transport of the other (enzymatically active) component into the cell. This is analogous to the situation for diphtheria toxin (14). We speculate that the MIF subunits described here may prove to correspond to an attachment piece and to a component that confers the biological activity. Our observation that one, but not the other subunit can inhibit the activity of intact MIF supports this possibility.

REFERENCES

1. Dvorak, H.F. (1974). *In* "The Inflammatory Process, vol. III" (B.W. Zweifach, L. Grant, and R.T. McCluskey, eds.), p. 292. Academic Press, New York.
2. Cohen, S. (1977). *Amer. J. Path. 88*, 502.
3. Waksman, B.H. (1979). *In* "The Biology of the Lymphokines" (S. Cohen, E. Pick, and J.J. Oppenheim, eds.), p. 585. Academic Press, New York.
4. Pick, E. (1977). *In* "Immunopharmacology" (J.W. Hadden, R.G. Coffey, and F. Spreafico, eds.), p. 163. Plenum Publishing Corp., New York.
5. Waksman, B.H. *Pharmacol. Rev.* (in press).
6. David, J.R. and David, R.R. (1972). *Progr. Allergy 16*, 300.

7. Rocklin, R.E., Remold, H.G., and David, J.R. (1972). *Cell. Immunol. 5*, 436.
8. Yoshida, T. and Reisfeld, R.A. (1970). *Nature 226*, 857.
9. Papageorgiou, P.W., Henley, W.L., and Glade, P.R. (1972). *J. Immunol. 108*, 494.
10. Yoshida, T., Kuratsuji, T., Takada, A., Takada, Y., Minowada, J., and Cohen, S. (1976). *J. Immunol. 117*, 548.
11. Yoshida, T. and Watanuki, M. (1968). *Med. Biol. (Tokyo) 77*, 131.
12. Reeves, J., Yoshida, T., and Cohen, S. (1973). *Immunol. Commun. 2*, 287.
13. Taylor, M.M., Burman, C.J., and Fantes, K.H. (1975). *Cell. Immunol. 19*, 41.
14. Pappenheimer, A.M., Jr. (1977). *Ann. Rev. Biochem. 46*, 69.

DISCUSSION

HADDEN: We have made similar observations in the guinea pig system using collodion bags with a 25'000 MW cut off, viz, that vacuum dialysis depletes MIF activity and reconstitution of the inactive dialysate and retentate restores activity. The phenomenon in the guinea pig system thus depends on the type of bag used.

COHEN M: Since the guinea pig MIF molecule is larger than the human MIF, it is not surprising that subunits would also be bigger. It's reassuring to know that our results may hold for another species as well.

HOLDEN: Has Cohen treated the macrophages with one component and then the other to determine whether they act sequentially or must act as a complex?

COHEN M: In the reconstitution experiments they were added simultaneously. The experiments suggested by Hadden will be performed in the near future.

FANTES: Taylor, Burman and Fantes (Cell. Immunol. 19:41, 1975) found that MIF activity apparent in supernatants of continuous human lymphoblastoid cell lines was completely lost on dialysis against fresh medium. The "active" supernatants were found to be greatly depleted of glucose and addition of glucose to such "exhausted" supernatants abolished most of the "MIF" activity. "MIF like" activity could be readily created by simply diluting full medium with physiological saline, i.e. artificially "depleting" the medium. Could some of Cohen's results be explained in this way?

COHEN M: No. Human MIF retains activity when dialyzed across spectropore membranes (3500 dalton cutoff) which allows free passage of glucose. Moreover, complete medium is present on both sides of our higher MW cutoff membranes. Finally, as I indicated, the dialysis data exclude removal of toxic metabolites as explanation for the observed effects. The reconstitution and competitive inhibition experiments are also difficult to reconcile with Fantes interpretation.

DAVID: Following Cohen's presentation at the 1979 FASEB meeting, Weiser took Con A -induced MIF active Sepharose fractions (65'000-23'000 MW) and produced lyophilized material in RPMI or MEM media. Half was dialyzed for 24 hr against 10-fold volumes of medium; dialyzed and undialyzed material was tested in 3 dilutions on guinea pig cells. There was no difference between the two. Cohen's data thus appears quite clear cut; we should exchange materials to resolve these discrepancies.

COHEN M: The differences in dialyzability of our MIF from long-term lines and SK/SD stimulated peripheral lymphocytes on one hand, and from David's Con A-stimulated cells on the other, may tell us something exciting about the mechanism of MIF action. We have found that the stability of the MIF subunit structure appears to be dependent upon salt concentration, with calcium an especially attractive candidate. For example, human MIF prepared in calcium-rich MEM medium is less readily dissociable than MIF prepared in (calcium-poor) RPMI. Calcium ions may thus stabilize the structure of human MIF. Similar changes in stability of subunit association may be involved in the interaction of MIF with the macrophage. In a certain sense, the dialysis bag may be a good model of the macrophage membrane, especially if it turns out that the insertion of a piece of mediator into the cell is necessary for expression of activity.

FARRAR: Has Cohen shown that the retentate exhibits a reduction in molecular weight after dialysis?

COHEN M: No, not yet.

MAYER: I cannot resist the temptation to look into the future by comparing Cohen's observations with those of Ferrata who showed in 1907 that complement comprises two distinct factors, C1 and C2. In the following 60 years, an additional 21 complement proteins were identified, not counting inhibitors and regulatory proteins, or low molecular weight cofactors, such as Ca^{++} and Mg^{++}.

COHEN M: If it should turn out that way, I hope that we will number them in order rather than C 1,4,2,3......

CHARACTERIZATION OF LYMPHOKINES FROM HUMAN MONONUCLEAR CELL CULTURES[1]

Ursula Otz
Sandor Lazary
Lawrence B. Schook[2]
Alain L. de Weck

Institute for Clinical Immunology
Inselspital
Bern, Switzerland

The purpose of our investigations has been to prepare and isolate from human activated lymphocytes sufficient amounts of lymphokines to prepare specific antibodies.

As a source of lymphokines we have used supernatants of Con A stimulated human lymphocytes[3]. The lymphocytes, isolated by gradient centrifugation, were cultured in the absence of serum in RPMI 1640 medium at the rather high concentration of 10×10^6 cells/ml and stimulated with 20 µg Con A/ml-Sepharose for 22 hr in the presence of 2×10^{-5}M 2-mercaptoethanol. In contrast to what had been observed previously with guinea pig lymphokines (1), especially MIF, we experienced difficulties in concentrating supernatants without losing MIF activity. Different procedures were tried to concentrate MIF activities. After dialysis for 24 hr the starting, strongly MIF active supernatants have completely lost activity (Fig. 1). Pressure dialysis also achieves no concentration of MIF activity since even 5 times concentrated supernatants have less activity than the starting solution. In fact, such experiments show that 80-90% of the

[1] *This work has been supported in part by the Swiss National Science Foundation (Grant Nos. 3.850.077 and 3.944.078)*
[2] *Recipient of Postdoctoral Research Fellowships awarded by National Cancer Institute, NIH (CA-0628-01) and Swiss National Fund (88.679-0.78)*
[3] *The supernatants have been prepared by the firm Biotest-Serum Institute GmbH, Frankfurt, Germany*

ISBN 0-12-213950-X

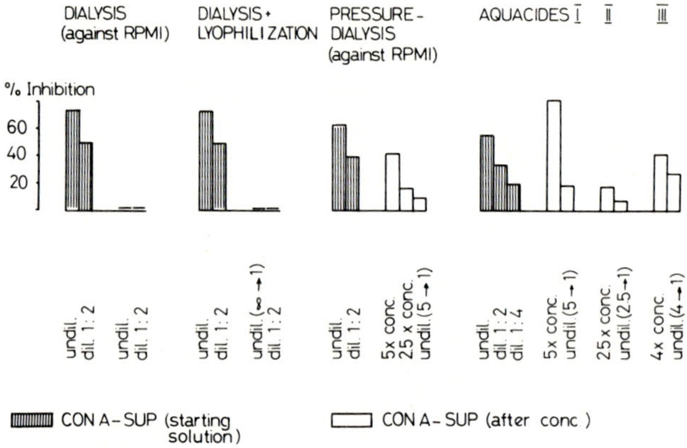

Fig. 1. Experiments to concentrate MIF active Con A supernatant without loosing the activity.

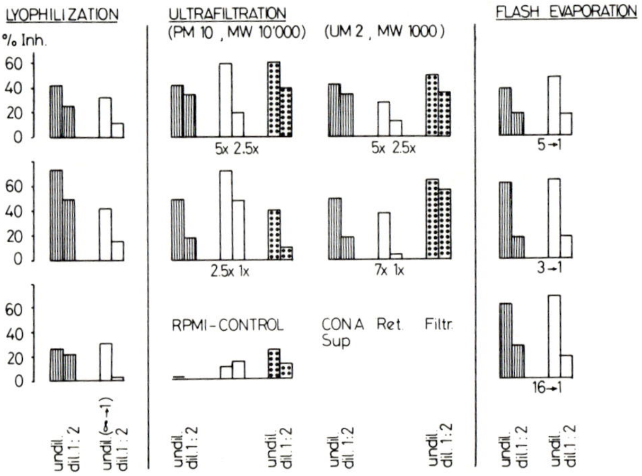

Fig. 2. Experiments to concentrate MIF active Con A supernatant without loosing the activity.

activity is lost upon 24 hr dialysis. Losses are also apparent when supernatants are concentrated by dialysis against aquacides. Lyophilization also appears to give some loss of activity in some samples, probably because it is difficult to dissolve the whole dried supernatant in small volumes of water (Fig. 2). Ultrafiltration on two different Amicon membranes, PM10 and UM2 shows the same phenomenon as dialysis, namely a loss of activity. Controls show that the membranes release no toxic substance neither into the retentate nor into the filtrate. Up to now the only method we found to achieve concentration of the active supernatant without loosing any MIF activity has been flash evaporation: even 16-fold concentration showed no loss of activity. From these experiments, we concluded that human MIF probably needs some low MW cofactor for its inhibitory effect.

For further purification, the supernatant concentrated by flash evaporation is dialyzed very briefly for 30' in order to reduce the salt concentration and then applied to a Biogel P100 column. Figure 3 shows the absorption profilesof the various fractions. All fractions are tested for MIF, LIF, MF, and LAF activity and pooled according to their activities. The pools obtained from Biogel P100 are then concentrated and desalted on Biogel P4. In this way we obtain fractions with fairly high protein concentrations. The pools represented in Figure 4 correspond to about half a liter of active supernatant. The protein content of the different pools measured by Folin-reaction is about 800 µg/ml for the LIF-Pool, 200 µg/ml for the LAF-Pool, 250 µg/ml for the MIF-Pool, and 300 µg/ml for the low MW pool. As shown in Figure 4, each pool showed many bands in SDS-PAGE and isoelectrofocusing. It is obvious that each pool represents a mixture of several proteins. The biological activities of the concentrated pools were also analyzed in order to find out whether the lymphokine activities can be found again after concentration and desalting. LIF activity is still in pool II which now contains MF also. However, we could no longer find MIF activity in any of the pools; probably because of the loss of the low MW cofactor. Most of LAF-activity is still found in pool III.

In the following step, we analyzed various antisera to human lymphokines, produced in the rabbit by immunization with PAGE gel slices[1]. The antibody 22 is made against a band of MW 28000; when used as immunosorbent this antibody retains

[1]The antisera have been prepared by C. Geczy (manuscript in preparation)

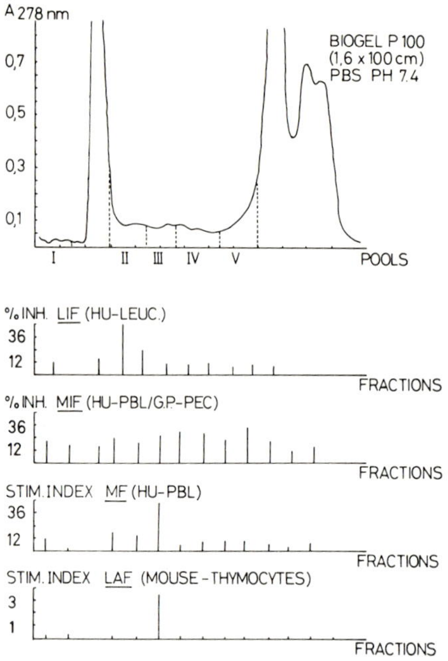

Fig. 3. Fractionation of Con A supernatant on Biogel P100.

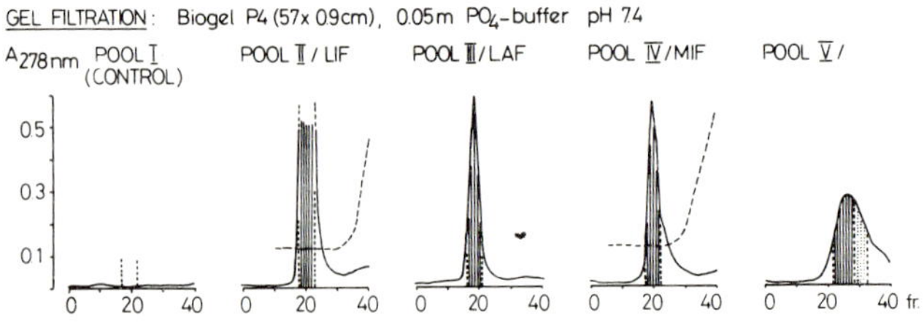

	POOL I (CONTROL)	POOL II / LIF	POOL III / LAF	POOL IV / MIF	POOL V /
PROTEIN (Folin):		~800 µg/ml	~200 µg/ml	~250 µg/ml	~300 µg/ml
MW (SDS-PAGE):		29 bands (100'000 – 15000)	12 bands (68000 - 14000)	4 bands (22000 – 13000)	2 bands (22000, 15000)
PI (IEF):		17 bands (4.6 – 8.0, 6.0)	17 bands (5.1 – 7.4, 5.6)	9 bands (5.1 – 7.5, 5.1, 6.2)	no band
BIOLOGICAL ACTIVITIES					
LIF (% Inh.)	-19 ± 6	26 ± 2	3 ± 5	-15 ± 5	-14 ± 2
MIF (% Inh.)	-12 ± 2	21 ± 7	-12 ± 7	0 ± 9	-27 ± 3
MF (SI)	1.2	6.6	1.5	1.4	1.7
LAF (SI)		26.8	29.3	6.22	1.6

Fig. 4. Characterization of the various chromatography pools.

the MIF activity from MIF active Con A supernatant (2). The antibody 23 is made against a band of MW 31000, antibody 25 is made against a band of MW 15000-20000. These antibodies, when tested in immunodiffusion with 10x concentrated Con A supernatant , with the various chromatography pools, with a concentrated control supernatant and with human serum, give various patterns of reactions (Table 1).

TABLE I. Antisera to Human Lymphokines Produced in the Rabbit

Antigens used in immunodiffusion	*#22 MW 28000*	*#22 absorbed with human AB serum Seph.*	*#23 MW 31000*	*#25 MW 15000-20000*
Con A-Sup. 10x conc.	*+ (1:20)[a]*	*± (undil)*	*+ (1:20)*	*+ (1:20)*
Pool II LIF	*+ (undil)*	*-*	*-*	*+ (1:10)*
LIF 4x conc.		*-*	*± (undil)*	
Pool III LAF	*+ (1:10)*	*+ (undil)*	*-*	*-*
LAF 4x conc.			*± (1:2)*	*+ (1:2)*
Pool IV MIF	*+ (1:10)*	*+ (undil)*	*+ (1:10)*	*-*
MIF 4x conc.				*-*
Pool V 4x conc.	*-*		*-*	*-*
Control-Sup 10x conc.	*+ (1:4)*	*-*	*-*	*-*
hu AB-Serum	*+ (1:32)*	*-*	*+ (1:2)*	*+ (1:4)*
RPMI 10x conc.	*-*		*-*	*-*

[a] *Immunodiffusion, antigen-dilution*

Obviously these antibodies react not only with defined lymphokines in the supernatant, but also with other proteins, which may be serum proteins produced by or not washed out from the cells. Immunoelectrophoretic patterns (results not shown) also suggest that the antisera contain antibodies directed a-gainst normal serum constituents as well as antibodies against proteins present in sizeable amounts only in activated supernatants or their fractions.

Since it obviously will be extremely difficult to produce monospecific anti-lymphokine antibodies by classical purification and immunization techniques, we have now endeavoured to produce anti-lymphokine antibodies with mouse hybridomas. In a first step, BALB/c mice were immunized with Pool IV MIF and antisera were investigated in immunodiffusion. We have obtained positive results with the different lymphokine pools. This time the antisera obtained do not react with human serum and preimmunization (normal) mouse sera are also negative. This indicates that the mouse is capable of producing antibodies against human lymphokines.

In order to measure anti-lymphokine antibodies in serum or hybridoma culture supernatants, we activated paper discs with CNBr and incubated the discs with Pool IV MIF; after several washings the discs were incubated with mouse anti-lymphokine serum and with radioactive Protein A. Specific binding by anti-lymphokine antibodies can be demonstrated (results not shown). Other ways to assess the presence of anti-lymphokine antibodies by RIA currently are being investigated.

In summary, it appears now feasible to isolate human lymphokines in sufficient amounts to achieve regular immunization and antisera, which contain anti-lymphokine antibodies as demonstrated by immunosorbent or neutralization techniques. However, this is still producing somewhat multispecific antibodies, which have to be absorbed; they will probably be poorly suitable for RIA. The last step in purification of human lymphokines might best be left to the mouse hybridomas producing monoclonal antibodies.

REFERENCES

1. Geczy, C.L., Friedrich, W., and de Weck, A.L., Cell. immunol. *19*, 65 (1975)
2. Geczy, C.L., Otz, U., and de Weck, A.L., Molecular Immunol. (1979) in press

DISCUSSION

LEONARD: In the flash evaporation step, how does Otz get rid of the 16-fold concentration of salt?

OTZ: After flash evaporation, the concentrated supernatant is dialyzed briefly for about 30 minutes, thus reducing the high salt concentration.

OGBURN: Did Otz find it necessary to inject her animals repeatedly in order to develop antibodies, and for how long?

OTZ: The mice were injected weekly, over a four week period.

SORG: Did Otz conduct any experiments to reconstitute MIF-activity with dialysate and retentate as Cohen had done in the work reported previously?

OTZ: Yes. Some degree of reconstitution can in fact be achieved. We can therefore confirm Cohen's results also with MIF from Con A-activated peripheral blood lymphocytes.

PURIFICATION AND SOME PROPERTIES OF GUINEA PIG MIGRATION INHIBITORY FACTOR[1]

Philip L. McCarthy

Department of Medicine
Robert B. Brigham Hospital
Harvard Medical School
Boston, Massachusetts

Eileen Remold-O'Donnell

Center for Blood Research
Boston, Massachusetts

Heinz G. Remold[2]

Department of Medicine
Robert B. Brigham Hospital
Harvard Medical School
Boston, Massachusetts

A lymphocyte mediator of cellular immunity, migration inhibitory factor (MIF), inhibits the migration of macrophages in vitro and is thought to confine them to sites of inflammation in vivo (1,2). Studies so far indicate that guinea pig MIF is biochemically indistinguishable from macrophage activating factor (MAF), a lymphocyte mediator that modulates the morphology, biochemistry and function of macrophages by enhancing their bactericidal and tumoricidal capabilities (3). This report reviews our recent findings on the heterogeneity of guinea pig MIF and presents some of its biochemical properties.

[1]*Supported in part by USPHS grant AI-12110-05 and a Grant-in-Aid from the American Heart Association.*
[2]*Recipient of an Established Investigatorship from the American Heart Association.*

ISBN 0-12-213950-X

MATERIALS AND METHODS

In the majority of the experiments lymphocyte cultures (24×10^6/ml) stimulated with concanavalin A (Con A) and from unstimulated lymphocyte cultures were subjected to sequential Sephadex G-100 gel filtration, sucrose density gradient electrophoresis, isoelectrofocussing in a pH gradient from pH 2.0-6.2, and further Sephadex G-75 gel filtration (4).

In the radiolabelling experiments, aliquots of 25 ml of the cell suspension containing 48×10^6 lymph node cells/ml obtained as previously described (5) were incubated with 20 μg/ml or without Con A as a control in the presence of 250 μCi/ml [^{3}H]-leucine according to the method of Sorg and Bloom (6). The supernatants were then fractionated as described above and analyzed by SDS-polyacrylamide gel electrophoresis (7) and fluorography (8). MIF assays were performed in parallel.

RESULTS

We could show that guinea pig MIF can be separated into two distinct molecular species. These two different forms are referred to as pH3-MIF and pH5-MIF on the basis of their different isoelectric points. Some of these properties are listed in Table I (9).

These results suggest that pH3-MIF is a carbohydrate-rich glycoprotein(s) which is relatively resistant to arginine-proteinase and requires sialic acid for its activity, whereas pH5-MIF is a carbohydrate-poor or carbohydrate-lacking protein which is proteinase sensitive. In this respect our results are at variance with the results of Klinkert and Sorg (10) who found that guinea pig MIF focuses at pH 5.2 and contains biologically active molecules with a molecular weight of 30,000, 45,000 and 60,000. In our pH5-MIF preparations we only find MIF activity with a molecular weight of 25,000-45,000. In addition, these authors find MIF with an isoelectric point (pI) of 3.1-4.1 containing material with a molecular weight of 30,000, 45,000 and 60,000. In contrast, in our hands pH3-MIF contains only active material with a molecular weight of 65,000 daltons.

TABLE I. Some Properties of pH3- and pH5-MIF

Properties	*pH3-MIF*	*pH5-MIF*
Isoelectric point	*3.0-4.5*	*5.0-5.5*
Apparent MW	*65,000*	*25,000-40,000*
Density determined by CsCl density gradient centrifugation	*denser than albumin*	*same density as albumin*
Susceptibility to trypsin	-	+
Susceptibility to neuraminidase	+	-
Susceptibility to chymotrypsin	+	+
Susceptibility to a macrophage-associated proteinase	-	+
Susceptibility to plasmin	-	-
Susceptibility to thrombin	-	-
Heat stability at 56°C for 30 min	*stable*	*stable*

Due to the low protein concentrations in our highly purified MIF preparations, activity could not be correlated with protein. We therefore performed studies in which we metabolically labelled lymph node supernatants. These [^{3}H]-leucine labelled supernatants were then fractionated as described above and the protein composition of the pooled active and control fractions was analyzed by SDS-gel electrophoresis and subsequent fluorography. pH5-MIF was found to contain multiple protein components with molecular weights ranging from 20,000 to 65,000. However, when pH3-MIF was analyzed by the above-mentioned method the following observations were made:

1) Proteins with a pI lower than 4.5 are not synthesized by normal lymphocytes, but are exclusively products of activated lymph node cells.

2) Fraction II from the isoelectrofocussing step containing pH3-MIF with a pI of 3.0-3.5 contains only a single labelled band with a molecular weight of 38,000 (Fig. 1). This fraction contains high MIF activity (47%, 37% and 46% inhibition in 3 experiments). This indicates that the single band represents pH3-MIF.

Fraction # I II III IV V VI VII VIII IX

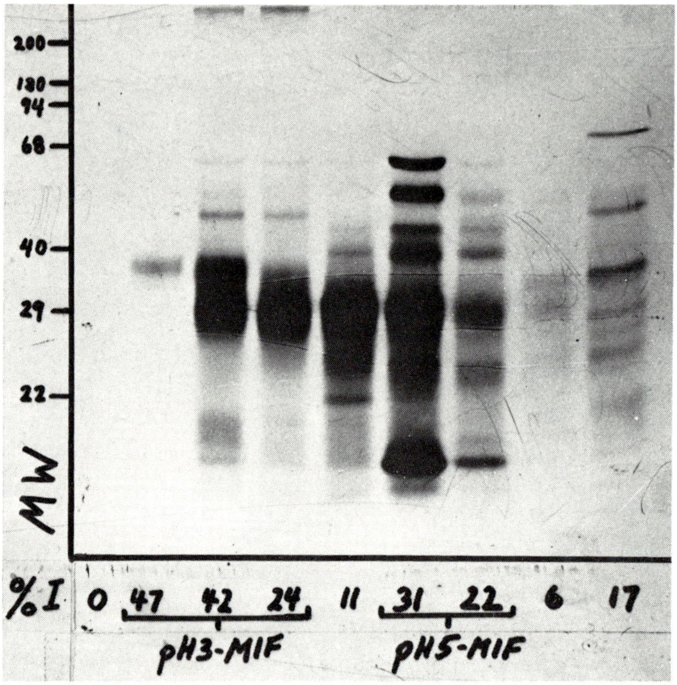

Figure 1. SDS-polyacrylamide electrophoresis of $[^3H]$-leucine labelled MIF containing fractions obtained by fractionation on a preparative isoelectrofocussing column. The radioactive proteins were made visible by fluorography. The pH gradient extends from fraction I with a pH of 3.0 to fraction IX with a pH of 6.0. The MIF activity of each fraction is recorded at the bottom. In total, 14 different radioactive polypeptides can be discerned. Note that fraction II with MIF activity of 47% has only one discernible protein band with a molecular weight of 38,000. The fluorograph is overexposed in order to make the band in lane II more visible. Molecular weight markers in thousands are indicated on the ordinate.

3) When this fraction II was rechromatographed on Sephadex G-75 columns, MIF activity cochromatographed with the single band indicating that the MIF activity is associated with the 38,000 dalton polypeptide ($K_d = 0.08$). This experiment demonstrates the apparent homogeneity of pH3-MIF and would be one of the first demonstrations of purification of a lymphokine to homogeneity. We are currently investigating whether these findings can be verified by other fractionation procedures.

REFERENCES

1. Bloom, B.R., and Bennett, B. (1966). *Science 153,* 80.
2. David, J.R. (1966). *Proc. Natl. Acad. Sci. 56,* 72.
3. David, J.R., and Remold, H.G. (1976). *In* "Immunobiology of the Macrophage" (D.S. Nelson, ed.), p. 401. Academic Press, New York.
4. Remold, H.G., and Mednis, A.D. (1977). *J. Immunol. 118,* 2015.
5. Remold, H.G., Katz, A.B., Haber, E., and David, J.R. (1970). *Cell. Immunol. 1,* 133.
6. Sorg, C., and Bloom, B.R. (1973). *J. Exp. Med. 137,* 148.
7. Laemmli, V.K. (1970). *Nature 227,* 680.
8. Bonner, W.M., and Laskey, R.A. (1974). *Eur. J. Biochem. 46,* 83.
9. Remold, H.G., and Mednis, A.D. (1979). *J. Immunol. 122,* 1920.
10. Sorg, C., and Klinkert, W. (1978). *Fed. Proc. Abs. 37,* 2748.

(Paper presented by Dr. J. David)

DISCUSSION

HADDEN: We have been able to show that MIF will adsorb to macrophage membranes. Accordingly I ask David how, for the pH 5 MIF, was degradation distinguished from adsorption and thus removal of activity?

DAVID: pH 5 MIF incubated with macrophages lost its activity; none was recovered in the supernatant. We do not believe this is due to absorption since when the macrophages are treated with DFP or other esterase inhibitors, the pH 5 MIF is recovered in the supernatant. One would therefore have to postulate that the active site of the esterase is the receptor for MIF.

WAKSMAN: Glycosylation could account for all the differences David has described, i.e. lower isoelectric point, sensitivity to neuraminidase and protection against some proteolytic enzymes, such as trypsin. Should one not get more specific information on sugars and/or degree of glycosylation in each presumptive molecule? This same question arises in connection with 24 hr and 48 hr human MIF described by David in a preceding paper.

DAVID: We have assumed that glycosylation and presence of sialic acid accounts for changes in pI and trypsin resistance. However, pH 3 MIF is no longer active after neuraminidase treatment, whereas pH 5 MIF is. This suggests to us that, (1) sialic acid is necessary on pH 3 guinea pig MIF in its action on macrophages, or (2) sialic acid is necessary for interaction of pH 3 MIF with an "enzyme", which then could convert it to pH 5 MIF. Without sialic acid it would not be converted to an active form.

PICK: Did David try using 2-DOG (2-deoxyglucose) or tunicamycin as inhibitors of glycosylation? They should eliminate the formation of pH 3 MIF. Secondly, did he consider using labelled glucosamine or fucose as internal labels to ascertain whether the pH 3 MIF would be preferentially labelled?

DAVID: We plan to carry out production of MIF in the presence of tunicamycin or 2-DOG to see if this blocks production of either form of MIF. We have considered labelling with sugars, but at present, only radioactive leucine was used in order to label both MIFs . MIF is not affected by fucosidase (fucose is a terminal sugar on the glycolipid receptor for MIF).

WOLSTENCROFT: I should like to know firstly, whether there is any consequential loss of activity in the pH 3 fraction due to the low pH and secondly, what recoveries of activity were achieved for the pH 3 and pH 5 MIF-active fractions?

DAVID: pH 3 MIF was obtained after 21 hr isoelectrofocussing; for part of the time it was at pH 3, and was then still active. We have not incubated it further at pH 3 to ascertain stability. It is difficult to get values of specific activity assessed as activity/mg protein since we must have a small amount of albumin present when collecting the fractions off the isoelectrofocussing column.

SALVIN: Is there an additive or synergistic effect on biologic activity when the two fractions are combined?

DAVID: I do not know whether there is a synergistic effect, when pH 3 and pH 5 MIF are added. This should be investigated.

MIZEL: Are pH 3 and pH 5 MIF irreversibly denatured by SDS? If not, has David determined whether SDS converts pH 3 to pH 5 MIF?

DAVID: We do not know. Mizel's is a good question. If either pH 3 or pH 5 MIF is not denatured by SDS, it should be possible to isolate the band and determine whether it is still active.

IDENTIFICATION OF FOUR LYMPHOCYTE ACTIVATION PRODUCTS OF GUINEA PIG AND THEIR CORRELATION TO MACROPHAGE MIGRATION INHIBITORY ACTIVITY

Wolfgang Klinkert
Clemens Sorg

Department of experimental Dermatology
University of Münster
Münster, Germany

Using a radioactive double-labelling technique it was possible to identify a great number of lymphocyte activation products (LAPs) which were synthesized either de novo or in increased amounts (1). From the LAPs three molecules were more prominent whose molecular weight could be determined at 60,000 (a), 45,000 (b), and 30,000 (c), and whose isoelectric point was determined at 5.2. It also could be demonstrated, that migration inhibitory activity was associated with the 45,000 molecule (b). Recently, an antiserum was raised against highly purified material from activated guinea pig lymphocyte culture supernatants which contained migration inhibitory factor (MIF). The antibodies if conjugated to a solid matrix specifically absorbed MIF from active supernatants (2). Furthermore, in extensive studies it was determined that the antiserum suppressed delayed type hypersensitive reactions in vivo and in vitro (3, 4). An analysis of the sereological specificity of the antiserum showed, that it reacted mainly with three lymphocyte activation products of a molecular weight 60,000, 45,000 and 30,000 which all had an isoelectric point of 5.2 (5). Furthermore, it could be shown that these molecules did not contain Ia or B_1 determinants,and that they were dis-

ISBN 0-12-213950-X

tinct from lymphotoxin (6) and that they also were produced by activated B-cells, L_2C leukemia cells and non-lymphoid cells such as growing fibroblasts (7). Here, we will describe the purification and some further biochemical characteristics of these products of activated lymphocytes which react with the anti-lymphokine serum and which are associated with macrophage migration inhibitory activity.

RESULTS

Supernatants from Concanavalin A (Con A) stimulated guinea pig lymph node cells, which were simultaneously labelled with H-3 leucine were chromatographed first on Sephadex G 75 and pooled fractions of a molecular weight range 70,000 - 20,000 were rechromatographed on Sephadex G 100. Distinct peaks of binding material could be identified at molecular weight ranges 60,000, 45,000, 30,000. In the following step pools of G 100 fractions in the molecular weight range of a, b and c were subjected to isoelectric focusing in polyacrylamide gels containing a pH gradient of 3,5 - 10. Most material of a, b and c focused at pH 5,2. This material was also found to react specifically with the anti-lymphokine serum. When peak fractions at pH 5,2 were collected and assayed in the macrophage migration test a, b and c contained significant inhibitory activity compared to identical fractions from non-stimulated lymphocyte culture supernatants which had been reconstituted with Con A before fractionation. With the preparations a, b and c some further characterizations were performed. Since it had been suggested earlier that the migration inhibitory factor of guinea pig was a glycoprotein (8) radiolabelled a, b and c were subjected to isopycnic centrifugation in a CsCl gradient.It was found that all material concentrated at a density of 1,278 g/cm^3 which was very similar to the density of radiolabelled albumin which was run in parallel. Since it has been reported that migration inhibitory activity was sensitive to neuraminidase treatment (8), a, b and c was also treated with neuraminidase from vibrio (comma) in a calcium containing buffer. When focused before and after treatment, no shift to an isoelectric point greater than 5,2 could be observed which would be expected if sialic acid would have been split off. However, in some preparations material with identical molecular weights but a pI of 3,5 - 4,5 was found which -after neuraminidase treatment- focused at pH 5,2 (7). This could be the molecular equivalent of the MIF activities, recently described by Remold and Mednis (9) with a pI 3 and 5. When material of preparations a, b and c was assayed for proteolytic activity using ^{14}C-labelled bovine serum albumin at pH 5,5 or 8 as substrate no degradation could be detected. For further information on the structure of the purified materials the following experiments were performed. Aliquots of purified a, b and c were treated with 8 M urea and fractionated by polyacrylamide gel electrophoresis (PAGE) without SDS. All three preparations contained only material with mw 30,000 and larger. When aliquots from the same preparations were treated with 8 M urea, SDS and 2-mercaptoethanol (2-ME) and were then analysed in presence of these agents, the profile did not change either indicating that molecules are probably not composed of non-covalently or disulfide linked subunits. More studies, however, are needed using stronger denaturing and reducing agents in order to settle this question definitely. In the course of these studies it was remarkable to observe, that the profiles were very similar in both systems, eventhough PAGE separates for size and charge where as SDS-PAGE separates for size only. It also showed high molecular weight material in preparation c which was similar in charge and size to that of preparation a and b but should have been removed by preceeding rechromatography on Sephadex. The resistance to urea, SDS and 2-ME showed that these materials were not simply aggregates. It rather appeared that material of pool c had the tendency to polymerize. This could be shown when different preparations of a, b and c were run on PAGE in presence of SDS and 8 M urea (10). Compared to marker proteins in parallel gels the molecular weights of peaks in preparation a, b or c were determined at 15,000, 30,000, 45,000, 60,000 and 82,000. It is remarkable that the preparation of pool c contained a 60,000 molecule as the major component eventhough molecules of this size had been removed before by repeated Sephadex chromatography. Furthermore, it was observed, that after purification steps according to size and charge all preparations contained material with a mw of 15,000. In a systematic search it was possible to detect the 15,000 mw material in cell lysates and in low amounts in stimulated culture supernatants. The isoelectric point of this molecule was determined at 5,2 which is identical with the pI of a, b and c. The 15,000 molecules also reacted with the anti-lymphokine serum and like the other three

Table 1

Chemical Properties of Migration Inhibitory Activities of Guinea Pig

	a	b	c	d
Molecular weight	60.000	45.000	30.000	15.000
Isoelectric point	5.2	5.2	5.2	5.2
after treatment with neuraminidase	5.2	5.2	5.2	n.d.
Density in CsCl gradient	1.278	1.278	1.278	n.d.
Inhibitory activity	+	+	+	+
after treatment with guanidin · HCl	+	+	+	+
" + 2 - ME	-	-	-	-
" + 2 - ME+I-acet.	-	-	-	-
Reaction with an anti-lymphokine serum	+	+	+	+

n.d. = not done; 2-ME = 2-mercaptoethanol; I-acet. = iodoaceticacid products of activated lymphocytes showed significant migration inhibitory activity compared to identical preparations from control non stimulated supernatants.

CONCLUSIONS

The data described and summarized in Table 1 are evidence that migration inhibitory activity is not associated with a single molecule but rather with a group of structurally related molecules. These findings have now been paralleled in detail by those obtained in the murine system. The molecular heterogeneity of migration inhibitory activity could be explained that the different molecules are oligomers of a common subunit of mw 15,000 which has a pI of 5.2. The generation of covalently linked oligomers could be brought about either by an autocatalytic mechanism, suggesting that MIF itself is an enzyme or by contaminating enzymes. While there are known examples for enzymes which can polymerize proteins, degradation to small molecules could be explained by contaminating proteolytic enzymes. However, we were unable so far to detect proteolytic activity in any of the preparations, nor was there any indication for a ligase like activity in the purified fractions.

REFERENCES

1. Sorg, C., and Bloom, B.R., J.exp.Med. 137, 148 (1973).
2. Geczy, C.L., Friedrich, W., and De Weck, A.L., Cell.Immunol. 19, 65 (1975).
3. Hentges, F., Geczy, C.L., Geczy, A.F., and De Weck, A.L., Immunology 32, 905 (1977).
4. Geczy, C.L., Geczy, A.F., and De Weck, A.L., J.Immunol. 117, 1824 (1976).
5. Sorg, C., and Geczy, C.L., Eur.J.Immunol. 6, 688 (1976).
6. Sorg, C., Geczy, C.L., GeczyA.F., Hämmerling, G.J., and Gateley, N., Z.Immun.-Forsch. 154, 44 (1978).
7. Sorg, C., and Geczy, C.L., J.Immunol. 121, 1109 (1978).
8. Remold, H.G., and David, J.R., J.Immunol. 107, 1090 (1971).
9. Remold, H.G., and Mednis, A.D., J.Immunol. 118, 2015 (1977).
10. Sorg, C., and Klinkert, W., Fed.Proc. 37, 2748 (1978).

CHARACTERIZATION OF MURINE MACROPHAGE MIGRATION INHIBITORY ACTIVITIES (MIF)

Clemens Sorg

Department of experimental Dermatology
University of Münster
Münster, Germany

Most information on the chemical and functional characteristics of MIF has been worked out in the guinea pig (1). Eventhough the mouse has been predominantly used for studies of various immune reactions, the information on the murine MIF is relatively scarce. Kühner and David (2) determined some characteristics of migration inhibitory activity in supernatants of Concanavalin A (Con A) stimulated murine spleen cells. The molecular weight was determined to be heterogeneous and was found within a range of 48,000 - 67,000 daltons. On the other hand Harrington determined the molecular weight of MIF produced in a mouse allograft model at 45.000 daltons with a pI of 5,0 - 5,5 (3). Earlier we reported on a double label technique which proofed useful in the analysis of guinea pig lymphocyte activation products (LAPs) (4) which had been adapted to the analysis of LAPs in Con A stimulated spleen cell cultures (5). Using this method it was possible to determine a series of LAPs according to their molecular size and their isoelectric point. No attempt was made however to correlate radiolabelled LAPs with the migration inhibitory activity. In the present study, we set out to determine the molecular characteristics (molecular weight and isoelectric point) of migration inhibitory activities in Con A stimulated supernatants of either spleen or thymus cells.

ISBN 0-12-213950-X

Balb C mice were used throughout. The culture conditions for MIF production have been described before (5). 24 h culture supernatants were concentrated 100 fold by rotary evaporation and were fractionated on 1,5 x 200 Sephadex G 100 columns using 0,01 Mphosphate buffer as eluant. Every second fraction was pooled and desalted on an ion exchange resin (AG 501 - X8 (D); Biorad) diluted with 2-fold concentrated MEM-Dulbecco, reconstituted with fetal bovine serum to 15 % and tested for MIF activity as described (6). Pools of the respective molecular weight ranges were concentrated and desalted as described above and subjected to isoelectric focusing in an ampholine gradient pH 3,5 - 10. Ampholines were removed either by desalting on an ion exchanger or on Sephadex G 25.

In the supernatants of stimulated spleen cell cultures several distinct peaks of inhibitory activity were found eluting at the molecular weight range of about 56,000 (a), 42,000 (b), 28,000 (c), and 14,000 (d). Activity -eventhough less consistent- was also found at higher molecular weight ranges. In non-stimulated control cultures only a minor amount of inhibitory activity at mw 56,000 was observed Similar results were obtained with stimulated and unstimulated thymocytes. However, the distribution of inhibitory activity over the respective molecular weight ranges appeared to be quantitatively different as compared to fractionated spleen cell cultures, showing main activities at 56,000 and 28,000 (a and c). When the materials of peak activity were pooled and subjected to isoelectric focusing in a pH-gradient of 3,5 to 10 inhibitory activity was found for all mw ranges (a - d) at pH 4,5 - 5,5. When the pools were split before focusing and one part was treated with neuraminidase (Vibro cholerae; Behringwerke AG) no significant shift to a higher pH was observed in the treated sample. Furthermore, the titer of activity in the treated sample was not significantly reduced compared to the untreated sample.

In extensive studies on MIF of guinea pig it was demonstrated that migration inhibitory activity is not attributed to a single molecule but rather to a group of molecules of different size (60,000, 45,000, 30,000, 15,000) and similar charge (pI 5,2) which correlate well with radiolabelled lymphocyte activation products whose physico-chemical characteristics had been determined the same (7). In studies on the chemical characterization of products of activated mouse lymphocytes, molecules with the characteristics of a, b and c had been identified (5). In those experiments a molecule with the characteristics of (a) was found to be produced predominantly which correlates well with the functional studies here, where it was found that in spleen cell cultures supernatants the main MIF activity is found at a mw range of about 56,000. Similar to the data in the guinea pig (8, 9) it was found, that murine MIF is insensitive to neuraminidase treatment (2), which allows the conclusion that sialic acid plays no functional role as a constituent of MIF. Furthermore, it appears that the MIFs focusing at pH 5,2 do not contain sialic acid at all or only in very low amounts. However, this might only be true for our culture conditions and there might also exsist a sialo-form of MIF as described before (10). In conclusion, our data allow to state that migration inhibitory activities are associated with a group of structurally similar molecules.

ACKNOWLEDGMENT

I wish to thank Mrs. Marlies Bacher for excellent technical assistance.

REFERENCES

1. Pick, E., in:Immunopharmacology (J.W. Hadden, R.G. Coffey, and F. Spreafico, eds.), p.163. Plenum, New York, 1977.
2. Kühner, A.L., and David, J.R., J.Immunol. 116, 140 (1976).
3. Harrington, J.D., jr. Fed.Proc. 34, 977 (1975).
4. Sorg, C., and Bloom, B.R., J.exp.Med. 137, 148 (1973).
5. Sorg, C., Eur.J.Biochem. 55, 423 (1975).
6. Neumann, CH., and Sorg, C., Eur.J.Immunol. 8, 582 (1978).
7. Sorg, C., and Klinkert, W., Fed.Proc. 37, 2748 (1978).
8. Klinkert, W., and Sorg, C., in: Proc. 12th Intl. Leucocyte culture conference (M.R. Quastel, ed.), Academic Press, New York, 1979, in press.
9. Ashworth, L.A.E., Eckersley, B.J., and Ford, W.H., Int. Arch.Allergy 48, 143 (1975).
10. Sorg, C., and Geczy, C.L., J.Immunol. 121, 1199 (1978).

DISCUSSION

COHEN S: Has Klinkert studied the stability of the monomers and polymers with respect to spontaneous aggregation and dissociation? This is important because it focuses on which is the active agent in vivo. In this regard, one might expect that the presence of macrophage membranes might facilitate either aggregation or dissociation. It is noteworthy that these polymers need not be limited to MW 60'000. We have reported that sera from patients with the Sezary syndrome have MIF with MW of 75'000 to 80'000 daltons.

KLINKERT: So far, we have not done experiments such as Cohen's, as we have only small amounts of biologically active MIF. We have also found radiolabelled material with a MW 82'000 which has not yet been assayed for MIF activity. On the other hand, in fractions of Sephadex chromatography we also find activity at higher MW ranges.

GECZY: How did Klinkert measure the proteolytic activity of his preparations? Did he add divalent metal ions, and at what pH did he measure activity?

KLINKERT: We have tried to measure the degradation of ^{14}C-labelled BSA and casein in PBS and Tris-buffers at pH 5.5 and 8. These buffers contained divalent metal ions (Ca^{++}, Mg^{++}). In contrast to different proteinases as controls, purified MIF-containing preparations did not degrade these substrates.

McDANIEL: What concentration of MIF is necessary to perceive activity in the bioassay? Is the supernatant concentrated or diluted? Human MAF must be diluted 10^3 - 10^4 fold to discern activity in a tumoricidal assay.

KLINKERT: We have concentrated our supernatants about 25-fold. In the MIF assay, we can dilute the activity to 1:16, but generally activity can be demonstrated only to 1:2 dilution.

SORG: As regards the assay of inhibition of plasminogen activator (IPA) in mouse supernatants, we routinely dilute our fractions from the column purification up to 1:256. This is necessary since we have to find the optimum. At high concentrations we sometimes find no activity which then is evident at higher dilutions.

PICK: What is Klinkert's explanation for the fact that 2-mercaptoethanol causes loss of activity since he does not assume that the MIF subunits are linked together by S-S bonds? With guinea pig MIF we have found that 2-mercapto-ethanol does not destroy MIF activity even in the presence of 8M urea and 6M guanidine hydrochloride unless we alkylate with iodoacetamide or acetylonitrile, whereupon activity is lost. Treatment of guinea pig MIF with 2-mercaptoethanol resulted in a decrease in molecular weight from more than 30,000 daltons to less than 30,000 daltons (as judged by passage through PM 30 membranes). However, dialysis of "less than 30,000 MIF" against medium resulted in the reappearance of "more than 30,000 MIF".

KLINKERT: Our explanation for such findings is that there could be inner-molecular S-S bonds which are necessary to form biologically active molecules. However, these S-S bonds seem not to be involved in subunit linkage as we are unable to split our MIF molecules into smaller subunits by reducing S-S bonds with 2-mercaptoethanol and alkylating them with iodoaceticacid in the presence of 8M urea.

de WECK: To supplement the data on mouse and guinea pig MIF which have been presented, I have a few short comments to make on the heterogeneity of human MIF. Analyzing a large number of individual human culture supernatants on Biogel P 100, MIF activity is regularly found around MW 25,000, but it is also present around 40-50,000 daltons and occasionally at higher MW such as 60-70,000 daltons. When human peripheral blood lymphocytes are cultured with Con A in the absence of 2-mercaptoethanol, activity is never encountered below 25,000 daltons. However, when the cells are cultured in the presence of 2-ME, MIF activity is regularly found in the 12,000-15,000 MW range. The isolated 25,000 dalton MIF-active molecule is not reduced in vitro by 2-mercaptoethanol to a 12,500 active molecule. Accordingly, I believe there now accumulates suggestive evidence in the three systems, man, mouse and guinea pig, that MIF activity is attributable to a family of molecules based upon a subunit of 12,000-15,000 daltons and capable of polymerization under conditions which we do not yet fully understand.

LEONARD: The papers by Klinkert and by Sorg have demonstrated heterogeneity of activity on gel filtration. In contrast, electrofocussing shows activity primarily at pH 5.

Is this a true picture, or is it due to destruction of activity at pH values other than 5? It would be interesting to mix pH 5 fractions with fractions at other pH values, e. g. 6 and 7, to determine whether or not the pH 5 activity persists.

KLINKERT: Leonard's proposal is a good one, but it is not too surprising, in our opinion, to find MIF activity only at pH 5 in isoelectric focussing.If our molecules are really oligomers of a common subunit with a molecular weight of 15,000 daltons and pI ∿5.2, all the oligomers should have the same pI.

MIZEL: Working with LAF, we have found that intracellular LAF has molecular weights of 15,000, 30,000, 45,000, 60,000 and 220,000 daltons. Is it possible that some of the heterogeneity of MIF molecular weights is due to the release of a number of intracellular precursor forms?

KLINKERT: It might be that cells release a number of intracellular precursor forms. If this is the case, we must assume that these molecules are capable of spontaneous association even after separation by Sephadex chromatography and isoelectric focussing, since we always find heterogeneity of MIF molecules in SDS-PAGE, even after the various purification steps. Another explanation could be the existence of a protein ligase-like activity which co-chromatographs.

PROPERTIES AND ISOLATION OF GUINEA PIG MACROPHAGE AGGLUTINATION FACTOR[1]

H. P. Godfrey

Department of Pathology
State University of New York at Stony Brook
Stony Brook, New York

Macrophage agglutination factor (MAggF) is a lymphokine found in culture supernates of mitogen and antigen activated guinea pig lymph node cells (LNC) whose activity is readily quantified by titration (Lolekha, Dray and Gotoff, 1971; Godfrey, 1976; Godfrey and Geczy, 1978). Supernates containing MAggF activity cause macroscopically visible clumping of viable peritoneal macrophages on culture tube walls after 4 hr which disappears after a further 8-12 hr of culture. The production of MAggF *in vitro* correlates well with *in vivo* manifestations of delayed hypersensitivity (Godfrey, 1976). Treatment of LNC with a specific anti-T cell serum and complement inhibits the elicitation of MAggF by antigen, indicating that T cells play an important role in elaboration of this lymphokine. Cell chromatography of LNC over anti-L chain containing substrates prepared by Dr. C. Koch removed 85% of B cells without affecting the titer of MAggF elicited by antigen, suggesting that any role for B cells in the elaboration of this activity is likely to be a limited one.

I. STABILITY OF MAggF TO FREEZE-THAW AND HEATING

Before any attempt could be made to purify MAggF activity from LNC culture supernates, it was necessary to establish its stability to freezing, thawing and heating. Freshly harvested

[1]*Supported by a grant from the Kroc Foundation.*

ISBN 0-12-213950-X

culture supernates containing MAggF activity were subjected to repeated freezing and thawing. Aliquots of culture supernate that had been frozen and thawed up to five times showed no decrease in activity in comparison to untreated aliquots. Repeated freezing and thawing of culture supernates from unstimulated cultures did not lead to appearance of MAggF activity. The heat stability of MAggF was evaluated by incubating aliquots of active fluids at various temperatures for various periods of time and comparing their activity with that of a freshly thawed aliquot. In confirmation of the report of Postlethwaite and Kang (1976), MAggF activity was found to be stable for 30 min at 56° and for 24 hr at 4° while undergoing dialysis.

II. PARTIAL PURIFICATION OF MAggF

Since MAggF had been previously shown to be antigenically distinct from MIF and from Ig (Godfrey and Geczy, 1978), and since it was clear that it was stable to both freeze-thaw and to dialysis, purification of this activity from LNC culture supernates appeared feasible. Three ml of ten-fold concentrated supernates from cultures incubated with or without PPD for 24 hr were dialyzed against PBS, pH 7.2, chromatographed over Sephadex G-200, and 10 ml fractions collected. Each fraction was tested for MAggF activity in duplicate and the optical density at 280 nm determined. Significant MAggF activity was found to be associated with molecules similar in size to IgG or somewhat larger. These observations confirm and extend those of Postlethwaite and Kang (1976).

Active fractions from the G-200 fractionation and comparable control fractions were then concentrated and aliquots of each were electrophoresed on a 4% polyacrylamide-0.5% agarose gel (2 mA/gel, pH 8.8). Gels were either stained with Coomassie brilliant blue or frozen, sliced into 1 mm sections and eluted with PBS. The eluents were assayed for MAggF activity and the results are shown in the upper part of Fig. 1 as geometric mean relative MAggF titer = MAggF $titer_D$/ MAggF $titer_C$ where D and C refer to fluids from cultures exposed to PPD ("D") or not exposed to antigen ("C"); the titers are shown on a logarithmic scale. Significant MAggF activity was associated with a peak of Rf = 0.53. The stained gel showed a faint band of protein at Rf = 0.50.
Under the conditions of electrophoresis that were employed, guinea pig IgG remained at the origin. The difference in Rf between MAggF activity and protein band is not significant

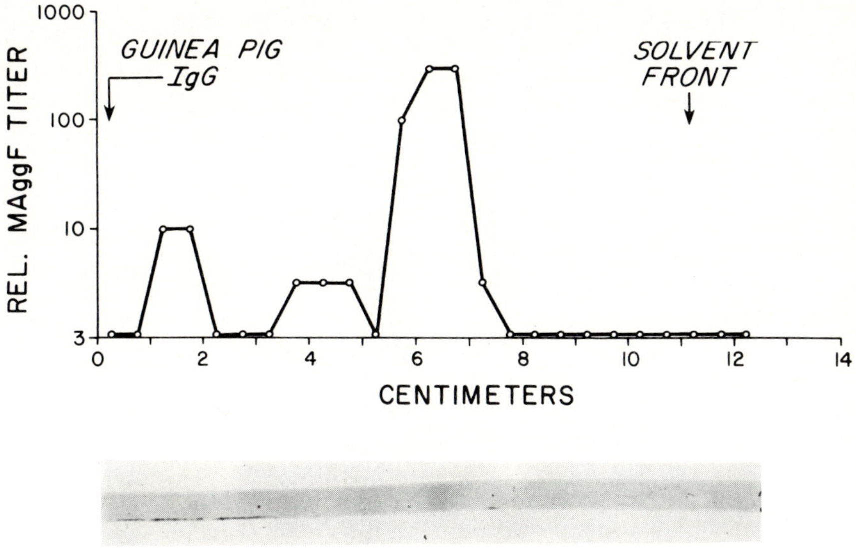

FIGURE 1. Acrylamide-agarose electrophoresis of concentrated active fractions and control fractions from G-200 Chromatography. Relative MAggF activity of eluted fractions is shown in upper panel, stained gel in lower. Note correspondence of peak of activity and stained band in gel.

($P < 0.5$) and it is therefore not unreasonable to suppose that the stained band is identical with the peak of activity. It would seem likely that MAggF could be separated from the other lymphokine activities present in LNC culture supernates, and amounts suitable for use in raising antibodies and for various biochemical studies prepared by this relatively simple two-step procedure. The availability of such materials will permit evaluation of the role of this lymphokine in *in vivo* manifestations of delayed hypersensitivity.

REFERENCES

Godfrey, H.P. (1976). *Immunology 30*, 685.
Godfrey, H.P., and Geczy, C.L. (1978). *J. Immunol. 121*, 1428.
Lolekha, S., Dray, S., and Gotoff, S.P. (1971). *J. Immunol. 104*, 296.
Postlewaite, A.E., and Kang, A.H. (1976). *J. Immunol. 117*, 1651.

DISCUSSION

DVORAK: What is the relation of Godfrey's material to the alveolar macrophage aggregation factor described by Myrvik that is thought to be hyaluronic acid? Is Godfrey's material a protein or could it also be hyaluronic acid?

GODFREY: I am uncertain of the relation of guinea pig MAggF to the material described by Myrvik and his collaborators. That substance was produced by antigen-stimulated lymphoid cells from rabbits sensitized with BCG, and its activity was assayed on normal rabbit alveolar macrophages. Rabbit MAggF caused relatively rapid (minutes) aggregation of macrophages at room temperature. This is certainly different from guinea pig MAggF activity which requires a 4 hr incubation at 37° C to effect clumping of peritoneal macrophages. The rabbit material was described as being larger than 400,000 daltons molecular weight and therefore much larger than guinea pig MAggF whose molecular weight is similar to that of IgG.

Guinea pig MAggF activity is destroyed by exposure to trypsin, indicating its protein nature. I do not know if it is sensitive to treatment with hyaluronidase.

PRODUCTION OF MIF BY MURINE LYMPHOCYTES[1]

Stanley Cohen
Nancy Adelman
Takeshi Yoshida

Department of Pathology
University of Connecticut Health Center
Farmington, Connecticut

The experiments described here were undertaken to define some aspects of lymphokine production in the mouse. Our initial studies involved the detection of Migration Inhibition Factor (MIF) by means of the agarose droplet technique. We found that there is variation in the MIF level produced by spleen cells from different inbred mouse strains in response to Con A or specific antigen stimulation in serum-free medium (1). We were able to demonstrate that BALB/c ($H\text{-}2^d$) and AKR ($H\text{-}2^k$) cells consistently secrete high levels of MIF and that DBA/2 ($H\text{-}2^d$) and C3H/He ($H\text{-}2^k$) elaborate marginal levels or no MIF. Thus, MIF production is not directly linked to the H-2 complex. In other words, the H-2 complex alone cannot be responsible for the observed strain variation in MIF production. This conclusion obviously holds only for those activating agents tested, and further generalization awaits studies utilizing batteries of antigens. Nevertheless, similarities in responses between mitogen and antigen activation that we found suggest that the strain differences in such responses is not the result of some peculiar activity of the Con A on the spleen cells. This is consistent with observations in other species on the identity of MIF induced by specific antigen or Con A (2).

We next determined that the variation in MIF activity observed did not simply reflect differences in the susceptibility of macrophages from the various strains to MIF. We

[1] *Supported by NIH grant no. AI-12477.*

ISBN 0-12-213950-X

found that MIF from any source affected macrophages from each strain to an equal degree. This ability of the Con A-induced MIF produced in one strain to inhibit the migration of macrophages from unrelated strains agrees with results from other studies where MIF was produced by antigen stimulation *in vivo* (3,4). These studies clearly show that the interaction of MIF with its target cell can transcend strain barriers.

In the above studies, we also observed that lymphocytes from C57BL/6 mice could not produce MIF, in contradistinction to reports in the literature (3-7). The main difference between the protocol we used and that of others was the absence of serum in our culture. We found that MIF could be generated by Con A-activated C57BL/6 lymphocytes, provided that the medium was supplemented with 2% heat-inactivated fetal calf serum (FCS). The action of the FCS was not due to an enhancement of the viability of the lymphocytes during culture, since incubation of cell-free supernatants from activated lymphocytes with FCS also led to the appearance of MIF activity. In the MIF agarose assay, 2% FCS itself in RPMI 1640 medium did not significantly inhibit migration compared to an RPMI 1640 medium without FCS. Furthermore, there was no significant difference between the migration in a conditioned (control cultured) medium containing 2% FCS as compared to conditioned medium alone. This demonstrates that FCS itself has no intrinsic migration inhibitory activity in the amount utilized, although Fox *et al.* (8) have demonstrated MIF in FCS in another system.

The precise role of FCS in this system is unknown. The following possibilities suggest themselves: 1) enzymes in the FCS activate a MIF precursor molecule; 2) proteins in the FCS may complex with the MIF molecule rendering it active; 3) FCS may destroy or inactivate an enhancing activity in the activated supernatants; 4) FCS may inactivate an inhibitor of MIF; and 5) a product of the stimulated lymphocytes may activate a molecule in FCS conferring MIF-like activity on the FCS molecule. Experiments are now underway in our laboratory to test these possibilities. Another possibility is that FCS might have, in some way, enhanced pre-existing sub-detectable levels of MIF in the C57BL/6-derived supernatants. This possibility is difficult to exclude unequivocally. However, we performed experiments using BALB/c cells, which as stated above are MIF producers. Addition of FCS in this situation did not lead to enhanced MIF production.

The mechanisms underlying the strain variation of MIF production are still unclear. It may well be the result of interplay among various activated lymphocyte products in addition to MIF. Alternatively, it may be due to quantitative differences in the capacity for cell activation or to qualitative differences in the mediators themselves (more active MIF in certain strains). In any case, this variation in lymphokine production may be partially responsible for the strain differences observed by others in the development of both delayed hypersensitivity and disease susceptibility in the mouse (9).

In order to obtain background data on MIF production to allow us to attack these problems, we next explored the relative ability of lymphocyte subpopulations to make MIF. T-cell enriched populations were obtained by passage of splenic and/or lymph node lymphocytes from BALB/c mice over glass wool columns. The cells eluted from the columns were more than 90% viable by trypan blue exclusion, and contained less than 4% of cells with C receptors and less than 0.5% macrophages on the basis of non-specific esterase staining. The original spleen cell population from immunized animals could be stimulated by Con A, or LPS, while the the T cell preparations could respond to Con A and PPD, but not LPS. Interestingly, the T cell response was macrophage dependent.

We next prepared B cell enriched populations by treating cell suspensions with a heterologous anti-T-cell antiserum and complement. The resulting populations demonstrated a 90% diminution in Con A mitogen responsiveness. In terms of surface Ig, and C receptor, the preparations showed greater than 95% purity for B cells. All starting populations and B cell-enriched populations produced MIF in response to LPS. The B cell preparations could not be stimulated with Con A. Both normal and immune B cells were found to produce MIF on challenge with PPD. However, no MIF was produced on challenging immune B cells with DNP-KLH. These results are consistent with our previous findings in the guinea pig (10).

The ability of the non-immune cells to respond to PPD with MIF production was dependent upon the removal of T cells. This suggests a suppressor function for murine cells similar to that we have found in the guinea pig (11).

The final set of experiments involved the use of cells from nude mice (nude mice on a BALB/c background). When cells from normal or immunized spleens or lymph nodes were stimulated with either DNP-KLH or PPD, no MIF activity was detected. However, LPS stimulation resulted in good MIF production. These experimental results demonstrate that, as is the case in other strains, LPS is a potent stimulator of MIF production in nude mice. The inability of the nude mouse cells to respond to PPD stimulation with MIF release may be the result of a regulatory effect exerted by the small T cell population present in these animals.

The results presented demonstrate that both T and B cells of murine origin can make MIF and that the stimulatory conditions appear to be similar to those in the guinea pig.

Further, in both species, B cell production of MIF appears to be under T cell control.
There are strain differences in the capacity of mouse lymphocytes to generate detectable MIF activity *in vitro*. Further experiments are necessary to pinpoint the relative contribution of T and B cells to this effect, both with respect to MIF production itself, and with respect to regulatory effects.

REFERENCES

1. Adelman, N., Cohen, S., and Yoshida, T. (1978). *J. Immunol. 121*, 209.
2. Remold, H.G., David, R.A., and David, J.R. (1972). *J. Immunol. 109*, 578.
3. Mortensen, R.F., Ceglowski, W.S., and Friedman, H. (1973). *J. Immunol. 111*, 657.
4. Al-Askari, S. and Lawrence, H.S. (1972). *Cell. Immunol. 5*, 402.
5. Harrington, J.T. (1975). *Cell. Immunol. 12*, 476.
6. Kuhner, A.L. and David, J.R. (1976). *J. Immunol. 116*, 140.
7. Neiburger, R. G. and Youmans, G.P. (1973). *Infect. Immun. 7*, 190.
8. Fox, R.A., Gregory, D.S., and Feldman, J.D. (1974). *J. Immunol. 112*, 1861.
9. Crowle, A.J. (1975). *Adv. Immunol. 20*, 197.
10. Yoshida, T., Sonozaki, H., and Cohen, S. (1973). *J. Exp. Med. 138*, 784.
11. Cohen, S. and Yoshida, T. (1977). *J. Immunol. 119*, 719.

DISCUSSION

WOOD: Has Cohen tested the various mouse strains for their ability to produce lymphokines other than MIF? Does the production of these lymphokines correlate better with skin reactions than does MIF?

COHEN: We are now testing the production of macrophage chemotactic factors but have not yet related these to skin reactions. I anticipate that the best correlation will be with macrophage and neutrophil chemotactic factor.

LANDY: To what extent do Cohen's findings reflect differences in inbred mouse strains with respect to (a) spleen cellularity (b) heterogeneity in cell types present in spleen, i.e., greater or lesser proportions of lymphocytic or macrophage cell types.

COHEN: The possibilities are:
(1) different cellular capacity for MIF production in different strains; (2) different proportion of inhibitors of MIF production or activity; (3) different proportion of lymphocyte subsets.
No data are available to allow a distinction between these possibilities. As I indicated in my report, macrophage differences do not seem to play a role.

KIRCHNER: Did Cohen rule out the possibility that an antagonist of MIF is produced by C57Bl/6 spleen cells. C57Bl/6 are usually quite active in producing certain other lymphocyte products such as interferon. An intriguing aspect of his observations is that he may be able to start an immunogenetic analysis whether MIF production is dependent on the H-2 locus.

COHEN: The data I presented suggest that the results are not due to concomitant migration enhancing activity or synergistic effects of the serum. It is, of course possible that the effect of serum is to selectively inactivate an MIF antagonist. However, if this were the case, then the C57Bl/6 is the unique possessor of such an antagonist. Mixing experiments utilizing supernatants of C57Bl/6 and other strains should allow us to examine this possibility.

The data thus far available do not show any direct H-2 dependency. Also, we found no evidence for H-2 associated antigens on the mediators themselves. The genetic restriction on lymphokine production is a largely unexplored area. In fact, this is the main reason why we developed an interest in a murine system.

DVORAK: The finding that C57Bl/6 mouse lymphocytes in serum-free medium release an inactive MIF precursor possibly activated by exposure to serum in vitro, is of particular interest to me in view of our earlier results (Hammond et al., Science, 1976; Roblin et al., PNAS (USA), 1978) indicating that SV40-transformed 3T3 cells behave in similar fashion. That is, when cultured in serum-free medium SV 3T3 cells secrete a mediator that can be activated to MIF by subsequent culture in serum. Our precursor co-chromatographed with plasminogen activator. Moreover, in our hands purified urokinase, incubated with serum, generated MIF-like activity. Does Cohen have data to indicate how his C57 precursor may activate a serum factor, or alternatively, how serum may activate his precursor, to yield active MIF?

COHEN: The possibilities are: (1) the serum activates a MIF precursor; (2) the serum inactivates a MIF inactivator; (3) the supernatant activates a MIF precursor in the serum; (4) the serum and supernatant each contribute molecules that act in concert; (5) the serum has a synegistic effect on a subdetectable quantity of MIF in the supernatant.

The data presented exclude (5) as a likely explanation. (1) - (4) all remain viable alternatives. For reasons of simplicity I prefer (3).

SALVIN: I would like to emphasize the fact that Cohen's results involve purely *in vitro* conditions, i.e., his MIF is produced *in vitro* by cells from sensitized animals with antigen or from non-sensitized animals with mitogen. On the other hand, we induce lymphokines by stimulation of sensitized mice with specific antigens. The results that Neta and I have obtained on the release of MIF by different strains of mice are thus different from those of Cohen.

COHEN: The differences may relate to different cellular sources of MIF in vitro vs in vivo situations; different mice (strain variants, differences in infectious history), differences in assay procedures or the effect of serum factors. We would have to exchange mice to investigate this problem.

PICK: We have different results from the ones Cohen reported. We get MIF production by C57Bl/6 mice induced by PPD and Con A. The cells responding to PPD appear to be B cells. I wonder whether these differences might be due to differences in the magnitude of intercurrent infections in mice involving Gram-negative bacteria serving as a source of LPS. This is based on the assumption that the active principle of fetal calf serum is in fact LPS. Has Cohen examined strains of mice resistant to LPS, such as C3H/HeJ, for their capacity to produce MIF in cultures containing fetal calf serum?

COHEN: I do not have data on B cell production of MIF by C57Bl/6. The difference in response to Con A may be, as Pick suggests, due to differences in the prior infectious history of the mice. We will try to obtain an LPS resistant strain, but to use it as a control we would have to hope that such mice do not make an active MIF on mitogenic stimulation, in analogy with C57Bl/6. Should they behave like BALB/c, the experiment would be vitiated.

USE OF *IN VITRO* IMMUNIZATION IN PRODUCTION OF MONOCLONAL ANTIBODIES AGAINST OSTEOCLAST ACTIVATING FACTOR: A METHOD WITH GENERAL APPLICABILITY TO LYMPHOKINES

Richard A. Luben[1]
Marjorie A. Mohler

Division of Biomedical Sciences and
Department of Biochemistry
University of California
Riverside, California 92521

I. INTRODUCTION

A major obstacle to functional and biochemical characterization of lymphokines has been the relative lack of simple, specific tests for quantitation of individual species. Most studies are dependent upon biological assays, which are time-consuming and often non-specific. Clearly, development of immunoassays would improve the situation. However, it has been difficult to prepare specific antisera against lymphokines because they are typically available only in very small amounts and often only in very impure form. In this report, we describe the application of techniques of *in vitro* immunization (1) and hybridoma production (2) to the development of immunoassays for the lymphokine osteoclast activating factor (OAF). We suggest that such techniques are uniquely suitable for production of antibodies against agents, such as lymphokines, which are available in limited quantities and/or as minor components of complex mixtures.

II. MATERIALS AND METHODS

OAF was obtained from PHA-activated human tonsil cultures as described previously (3). The culture medium was concentrated by ultrafiltration and fractionated on Sephacryl S-200. Active OAF fractions were subjected to further purification

[1]*Supported by ACS Grant BC-263, Nat. Found. Grant 5-152, USPHS Grants RR09070 and DE00057.*

ISBN 0-12-213950-X

using DEAE-Sephacel and polyacrylamide gel electrophoresis (3). For immunization of animals, the segments of polyacrylamide slab gels which contained OAF activity (Rf = 0.6) were homogenized in phosphate buffered saline using a glass-teflon homogenizer. The suspension (approx. 50% gel by volume) was injected subcutaneously into BALB/c mice at weekly intervals for three to four weeks using approximately 10 μg OAF per injection. Two days after the final injection, spleen cells were isolated for hybridization (2).

In vitro activation of spleen cells from BALB/c mice was carried out using a modification of the system of Andersson et.al. (1). Spleen cells were cultured at 10^6 cells/ml in a medium consisting of 50% fresh Eagle's MEM with 20% fetal bovine serum, 5 x 10^{-5} *M* β-mercaptoethanol, and 2 *mM* glutamine; and 50% conditioned medium from BALB/c mouse thymocytes. To furnish conditioned medium, thymocytes were cultured at 3-5 x 10^6 cell/ml in the same Eagle's MEM medium as above; after 48-72 hours the medium was removed, sterilized by filtration and used immediately for *in vitro* activation. The antigen used in these experiments was either highly purified OAF or pooled S-200 fractions. Both were added to the spleen cell culture medium at concentrations equivalent to approximately 1 μg OAF per ml. Spleen cells were cultured in the presence of antigen for four days without a change of medium, and were then hybridized.

Hybridizations were carried out with the mouse plasmacytoma cell line 45.6TG1.7 (4) obtained from the Cell Distribution Center of the Salk Institute. Spleen cells (either freshly isolated or from *in vitro* activation cultures) and plasmacytoma cells were washed twice in serum-free Eagle's MEM, then fused using PEG 1000 as described previously (2). Hybrids were selected by treatment of cultures with HAT (5). Hybrid cells which produced anti-OAF activity were cloned and re-cloned by limiting dilution in conditioned medium from parental plasmacytoma cells.

To assess the anti-OAF activity of hybridoma clones, the culture medium was collected, concentrated by ultrafiltration and adsorbed with DEAE-cellulose to remove most non-immunoglobulin proteins. The isolated fraction was then incubated with purified OAF at the indicated dilutions for 12-18 hours at 0° C. In some experiments, the incubated mixture was then assayed directly; in other experiments the samples were treated with S. aureus protein A prior to assay (6). The remaining OAF activity after incubation with hybridoma media was assayed by a bone resorption assay as described previously (3). The reduction of activity by anti-OAF antibodies was estimated by comparison against equal concentrations of OAF which had been incubated with medium from parental plasmacytoma cells. A computer program for parallel-line bioassay was used to quantitate results.

To furnish radioactive OAF as a tracer in RIA experiments, purified OAF was iodinated using an insolubilized glucose oxidase/lactoperoxidase system.

III. RESULTS

Spleen cells from mice immunized against OAF served as effective parental cells in production of hybridomas (Table 1). In a typical experiment involving the hybridization of 10^8 cells from a single spleen, viable hybrids were obtained in 75-90% of the culture wells, with the hybridization frequency estimated as between 10^{-5} and 10^{-4}. In successful experiments 10 or more of the isolated hybrid clones could be shown to produce anti-OAF antibodies, with activity titers ranging as high as 1:100,000 for minimal blocking of OAF-induced bone resorption.

A substantial disadvantage of using *in vivo* immunization was that this technique required multiple doses of microgram quantities of OAF. Each 10 μg dose administered represented the equivalent of approximately 100 liters of supernatant from

TABLE 1. Anti-OAF Activity Produced by Hybridoma Clones[a]

Clone number	*Percentage OAF activity recovered at the indicated dilutions*		
	1:100	*1:1000*	*1:10,000*
AE-14-1	*86*	*97*	--
AE-14-2	*10*	*56*	*98*
AE-14-3	*100*	--	--
AE-14-4	*1*	*19*	*72*
AE-14-5	*100*	--	--
AE-14-6	*90*	--	--
AE-14-7	*3*	*21*	*39*
AE-14-8	*23*	*68*	*95*

[a]*Hybridoma supernatants were assayed for anti-OAF activity as described in the text. Clones presented were chosen sequentially from a single experiment as a representative sample. The symbol (--) indicates that this dilution was not tested.*

TABLE 2. Comparison of In Vivo and In Vitro Immunization For Production of OAF-Specific Hybridomas

Expt. No.	*Immunization Method*	*Positive Cultures*[a]	*Maximum Titer*[b]
1.	*in vivo*	13/48	1:1000
2.	*in vivo*	9/48	1:100,000
3.	*in vivo*	22/96	1:10,000
4.	*in vitro*	24/48	1:3000
5.	*in vitro*	31/48	1:100,000
6.	*in vitro*	46/96	1:10,000

[a]*Number of initial hybrid cultures producing anti-OAF activity in screening experiments, vs. number of cultures initially established after cell fusion. Each active culture contains between 1 and 100 hybrid clones.*

[b]*Maximum dilution of supernatants producing anti-OAF activity.*

activated tonsil lymphocytes (3) and therefore necessitated a major purification effort. In order to conserve antigen as well as time, we investigated the possibility that activated lymphoblasts suitable for hybridization could be obtained from single doses of antigen administered to spleen cells *in vitro*. Such experiments have in the past proved to be effective for production of antibody-forming cells specific for a wide variety of antigens (1). The system of Andersson, et.al. (1) was particularly attractive for this purpose, as this system has been shown to allow antigenic activation to antibody production of a very broad variety of B-lymphocyte precursor cells. Moreover, it has been shown that the blasts formed by activation in this system can be used as parental cells for production of hybridomas specific for the immunizing antigen (7). In our studies, we found that use of MEM and of conditioned medium from unpurified thymocytes gave better yields of specific hybridomas than the conditions described by Andersson (1, 7). Using this modified system, we immunized spleen cells *in vitro* with OAF for four days, then hybridized the cells with 45.6TG1.7 cells. The results (Table 2) indicate that *in vitro* immunization was at least as effective in producing anti-OAF hybridomas as was *in vivo* immunization. Although there were fewer total viable spleen cells after four days in culture (2-5 x 10^7 cells as opposed to 10^8 cells in a freshly isolated spleen), we obtained roughly the same total number of hybrids in a given experiment (1000-5000 individual colonies estimated, after HAT selection). Moreover, the number of hybridomas producing anti-OAF activity was consistently higher: for example, in a typical experiment positive anti-OAF activity was found in 25-30 individual clones, as opposed to the 10 or so expected in experiments using spleen cells from animals immunized *in vivo*.

To design radioimmunoassays for OAF, the antibody fraction from hybridoma clone AB-14 was isolated by pooling 4 liters of culture medium, concentrating by ultrafiltration, and fractionating the resulting material on a column of DEAE-Affi-Gel Blue (Bio-Rad). The isolated immunoglobulins were incubated with ^{125}I-labeled OAF at pH 7.4 in 0.2 *M* phosphate buffer containing 1 mg/ml bovine serum albumin. The incubation was continued at 0° C overnight, and then protein A was added to precipitate antibody molecules. It was determined that the AB-14 antibody could bind approximately 18,000 cpm of ^{125}I-OAF at a dilution of antibody equivalent to 1:100,000 relative to the original culture medium. When purified, unlabeled OAF was added to the incubation (Fig. 1), the ^{125}I-OAF was displaced. Minimum displacement was at approximately 1 ng/ml. Using this system, 3-5 ng/ml was the lowest level at which purified OAF could consistently be measured with precision.

We had shown previously (8) that, by ultrafiltration and polyacrylamide gel electrophoresis, a fraction biologically identical to OAF could be isolated from human myeloma cells (RPMI 8226) and from the serum of patients with myeloma. Using OAF fractions isolated in this manner, we were able to show (Fig. 1) that the OAF from these sources competed for ^{125}I-OAF binding to the AB-14 antibody essentially identically to authentic purified OAF. Moreover, the AB-14 antibody blocked the biological activity of OAF isolated from both myeloma cells and myeloma serum (data not shown), indicating that OAF from these sources has identical immunoreactivity with purified OAF from tonsil cells.

IV. DISCUSSION

These results demonstrate that monoclonal antibodies against OAF can be produced effectively, using microgram quantities of antigen, by means of the techniques of hybridoma production. These antibodies were used to design an immunoassay for OAF, which we then used to demonstrate that OAF isolated from tonsil cells shares apparently identical immunologic specifity with OAF isolated from human myeloma cells and from the serum of patients with myeloma.

The major advantages of the hybridoma production technique as applied to lymphokines are that this technique allows the use of weak, scarce or impure antigens, which are the current states of availability of many lymphokines. Hybridoma production, once mastered, is sensitive and reliable, allowing the production of a significant number of clones secreting a few micrograms of antigen. Moreover, since cloning of the hybridomas produces monoclonal cell populations secreting homogeneous antibody profiles, the initial antigen need not be in homogeneous form as long as suitably specific tests are available for detecting clones producing the desired antibodies. These and other factors argue that use of hybridoma production should be the method of choice for isolation of antibodies against lymphokines.

When coupled with *in vitro* immunization, as in this study, the hybridoma technique can be used to produce a series of specific antibodies against a given factor within several weeks of the original isolation of antigen. In addition, *in vitro* immunization appears to allow a somewhat higher frequency of production of specific hybridomas than does *in vivo* immunization. This observation is based not only on the present study, but on previous observations by others (1) that the function of T-suppression seems to be abolished *in vitro* for most antigens, allowing a significantly enhanced response in terms of the number of antibody-producing lymphocyte clones produced. It should be pointed out that with the techniques used here, production of antibodies against lymphokines need not be a long-delayed phase of the research project. Antibodies produced at an early stage of the characterization of a lymphokine can be used in turn to facilitate both purification and evaluation of function in subsequent studies. Thus, the judicious use of hybridoma production techniques should allow more rapid advances in knowledge of the nature and functions of lymphokines *in vivo*.

REFERENCES

1. Andersson, J., Coutinho, A., Lerhardt, W., and Melchers, F. (1977). *Cell 10*, 27.
2. Galfre, G., Howe, S. C., Milstein, C., Butcher, G. W., and Howard, J. C. (1977). *Nature 266*, 550.
3. Luben, R. A. (1978). *Biochem. Biophys. Res. Commun. 84*, 15.
4. Margulies, D. H., Kuehl, W. M., and Scharff, M. D. (1976). *Cell 8*, 405.
5. Littlefield, J. W. (1966). *Exptl. Cell Res. 41*, 190.
6. Goding, J. W. (1978). *J. Immunolog. Methods 20*, 241.

7. Andersson, J., and Melchers, F. (1978). In *"Current Topics in Microbiology and Immunology"* (F. Melchers, M. Potter, and N. Warner, eds.), p. 130. Springer, Berlin.
8. Luben, R. A. (1979). *Cellular Immunology (in press).*

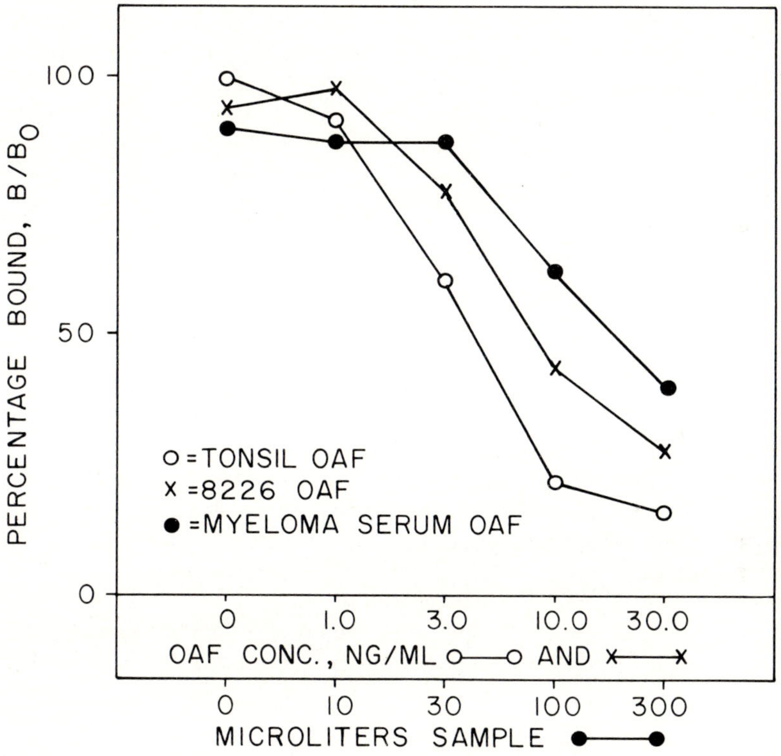

FIGURE 1. Competition for binding of ^{125}I-labeled OAF to antibody by OAF from various sources. Unlabeled OAF, from tonsils, RPMI 8226 cells or serum from a myeloma patient, was added to an incubation mixture containing antibody AB-14-12 at 1:100,000 dilution and labeled OAF. The added concentrations of OAF are expressed as ng/ml for tonsil OAF and 8226 OAF, but as microliters of sample for the myeloma serum OAF since the sample was only partially purified (ref. 8).

DISCUSSION

OPPENHEIM: This report represents a very promising approach to the purification of lymphokines. I have 2 questions: (1) how much antigen is required for Luben's in vitro generation of anti-OAF producing cells? (2) when he uses impure antigens to obtain hybridoma clones, does not his yield of clones decrease due to antigenic competition?

LUBEN: We have used as little as 1 microgram of OAF to produce hybridomas, but I suspect that we could have managed with considerably less than that. We have not really tried to examine just how low in dosage we could go. When one uses impure antigen he gets a lot of clones secreting antibodies against the contaminants in that preparation. But that does not really seem to decrease the net yield of specific anti-OAF hybridomas; it just makes the screening process somewhat more critical. When one realizes that we are screening for 20 or 30 specific anti-OAF clones out of perhaps 10,000 total hybrid clones, it does not really make that much difference that more or fewer of the 10,000 are directed at antigens other than OAF. The key to the process is, ultimately, having a good specific screening test for whatever antibodies one is seeking.

MERGENHAGEN: Does Luben have any data on the spectrum of lymphokine activities that can be neutralized by anti-OAF monoclonal antibodies?

LUBEN: We have examined a few, including chemotaxin and MIF, and have not found any cross-reactivity with anti-OAF. However, this is not to say that OAF might not share determinants with still other lymphokines.

MUNDY: A difficult problem with the interpretation of these interesting results is that the material Luben is calling OAF differs both biochemically and biologically from the bone resorbing factor that has been described by our own group and by others. Thus, what he is calling "OAF" generically, and now measuring by its immunoreactive behavior is not the same lymphokine that the other workers in this field call OAF. I think it is vital to define lymphokines precisely by their biological behavior to avoid confusion with results obtained using non-biological assays.

LUBEN: I do not agree with Mundy that the molecule we are studying is all that different from the OAF preparations used by other groups. Unlike others, we have purified the molecule to essential homogeneity. We know a considerable amount about its chemistry and mechanisms of action on bone. We have also shown that this molecular species is produced by human myeloma cells *in vitro* and *in vivo*. The radioimmunoassay and other data demonstrate that this molecule is present in the serum of patients with myeloma. Therefore, I would say that the burden of proof is really on the groups using impure OAF preparations to demonstrate just what molecular species they are studying and whether or not those molecules play a role in disease. I think that in the final analysis we have to get away from looking just at unpurified biological activities and start specifying just what molecules we are dealing with when we talk about lymphokines.

EPSTEIN: Can Luben use his radioimmunoassay to monitor OAF serum levels as a reflection of tumor cell burden and/or efficacy of chemotherapeutic regimen in patients with multiple myeloma?

LUBEN: We are currently studying those issues, but we do not have any additional data to report at this time.

LEONARD: With hybridoma-produced monoclonal antibodies, Luben is now in a position to determine what fraction of the starting antigen is actually OAF. Has he done that? In detecting hybridoma antibody, what is the proportion of IgM and IgG producers?

LUBEN: First of all, our starting antigen for most of these experiments *was* homogeneous purified OAF, so we do not need to pose Leonard's question. However, it is important to realize that one does not really have to have pure starting antigen in order to raise monoclonal antibodies, as long as one can specifically detect the presence of hybridomas secreting antibodies of the desired activity. On the other hand, one does have to have pure antigen to design an immunoassay, of course. Secondly, when we use *in vivo* immunization, we get mostly IgG antibodies. With *in vitro* immunization, as many as half the clones are secreting IgM, the rest are mainly IgG.

SORG: What happens when Luben precipitates his ^{125}I-labelled OAF with his monoclonal antibody, dissolves the complexes and analyzes them as SDS-PAGE; would he get a single homogeneous peak?

LUBEN: We have not done that particular experiment yet. The competition of unlabelled OAF with the antibody-bound labelled OAF occurs at about the same dilutions as antibody blocking of biological activity. This suggests that labelled OAF and unlabelled OAF are binding with the same affinity and that they are probably the same molecule.

GRANGER: The amount of antigen necessary to induce antibodies may vary depending upon the antigenicity of the various lymphokines studied. OAF is a small molecule and may be a relatively poor antigen. For example, 100 ng of human α-LT (lymphotoxin) provides a good antigenic stimulus for the rabbit. Accordingly, I would expect Luben's method to work very well with much less material when applied to other lymphokines. Once obtained, it must be determined that the antibody active site is directed towards the actual protein portion of the molecule, before comparisons between lymphokines can be made. Many lymphokines are glycoproteins, consequently they may show common carbohydrate moieties but have different protein backbones.

LUBEN: Yes, I agree with Granger. OAF is not a very immunogenic molecule and it is likely that much less antigen would suffice for other lymphokines, especially when *in vitro* immunization is used. In order to assess specificity, it is certainly advantageous to prepare a broad range of anti-lymphokine hybridomas rather than being satisfied with only one or two.

de WECK: I would expect it might prove advantageous to use small amounts of purified antigen in order to assure recruitment of high affinity clones for RIA. Do Luben's hybridoma antibodies actually precipitate antigens? On purely theoretical grounds they should not.

LUBEN: One should always try to investigate just how little antigen can be used for these immunizations, for the very reasons given by de Weck. Like others, we find that monoclonal, monospecific antibodies are not generally useful as direct precipitating agents. This means that they can not be used for Ouchterlony double diffusion plates, radial immunodiffusion or the like unless they are used in the presence of secondary precipitating antibodies. This is probably because the monospecific nature of the molecules prevents formation of large crosslinking complexes. This is a good example of the many modifications in thinking that one must undergo when dealing with hybridomas rather than classical antisera.

MAYER: One of the important issues in lymphokine research concerns the discrimination between a lymphokine measured as a "biologic activity" and a lymphokine measured as a "chemical substance or activity". OAF or MIF or LT are "activities" that are mediated by *one or several* substances. By contrast, immunoassay with monoclonal antibody measures a *single* one of the substances involved in mediating a given lymphokine "activity".

LYMPHOKINE ACTIVITIES IN SUPERNATANTS FROM HUMAN LYMPHOID CELL LINES[1]

Lawrence B. Schook[2]
Ursula Otz
Sandor Lazary
Alain L. de Weck

Institute for Clinical Immunology
Inselspital
Bern, Switzerland

Jun Minowada

Roswell Park Memorial Institute
Buffalo, New York

I. INTRODUCTION

Classical approaches in the production of human lymphokines (LK) have involved the stimulation of PBL either specifically by antigen or non-specifically through mitogen stimulation (1,2). One problem in using such unfractionated cell populations is a "ping-pong" effect in which stimulated cells foster the indirect production of LK and monokines from other cells (3). This phenomenon leads to large variations in the production and pattern of LK activities in supernatants from various individuals (4). In an attempt to produce large amounts of supernatants containing more restricted LK activities we have systematically assayed 24 human lymphoid cell lines (LCL) for 9 various factors.

[1] *This work has been supported in part by the Swiss National Science Foundation (Grant No. 3.850.077)*
[2] *Recepient of Postdoctoral Research Fellowships awarded by National Cancer Institute, NIH (CA-0628-01) and Swiss National Fund (88.679-0.78). Present address: Department of Microbiology, University of Michigan, Ann Arbor, MI*

ISBN 0-12-213950-X

TABLE I. MIF Activities in Lymphoid Cell Lines[a]

Cell Lines		No Serum	10% Serum
Normal B	B-23-3	24±10	27±14
	B 66	39± 5	43± 5
	B 89	35± 4	26± 6
	RPMI 1788	77± 4	61± 7
	SN 1036	44± 6	23± 2
	B-411-4	34± 8	44± 6
	B 70	35±11	46± 6
	B 85	38±19	38± 9
	RPMI 8392	32± 8	43±15
	B 76	9± 9	23±13
B cell ALL	BALL-1	20±11	17±11
	BALM-2	22±16	30± 9
	NALM-6	3± 4	3± 5
B cell Lymphoma	B 35-M	35± 8	22±11
	B 46-M	57± 8	46±13
	U-698-M	27±13	18±10
T cell ALL	MOLT-4F	33±13	30±13
	RPMI 8402	30± 9	22±14
	HPB-ALL	17±12	28± 7
CML-BC	K-562	33±13	40±16
	NALM-1	17± 2	17± 7
Null cell ALL	NALM-16	19± 8	18± 7
	Reh	40± 4	8± 6
	NALL-1	23±12	15±10

[a]Values represent the mean % inhibition of 3 experiments (done in duplicate) ± S.D. for undiluted supernatants

II. RESULTS

LCL supernatants were prepared from 500 ml spinner cultures containing 2 x 10^6 cells/ml. After 22 hr of incubation in RPMI 1640, with or without 10% FCS, the supernatants were collected, aliquoted, and maintained at -70'C until assayed.

A. *Migration Inhibitory Factor (MIF)*

The greatest MIF activity was found associated with the B cell lines RPMI 1788, SN 1036, and the B cell Lymphoma B-46-M (Table I). Activity was also observed in these lines following subsequent dilutions. Although activity was detected with the T cell lines, little remained after dilution. Impressive was the finding that MIF activity was produced using serum-free culture conditions and was even higher than when FCS was supplemented into the culture medium for the above mentioned B cell lines.

B. *Mitogenic Factor (MF), Macrophage Cytotoxic Factor (MCF), Leukocyte Inhibition Factor (LIF), and Interferon (IF)*

MF activity for human PBL was detected in serum-free supernatants of the B cell B 85; B cell Lymphoma B 46-M and U-698-M; and the T cell ALL MOLT 4-F and HPB-ALL (Table II). These lines also caused a strong mitogenic response when tested using mouse thymocytes. Similar results were observed when supernatants produced with FCS were tested. However, unlike MIF, MF appears to be slightly higher in serum containing culture medium. MCF activity, enhancement of BALB/c macrophage killing of tumor cell EL4, was highest in the B cell lines B-66, B-411-4, and the B cell Lymphoma B 46-M. FCS supplemented supernatants gave similar, albeit, slightly higher values. LIF assayed using a fibrin drop method was present in the Null cell lines NALM-16 and Reh under serum-free conditions. FCS-supplemented supernatants appeared to stimulate migration suggesting the presence of chemotactic activity. IF was found only in supernatants from several of the EBV antigen positive B cell lines, was stable at pH 2.0, and was present in equal titers whether produced with or without serum.

TABLE II. MF, MCF, LIF, and IF Activities in Serum-free LCL Supernatants

Cell Lines		MF[a]		MCF[b]	LIF[c]	IF[d]
		PBL	C57			
Normal B	B-23-3	2.2	1.5	25.9±1.1	2±12	0
	B 66	1.1	5.5	51.1±0.8	10± 9	8
	B 89	2.1	3.0	34.5±2.2	-5±16	0
	RPMI 1788	1.7	7.5	33.4±0.6	6±18	2.5
	SN 1036	2.0	2.8	26.6±0.9	16± 7	16
	B-411-4	1.3	17.2	51.5±1.6	2±13	25
	B 70	1.9	3.6	36.0±8.8	14± 3	16
	B 85	6.1	9.5	37.8±7.7	-16± 4	0
	RPMI 8392	1.3	3.1	36.6±1.1	1±16	25
	B 76	1.0	2.7	38.8±5.9	16± 5	16
B cell ALL	BALL-1	1.0	8.8	31.2±5.9	19±12	0
	BALM-2	3.0	2.1	34.9±3.1	15±16	0
	NALM-6	1.3	2.2	24.6±0.5	17±19	0
B cell Lymphoma	B 35-M	2.2	7.8	32.7±0.8	0±16	0
	B 46-M	6.3	11.7	51.2±0.5	5± 6	25
	U-698-M	3.6	10.7	31.4±0.2	9± 4	0
T cell ALL	MOLT-4F	3.8	12.8	32.2±1.8	6±14	0
	RPMI 8402	1.6	4.1	30.5±1.1	-3± 3	0
	HPB-ALL	3.5	14.8	28.6±1.4	2± 1	0
CML-BC	K-562	2.8	12.2	40.4±0.1	10± 7	0
	NALM-1	1.0	1.0	29.8±0.1	6± 2	0
Null cell ALL	NALM-16	2.9	11.4	39.0±13	24±13	0
	Reh	1.1	2.3	28.1	31±12	0
	NALL-1	2.1	7.0	35.8±16	10± 5	0

[a] S.I. for human PBL and C57Bl/6 thymocytes, mean of 2 expts. (triplicate)
[b] % ^{51}Cr release ± S.D. (triplicate); medium control, 25.4±0.3
[c] Mean % inhibition for 2 expts. (triplicate) ± S.D.
[d] Titer (reference Units/ml)

C. *Colony Stimulating Activity (CSA), Vascular Permeability Factor (VPF), Skin Reactive Factor (SRF), and Lymphocyte Activating Factor (LAF)*

CSA was not detected in any supernatants when tested on frozen bone marrows. Experiments using fresh marrows showed these supernatants to be cytotoxic and suppressing the spontaneous colony formation. LAF, enhancement of the mouse thymocyte PHA response, was absent as would be expected if a monokine is origin. SRF and VPF were not detected using unconcentrated supernatants.

ACKNOWLEDGMENTS

The authors wish to thank Dr. E. Kniep, Max Planck Institute for Immunobiology, for performing the MCF assays and Dr. V. Edy, Theodor Kocher and Sloan-Kettering Institutes for determination of the IF titers.

REFERENCES

1. Horvat, M., Havemann, K., Sodomann, C.P., and Burger, S., Int. Arch. Allergy *43*, 466 (1972).
2. Rocklin, R., Remold, H.G., and David, J.R., Cell. Immunol. *5*, 436 (1972).
3. Oppenheim, J.J., Mizel, S.B., and Meltzer, M.S., *in* "Biology of the Lymphokines", p. 291 (S. Cohen, E. Pick, and J.J. Oppenheim, eds.). Academic Press, New York, 1979
4. Schook, L.B., Otz, U., Lazary, S., and de Weck, A.L., Z. Immun. Forsch. *115*, 59 (1978).

DISCUSSION

SMITH: Was the test for mitogenic factor activity performed with or without a T-cell lectin?

SCHOOK: Without.

LEON: Did Schook determine whether any of the activities that he measured were produced at a particular stage of the cell cycle by using reagents such as hydroxyurea?

SCHOOK: No, we did not use inhibitors of the cell cycle to determine at what stage of the cell cycle these factors were produced. However, studies done by other groups (Waksman et al.) have shown LKs to be produced during the G_1 phase of the cell cycle.

VILCEK: Was the interferon produced in the various cell lines characterized as to its species, i.e. was it "leukocyte", "fibroblast" or "type II" interferon? How was the interferon assayed?

SCHOOK: The IF produced by the various cell lines was stable at pH 2.0, implying that it was predominantly of type I. The IF was assayed by challenging CCL 23 cells with Semliki Forest virus and the titers were determined by comparison with an international standard.

EPSTEIN: Would Schook please comment on whether the mechanism of induction of the mediators relates to the presence of the EBV virus genome?

SCHOOK: There appears to be no direct correlation between the production of mediators and the presence of the EBV virus genome. As I mentioned, however, only EBV antigen-positive cells produced interferon but not all positive cells had IF activity associated with their supernatants.

PAPERMASTER: In partial response to the query by Epstein, I would point out that differences in activity for a given factor ought best to be compared on a specific activity basis such as per mg of protein or dilution from a starting volume. Induction of lymphokine activity in cultured lines is elusive in the sense that most cell lines produce lymphokines constitutively, either as a result of transformation or mitogen induction during original establishment of the cell line itself. But for practical purposes, producer cell lines synthesize lymphokines at a relatively constant rate.

den HOLLANDER: We have definitely demonstrated LIF activity in RPMI 1788 cell line supernatants with both pig and human polymorphonuclear cells as targets. These also contain SRF. The difference might be due to the fact that Schook has used unconcentrated supernatants while we use ultrafiltered material.

FANTES: We too have analyzed supernatants from several human lymphoblastoid cell lines for MIF activity and found them to be "active" (Taylor, Burman, Fantes; Cell. Immunol. *19*:41, 1975). However, on dialysis against fresh medium these activities virtually disappeared. We found moreover that more actively metabolising cells showed greater apparent MIF activities, which seemed to be correlated with glucose depletion of the media.

YOSHIDA: Apart from the problem of concentration, one has to consider, for each cell line, the age of the cultures before concluding that there are differences among cell lines in the spectrum of lymphokines produced. For example, it has been our experience that a good MIF producer cell line becomes a poor producer when cultures are set up from the later generations of that cell line. Therefore determination of the spectrum of lymphokine activities produced by a cell line from data obtained with a single batch of supernatant could well be misleading. As far as physicochemical characteristics are concerned, we could not detect any difference between antigen-stimulated human MIF and the lymphoid cell line product. Anti-guinea pig MIF antiserum did not react with either of these materials.

de WECK: In terms of identity between cell line MIF and peripheral blood lymphocytes (PBL) MIF, we can state that RPMI 1788 MIF, PGLC 33 MIF (from Philip Glade) and PBL MIF give in immunodiffusion a line of identity with anti-MIF serum prepared by immunization with PBL MIF. Of course, this only shows that the same material is present in all three purified fractions but not necessarily that this material is active MIF.

LUBEN: We have looked at several lymphoid cell lines for the nature of the OAF produced. As I indicated previously, RPMI 8226 produces OAF which is chemically and immunologically identical to OAF from activated tonsil cells. We have also shown that OAF from other B cell lines such as Raji and IM9 is the same species. Thus, in these cases at least, the molecule produced by cell lines is the same as that produced by normal cells.

LANDY: The culture conditions used in work with established lymphoblastoid cell lines almost invariably are poised for optimal cell replication. There are, however, ample indications that lymphokine production can occur in the absence of replication and is not necessarily correlated with it. Therefore what we have thus far seen in surveys of such lines could well be an entirely non-optimal situation. These findings in no way reflect a realistic view of the capabilities of these lines.

WARE: Certain B cell lines (PGLC-33h) produce alpha-lymphotoxins (LT) that are biochemically and immunologically identical with those produced by normal lectin-stimulated cells. However, these cell lines only produce α-LT molecules, whereas normal cells produce a heterogeneous mixture of LT molecules (complex, α, β, and γ). Thus these cell lines can be used as a "simplified model system" to study the various properties of α-LT.

de WECK: A further advantage of using lymphoid cell lines, apart from those identified thus far, is the absence of monocytes and monokines, thereby avoiding the usual "ping pong" effect observed when PBL are used. As far as optimal conditions for production of individual lymphokines is concerned, such as time and concentration of cells for example, preliminary kinetic experiments certainly indicate that optimal conditions will have to be worked out for each cell line.

MOUSE BONE MARROW MACROPHAGES AS INDICATOR CELLS FOR ASSAYING MURINE MIGRATION INHIBITORY FACTOR AND ITS PURIFICATION INTO TWO MOLECULAR SPECIES

V. Klimetzek, D. Bout, A.L. Kühner, H.G. Remold, and J.R. David

Harvard Medical School
Boston, Massachusetts

INTRODUCTION

To measure the activity of murine MIF usually peritoneal exudate cells (PEC) are used. We demonstrate in this study that bone marrow macrophages (BM MØ) cultured on Teflon coated plates (TC plates) can be used as an alternative source of MØ for large scale MIF assays. Using these cells, MIF activity from Con-A stimulated lymph node cell supernatants was monitored after Sephadex G-100 filtration, sucrose density electrophoresis and isoelectric focussing. Two MIF species were recovered, suggesting that mouse MIF is similar to guinea pig MIF in this respect (Remold and Mednis, 1977).

METHODS

Petri dishes (ø 100 mm, Falcon No. 3003) were sprayed with a Teflon aerosol (Crown Ind. Prod.) until they were covered with a thin film. The plates were air dried and sterilized by UV light. Prior to use, the plates were washed twice with Dulbecco's MEM containing 5% FCS.

BM cells from C57BL/6 mice were cultured for 8 to 16 days on TC plates in Dulbecco's MEM containing 15% FCS plus 5% HS and 20% L-cell supernatant (Meerpohl *et al.*, 1976). To remove the attached BM MØ the TC plates were incubated for

ISBN 0-12-213950-X

10 min at 4°C. After removing the supernatants and washing once with Dulbecco's PBS, 15 ml D-PBS containing 1.5% FCS and 0.3 ml of 0.1 M EDTA (pH 7.2) was added. After 15 min the MØ were removed by rinsing the plates with a syringe.

MIF-rich and control supernatants from lymph node cells were produced by C57BL/6 mice as described by Kühner and David (1976). The lyophilized supernatants were filtered through Sephadex G-100 columns and MIF containing fractions were pooled. Their fractionation by sucrose density electrophoresis and isoelectrofocussing in a sucrose gradient was performed as described before (Remold and Mednis, 1977).

The MIF assay was performed as described by Kühner and David (1976) using BM MØ as indicator cells.

RESULTS AND DISCUSSION

From one mouse 5-6 x 10^7 BM cells could be recovered. When the cells were grown for 8-16 days in the presence of conditioned medium about 1.8-2.2 x 10^8 BM MØ were recovered. In order to get the same amount of oil-induced PEC 10-15 mice are needed. Therefore the BM MØ represent an ideal alternative source of MØ, if they could be recovered from the culture dishes. When the BM cells were grown on TC plates the attached MØ could be removed with a yield of 90-95% after 15 min incubation in 1 mM EDTA. The viability was greater than 95%. Comparative studies showed that the detached MØ had the same functional and biochemical characteristics as MØ grown on plastic dishes. Eight to sixteen days in vitro cultivated MØ were esterase positive and peroxidase negative cells, which resembled inflammatory exudate MØ elicited with thioglycollate. They secreted high amounts of neutral proteinases and showed high pinocytic activity. These 8-16 days old MØ were also highly responsive to crude MIF supernatants. The degree of the MIF response was not related to the age of the cells.

In the following study BM MØ were used to monitor the purification of murine MIF. When MIF-containing and control lymph node supernatants were filtered through Sephadex G-100 columns, MIF activity was recovered in a broad mol. wt. range of 25,000 to 70,000. The active fractions were pooled, concentrated and subjected to sucrose density gradient electrophoresis. MIF activity was recovered as a single peak in the post-albumin region. The fractions from this peak were then pooled and subjected to isoelectrofocussing in a pH gradient ranging from pH 2-6. Two peaks of MIF activity were recovered. One focussed between pH 3 and 4.3 and the other between pH 4.6 and 5.2. Thus, mouse lymph node cell MIF like guinea pig MIF (Remold and Mednis, 1977) can be fractionated into two closely related species.

REFERENCES

Kühner, A.L., and David, J.R. (1976). *J. Immunol.* 116, 140.

Meerpohl, H.G., Lohmann-Matthes, M.L., and Fischer, H. (1976). *Eur. J. Immunol.* 6, 213.

Remold, H.G., and Mednis, A.D. (1977). *J. Immunol.* 118, 2015.

PURIFIED HUMAN MIF: EFFECTS ON OXIDATIVE METABOLISM AND SURFACE ARCHITECTURE OF EFFECTOR CELLS

Lutz H. Block
Harry A. Bernheim
Karen Wenc

Department of Internal Medicine
Yale University
New Haven, Connecticut

Herbert Jaksche

Sandoz Forschungsinstitut Ges.m.b.H.
Vienna, Austria

I. INTRODUCTION

Previous studies have revealed various functional, biological and metabolic effects of partially purified MIF on its target cells (mononuclear phagocytes) after a 3-day incubation. These partially purified MIF preparations contain considerable amounts of contaminating proteins, and it still remains unclear whether the MIF molecule or another protein is responsible for the reported effects. However, purified MIF provides an opportunity not only to clarify this ambiguity, but also to investigate its effect on both the macrophage membrane and the oxidative metabolisms of these cells.

II. MATERIALS AND METHODS

A. Purification of MIF

MIF was purified from supernatants of Concanavalin A-activated human lymphocytes by gel filtration on Sephadex G100 and preparative isotachophoresis according to Block et al.,1978. Preparation of guinea pig peritoneal macrophages and migration inhibition test was performed according to David and David,1970.

ISBN 0-12-213950-X

B. Electron Microscopic Techniques

For scanning electron microscopy, 4 mm diameter glass coverslips were placed in the migration chambers. The macrophages migrated onto the coverslips under the same experimental conditions as described previously (David and David,1970). Prior to fixation, the coverslips were mounted in a special Teflon holder immersed in Hank's buffer. When in place, the coverslips formed the base of a cylinder which retains a small amount of fluid when the holder is moved from one solution to the next. Cell preparations were processed according to Biemesderfer et al.,1978.

C. Oxygen Consumption Measurement

Guinea pig peritoneal macrophages were incubated for 14 hrs in plastic petri dishes at 37°C, 5 % CO_2. Purified MIF (10^{-7}M) and control material in Eagle's minimal Essential Medium (MEM) containing 10% heat-inactivated guinea pig serum were added at zero time. Following incubation, cells were collected, washed twice in MEM (500 g x 10min) and resuspended in Hank's Balanced Salt Solution (HBSS). Oxygen consumption was measured with a Clark oxygen electrode as described by Root and Stossel,1974, at a concentration of 1 x 10^7 cells suspended in 3 ml HBSS.

III. RESULTS

After a 14 hour incubation period with 10^{-7}M MIF, macrophages show broad, sheet-like processes that extend over the entire cell surface (Fig.1). In cross sections observed via transmission electron microscopy, these processes appear as filipoidal extension protruding a great distance from the cell surface.

Supernatants of stimulated lymphocytes containing MIF were found to activate phagocyte function following a 24 hour incubation period. In contrast, the duration of macrophage activation by partially purified MIF was 2-3 days (David,1975). If MIF should serve a regulatory role in the mechanisms of cell-mediated immunity, its stimulatory effects on macrophages function should be detected after shorter time intervals.

When exposed to purified MIF (10^{-7}M) for 14 hours macrophages were found to have an approximately four-fold increase in O_2 consumption (Table 1), indicating an increase in their oxidative metabolism.

TABLE I. Oxygen consumption of MIF-treated macrophages

Treatment	O_2 Consumed μ moles/10^7 cells $\pm$ S.D.
MIF (10^{-7}M)	103.4 $\pm$ 12.4
Control supernatants	22.6 $\pm$ 16.7

IV. SUMMARY AND CONCLUDING REMARKS

Previous studies have shown that partially purified preparations of MIF are capable of affecting the morphology and oxidative metabolism of macrophages. Here, for the first time, we report that these effects can be duplicated by purified MIF. In addition, our studies clarify controversial claims concerning the time course of activation of macrophages by MIF in vitro. Our finding that MIF affects oxidative metabolism of macrophages within a relatively short period of time (14 hrs.) indicates that MIF plays an important role in host defense systems. The contrast between the kinetics of macrophage activation by purified MIF and partially purified MIF might be explained by the enhanced effectiveness of purified MIF itself, or by antagonistic effects of contaminating proteins present in the preparation of partially purified MIF.

Membrane-associated phenomena which lead to increased oxygen consumption with subsequent generation of O_2 and H_2O_2 in phagocytes have been presumed by Root et al.,1975. The pronounced effect of purified MIF on the plasma membrane may therefore be related to changes in the metabolic activity of macrophages after binding of MIF to its specific receptor. The subsequent increase in metabolic activity could explain the enhanced microbicidal activity of mononuclear phagocytes after exposure to MIF.

c b a

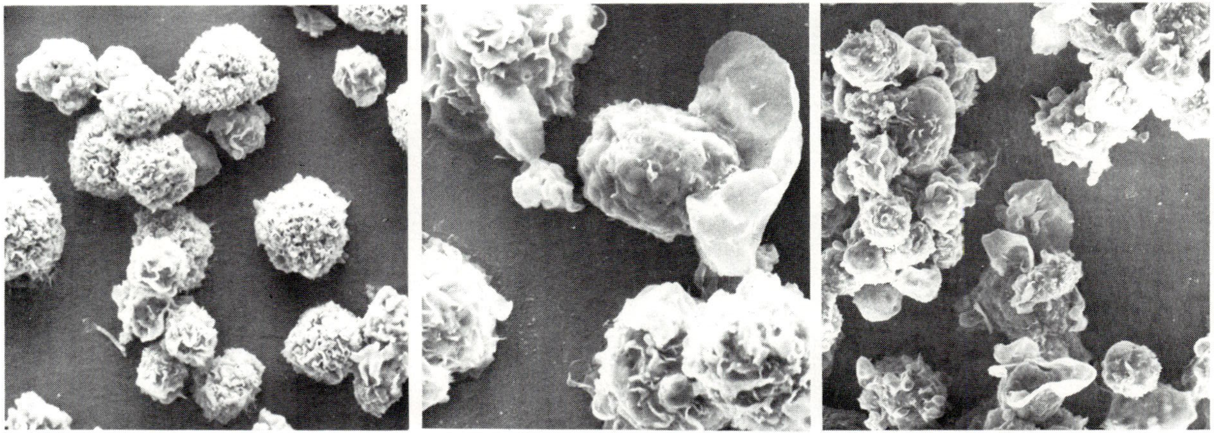

Fig. 1. Representative scanning electron micrographs of (a) mononuclear phagocytes treated with MIF (10^{-7}M) after 14 hrs. of incubation x2200, b) x4000, c) cells treated with control supernatants x2400.

REFERENCES

Biemesderfer, D., Block, L.H., Male, P., and Kashgarian, M. (1978). Scanning Electron Microscopy II, 333.

Block, L.H., Jaksche, H., Bamberger, S., and Ruhenstroth-Bauer, G. (1978). J. Exp.Med. 147, 541.

David, J.R., (1975). *In* "The Phagocytic Cell In Host Resistance" (J.A. Bellanti and D.H. Dayton, ed.), p. 143. Raven Press.

David, J.R., and David, R.A. (1970). *In* "In Vitro Methods In Cell-Mediated Immunity" (B.R. Bloom and P.R. Glade, ed.), p.249. Academic Press, N.Y.

Root, R.K., Metcalf, J., Oshino, N., and Chance, B. (1975). J.Clin.Invest.55, 945.

Root, R.K., and Stossel, T.P. (1974). J. Clin. Invest. 53, 1207.

DISCUSSION

BENDIXEN: The concentration of human MIF used may very well be without adequate correlation to MIF concentrations operative under biological conditions in the tissues. EM studies and studies of oxidative metabolism should be repeated at molar concentrations of 10^{-7}, 10^{-8}, 10^{-9}, perhaps even less. Have such experiments been made?

BLOCK: Because of limited availability of preparative amounts of purified human MIF, we were unable to vary the MIF concentration in our studies, but we plan to perform those experiments.

WEBB: I am concerned about the level of purification of Block's material. He showed a purification of 300-fold from supernatants. Is this material necessarily pure?

BLOCK: Yes. By using basically a two step method, column chromatography on Sephadex G 100 and preparative isotachophoresis, we have achieved an approximately 300-400 fold purification of human MIF.

WEBB: I would consider it very unlikely that this material is pure. Most proteins which are biologically active require purifications of several thousand fold in order to reach homogeneity. An example is interferon which requires intensive purification ($\sim 10^5$ fold) and has a specific activity in the picogram range. Until one can demonstrate lack of heterogeneity by chemical and biological criteria, it is difficult to draw conclusions concerning mechanisms of action.

BLOCK: There are two points to be made. Preparative isotachophoresis may not be the most appropriate method for purification of specific activity of the MIF protein, e.g. it might destroy the molecule and/or we may have lost considerable amounts of a "cofactor" which contributes to MIF effect on the target cells. In addition, in referring to the purification of MIF, one has to consider the fact that the capillary assay is used as the criterion for detection of its biological activity. This test is semiquantitative and relatively insensitive. Therefore, in absence of an MIF-RIA one cannot satisfactorily calculate the degree of purification of MIF.

SORG: A number of investigators assay for human MIF using heterologous macrophages. Is there not a certain species specificity of MIF, since, as reported by David et al. several years ago, using guinea pig macrophages, human MIF-containing supernatants have to be concentrated 10-fold?

BLOCK: I am aware that there are species specificities regarding the effects of lymphokines. It has been shown by various laboratories that one can test biological activity of human MIF on guinea pig macrophages, however, homologous systems appear more appropriate.

DAVID: Presently we make human MIF with (1) more cells, (2) Con A, (3) no serum. This is different from earlier studies of Rocklin using (1) less cells, (2) specific antigen, (3) presence of serum. Rocklin has shown that human monocytes are more sensitive to human MIF than guinea pig macrophages. However they are more difficult to come by.

de WECK: Human and horse monocytes are certainly better targets than guinea pig macrophages for human MIF (Friedrich et al. Int.Arch.Allergy 50: 142, 1976)

LITTMAN: We confirm that human MIF is 25,000 MW and has a pI of 3.5, using purified SK-SD stimulated lymphocyte culture supernatants. Block's material is Con A stimulated. Could he compare his results with those of David's laboratory? They have found two human MIFs with pI's of 3.5 but their pH 3 MIF was 68,000 daltons. How are these differences explained?

BLOCK: Isoelectrofocussing of our Con A-induced human MIF revealed a pI of 3.5-4.0. This material appears almost homogeneous when assayed with analytical gel electrophoresis on 10% polyacrylamide gel. As I do not know the stage of purity of David's pH 3 and pH 5 MIFs, I cannot formally exclude the possibility that one of the two MIFs might just mimic MIF action.

DAVID: We have not yet analyzed our pH 3 or pH 5 human MIF for the number of protein bands on SDS-PAGE. However, studies on guinea pig MIF which is internally labelled show *many* bands in the entire pH 3 and pH 5 fractions. I doubt that the pH 3 human MIF is homogeneous. I believe that this problem is an example where there is needed an exchange between laboratories of crude and purified fractions of human MIF to resolve these unexplained differences.

LEONARD: I am interested in the morphological changes Block observed at 14 hr. Does he observe such changes at 14 hr when he exposes cells to MIF for 2-6 hr, washes, and replaces with fresh medium?

BLOCK: Since we were interested in establishing a new SEM-method for scanning of MIF-induced effects on the surface of macrophages *without* disruption of the monolayers, we had to choose an overnight incubation period. We were therefore unable to look at earlier effects of MIF on the surface characteristics of target cells.

BIOCHEMICAL STUDIES ON THE FUCOSE-BINDING ABILITY OF MURINE MACROPHAGE MIGRATION INHIBITION FACTOR (MIF)

James A. Braatz
Lena W. Redmon
Howard T. Holden

Laboratory of Immunodiagnosis
National Cancer Institute
Bethesda, Maryland

I. INTRODUCTION

This report summarizes our evidence for an interaction between mouse MIF and L-fucose. We have found that mouse MIF will bind to fucose covalently attached to Sepharose beads and that MIF isolated in this manner can be radioiodinated and shown to bind to mouse macrophages. This type of interaction may form the basis of a radioreceptor binding assay for MIF. As an alternative to this approach we are also investigating the binding of *Lotus* lectin, a fucose-binding protein, to mouse macrophages and to fucose-Sepharose beads. Such binding would be expected to be inhibited by MIF if both the lectin and the lymphokine bind to the same site.

II. RESULTS AND DISCUSSION

Previous work has shown that MIF from fetal calf serum or antigen-stimulated guinea pig PEC (Fox and MacSween, 1974) and human leukocyte migration inhibition factor (Bendtzen, 1975) will bind to fucose affinity adsorbents. As shown in Fig. 1, we have been able to adsorb mouse MIF to fucose-Sepharose gel and subsequently elute the activity with high concentration of L-fucose. In this experiment, two adsorptions were required for complete removal of MIF activity from the supernatant and

ISBN 0-12-213950-X

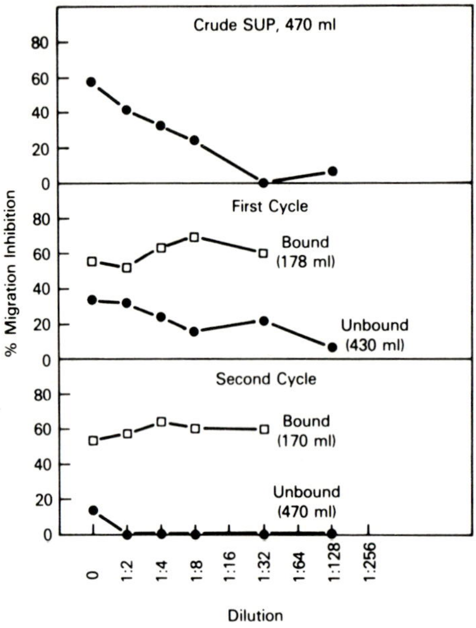

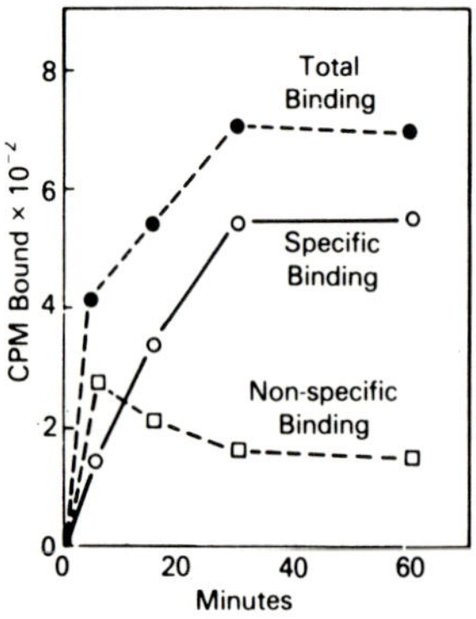

Figure 1 (left). Complete removal of MIF activity with two adsorptions to fucose-Sepharose. MIF generated with Con A in the absence of serum (470ml) was mixed with fucose-Sepharose 4B (80ml) at 4°C for 2.5 hours. The bound fraction was eluted with 2 volumes of 0.2M fucose and the adsorption was repeated.

Figure 2 (right). 5 x 10^6 WEHI-3 cells in 300ul PBS containing 10mg BSA were incubated with ^{125}I-labeled fucose affinity purified MIF in 400ul microcentrifuge tubes at 22°C. After centrigugation the cell pellet was counted for radioactivity. Input = 2300cpm.

although difficult to quantitate, most if not all of the activity was released by fucose. Less than 0.02% of the protein applied was recovered in the MIF active fractions which, after radioiodination, appeared heterogeneous on sodium dodecyl sulfate as well as non-detergent acrylamide gel electrophoresis.

Studies similar to these indicate that MIF can also bind to sugar affinity adsorbents prepared with N-acetyl-D-glucosamine, but not with D-glucose.

Affinity-purified and radioiodinated MIF can be bound to mouse macrophages as indicated in Fig. 2. The binding reached a plateau after 30 min at 22°C, with approximately 24% of the labeled preparation bound to the cells. We plan to further characterize and refine these binding studies with a major emphasis on optimizing the specific MIF-receptor interactions. We would then attempt to inhibit these interactions with MIF,

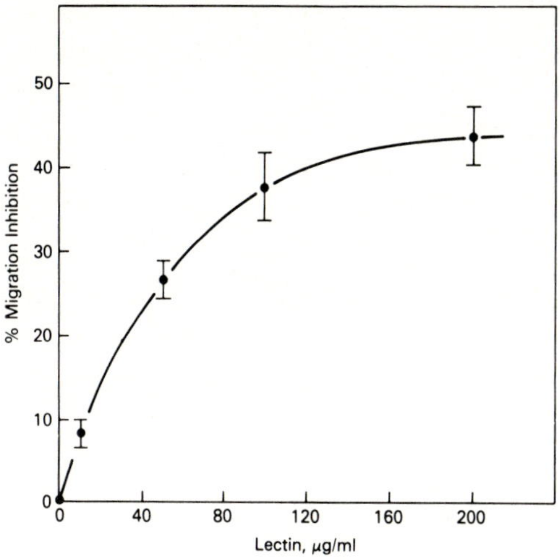

Figure 3. Inhibition of macrophage migration by Lotus lectin. Cells (2 x 10^7) were incubated at 22°C for 1.5 hours with lectin then washed prior to migration. Viability remained at 85-90% at all concentrations of lectin.

thereby laying the foundation for a radioreceptor binding assay for MIF.

As an alternative to this approach, we are trying to take advantage of the similarities between MIF and the fucose-binding lectin from *Lotus*. Both can be shown to bind to fucose-Sepharose gels as well as to mouse macrophages. Furthermore, as shown in Fig. 3, this lectin can inhibit migration of mouse PEC and may therefore be binding to the MIF receptor. If this is the case, then radiolabeled lectin bound to these receptors might be displaced by suitable MIF preparations. Similarly, fucose-Sepharose gels might serve as a convenient source of binding matrix for subsequent displacement by MIF.

In any case, it is obvious that several avenues can be pursued for developing a radioreceptor assay for MIF which could substitute for the less quantitative cell migration assay currently in use. A new assay of this type would contribute significantly to studies involving MIF and facilitate its purification and subsequent characterization.

REFERENCES

Bendtzen, K. (1976). *J. Immunol. Methods 11*, 147.

Fox, R.A., and MacSween, J.M. (1974). *Immunol. Comm. 3*, 375.

DISCUSSION

ZSCHIESCHE: Braatz stated that the fucose-binding lectin from *Lotus tetragonolobus* might attach to the same receptor as MIF on macrophage membranes. Does he have any more direct evidence for this assumption? According to our experience, it is much more difficult to prevent by α-L-fucose the migration inhibitory effect of this lectin than MIF.

BRAATZ: We have no direct evidence that both bind to the same receptor on the macrophage surface and we also find it more difficult to inhibit lectin than MIF with fucose. This assumption is based primarily on the ability of lectin to elicit the same response as MIF.

ZSCHIESCHE: One has to consider that the hypothetical receptor for MIF contains α-L-fucose only at the terminal position and, that physiologically it is an oligosaccharide (as far as the carbohydrate part is concerned). Did Braatz test di- or trisaccharides for their blocking activity in the MIF assay?

BRAATZ: No. Only monosaccharides have been tested so far.

OPPENHEIM: My questions for Braatz deal with the utility of fucose binding of MIF as a tool for its purification:
(1) Can he obtain purity of MIF with such an approach?
(2) Does serum in supernatants interfere with the binding of MIF?
(3) Do other lymphokines bind to fucose and contaminate the MIF?

BRAATZ: (1) In one experiment we started with 450 mg of protein. After adsorption to fucose-Sepharose, this was reduced to about 80 micrograms and it still had good MIF activity. However, this is still heterogeneous as indicated by SDS and non-detergent gel electrophoresis after radioiodination.
(2) We have performed these adsorptions successfully in the presence or absence of fetal calf serum.
(3) We do not know whether other lymphokines bind, but have plans to assay these fractions for other activities.

SCHUURS: How does Braatz bind the sugars to the Sephadex? Is he using a spacer?

BRAATZ: We effect binding through ether linkages using epoxy-activated Sepharose 4B. This gel matrix has a spacer equivalent to a C12 unit.

COHEN S: Fucose inhibits several lymphokines in addition to MIF, so that one would have to be careful that the assay was detecting MIF only. Also, lotus lectin may be a poor model for fucose-lymphokine binding as non-fucose binding lectins also block migration by non-specifically affecting membrane "stickiness".

BRAATZ: Yes, we also hope to learn more about the nature of the carbohydrate binding site from these studies and hopefully this would allow us to prepare more specific sugar adsorbents.

de WECK: Guinea pig macrophages are inhibited in their migration by various heterologous sera. This is due in part to heterophilic antibodies which can be absorbed by other cells like erythrocytes. It should be noted that L-fucose also inhibits these antibodies.

ZSCHIESCHE: Working with a microbial growth inhibitory factor, induced by tilorone in mice in vivo, we found that its effect on macrophages (inhibition of intracellular growth of Corynebacterium kutscheri) could also be blocked by α-L-fucose.

ROCKLIN: It needs to be emphasized that inhibition of mediator activity by a particular sugar is of itself insufficient evidence to implicate its presence in the lymphokine receptor. One needs also to demonstrate that the specific glycosidase will also block the mediator effect on the target cell following pretreatment of the latter by the former.

HUMAN LEUKOCYTE INHIBITORY FACTOR (LIF): TWO DISTINCT MOLECULAR SPECIES

Ross E. Rocklin[1]
Alan P. Brown

Department of Medicine
Harvard Medical School
Robert B. Brigham Hospital
Boston, Massachusetts

Human lymphocytes stimulated by concanavalin A produce a lymphokine that has been termed leukocyte inhibitory factor or LIF (1, 2). LIF selectively inhibits the migration of polymorphonuclear (PMN leukocytes (3). Recent studies have demonstrated that LIF has the properties of an esterase by virtue of its sensitivity to certain serine esterase inhibitors such as diisopropylphosphofluoridate (DFP), phenylmethylsulfonylfluoride (PMSF), and a benzamidine derivative (1, 2, 4, 5). Furthermore, LIF preparations contain hydrolytic activity for certain synthetic arginine ester substrates (4, 6-8).

In the present studies, we have pursued the purification of LIF by means of an isoelectric focusing technique. We report the finding of two molecular species of LIF that differ with respect to their isoelectric points but which have similar m.w. and which are both sensitive to DFP (9).

MATERIALS AND METHODS

LIF was prepared by previously described methods (1). PMN leukocytes were obtained from donors by Ficoll-Hypaque gradient centrifugation of leukocyte-rich plasma (10).

[1]*Present address: Tufts-New England Medical Center, Boston, Massachusetts.*

ISBN 0-12-213950-X

The final cell pellet was packed into capillary tubes. Lyophilized normal and active supernatants from 300 to 500 ml of starting material were reconstituted to 2 ml and applied to 2.5 x 100 cm columns containing Sephadex G-100 (1). Fractions were pooled and concentrated to 1/100 the volume of the original lymphocyte supernatants. Fraction III (Kd 0.09 to 0.19) contained material eluting with the albumin (68,000 daltons) peak and had LIF activity as demonstrated previously (1). Active and normal Fraction III supernatants from Sephadex G-100 chromatography were subjected to isoelectric focusing with a LKB 8102 Ampholine electrofocusing, 440 ml capacity, apparatus (LKB Producter, Bromma, Sweden)(11). The pH of the tubes was determined and tubes were pooled into larger fractions for testing.

After isoelectric focusing, LIF-containing fractions and their corresponding normal fractions were subjected to gel filtration on G-75 Sephadex (calibrated columns kindly provided by Heinz Remold and Alma Mednis, Harvard Medical School)(11).

Control and LIF fractions of 1 to 2 ml volume in medium TC-199 were incubated with various concentrations of DFP for 30 min at 37^{0}C (4). After incubation, the preparations were dialysed extensively against Tris HCl buffer for 18 hr and then against TC-199. Untreated control and LIF fractions were treated similarly except that no DFP was added.

RESULTS AND DISCUSSION

LIF-containing and control supernatants were subjected to isoelectric focusing after a preliminary separation on Sephadex G-100. Two peaks of LIF activity were reproducibly recovered. LIF activity was recovered in the pH 5.0 to 5.5 fraction in 10/10 experiments. In 9/10 experiments LIF activity was detected in either the pH 8.0 to 8.5 or pH 8.5 to 10.0 fraction. No significant LIF activity was detected in the other fractions. Data from three representative experiments are illustrated in Figure 1. The pH 5.0 to 5.5 fraction contained approximately 15% of the protein applied to the column and the pH 8.0 to 8.5 contained about 5%. No significant difference in protein content was found between supernatant fractions obtained from Con A-stimulated and unstimulated lymphocytes.

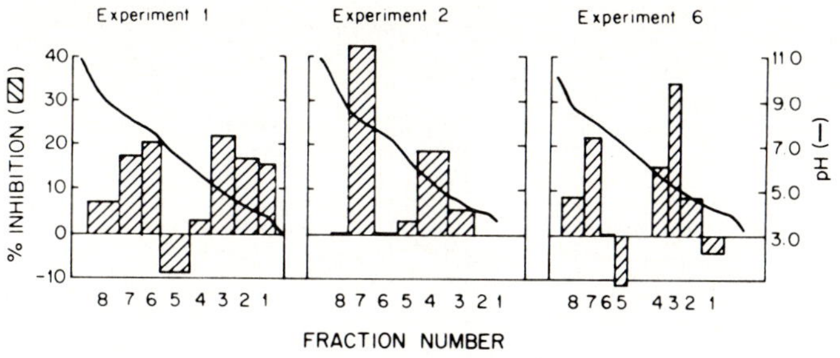

FIGURE 1. Isoelectricfocusing of LIF in a gradient from pH 4.0 to 10.0. Three typical experiments of ten performed are shown. The fraction number is indicated on the abscissa, and the per cent inhibition (bars) and the pH of the fractions (solid line) are shown on the ordinate.

After isoelectric focusing, pH 5.0 and pH 8.5 fractions containing LIF activity and corresponding normal fractions were rechromatographed on Sephadex G-75 columns (Fig. 2). The latter provides greater resolution than the Sephadex G-100 columns employed in the preliminary purification step. In two experiments, both the pH 5.0 and the pH 8.5 LIF eluted in the Kd range of 0.032 to 0.076 corresponding to an apparent m.w. of approximately 68,000 to 75,000. No significant LIF activity was detected in any of the other fractions.

Both pH 5.0 and pH 8.5 LIF were examined for their sensitivity to DFP. In six of six experiments, pH 5.0 LIF activity was significantly reduced (>50%) by incubation with 10^{-3}M DFP. In four of six experiments with pH 8.5 LIF, the LIF activity of untreated material was reduced just by incubation at 37^{0}C for 30 min. In two experiments where pH 8.5 LIF activity was recovered in untreated fractions, 10^{-3}M DFP reduced the LIF activity by more than 50%. Data from these two experiments are shown in Fig. 3.

These experiments demonstrate that LIF activity can be separated into two components having distinct isoelectric points of approximately 5.0 and 8.5. Both molecular species had similar elution patterns on Sephadex G-75 and therefore share an apparent m.w. of 68,000 to 75,000. This agrees with previous published reports of an apparent m.w. of 68,000 as determined by Sephadex G-100 gel filtration (2, 3). Furthermore, the finding that LIF is comprised of at least two heterogeneous molecular species is consistent with the documentation of heterogeneity among other lymphokines such as MIF and lymphotoxin (11-13). In addition, our data

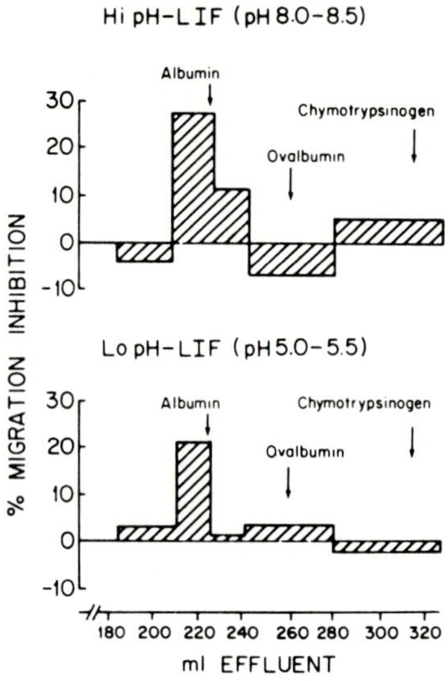

FIGURE 2. Sephadex G-75 gel filtration of the two LIF activities. After isoelectricfocusing, partially purified active and control fractions were chromatographed on G-75 columns.

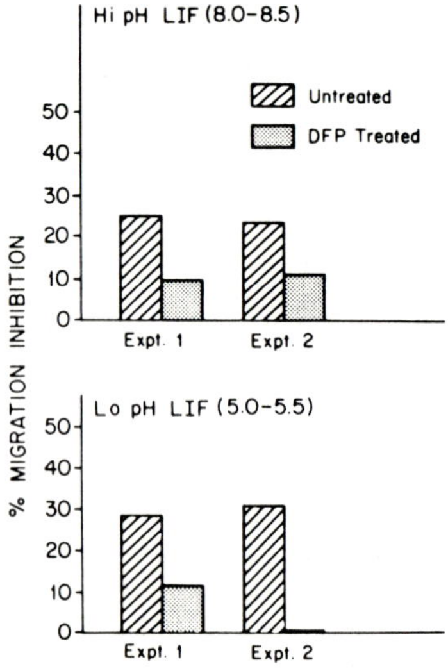

FIGURE 3. DFP sensitivity of the two LIF activities. Results of two experiments are shown in which activity in untreated fractions was preserved. Active fractions recovered after isoelectricfocusing were incubated at 37^{0}C for 30 min with or without the addition of 10-^{3}M DFP. The fractions were then dialysed extensively before assay.

demonstrate that both LIF activities are DFP sensitive and are consistent with previous data (4). The pH 8.5 LIF activity was often labile during the 30-min 37°C control incubation without DFP being present. This heat lability may only be apparent in highly purified fractions, despite the addition of albumin in an attempt to reduce non-specific loss of activity. This observation may explain in part the conflicting reports concerning the lability of LIF at 56°C (1, 2). The relationship between the two LIF species is currently under investigation.

REFERENCES

1. Rocklin, R.E., *J. Immunol. 114,* 1161 (1975).
2. Bendtzen, K., *Acta Pathol. Microbiol. Scand. (C), 84,* 471 (1976).
3. Rocklin, R.E., *J. Immunol. 112,* 1461 (1974).
4. Rocklin, R.E., and Rosenthal, A.S., *J. Immunol. 119,* 249 (1977).
5. Bendtzen, K., *Scand. J. Immunol. 6,* 125 (1977).
6. Bendtzen, K., *Scand. J. Immunol. 6,* 133 (1977).
7. Bendtzen, K., *Scand. J. Immunol. 6,* 1055 (1977).
8. Rocklin, R.E. and Urbano, A.M., *J. Immunol. 120,* 1409 (1978).
9. Rocklin, R.E., and Brown, A.P., *J. Immunol. 122,* 1059 (1979).
10. Boyum, A., *Scand. J. Clin. Lab. Invest. 21 (Suppl.97),* 77 (1968).
11. Remold, H.G. and Mednis, A.D., *J. Immunol. 118,* 2015 (1977).
12. Hiseredt, J.C., Prieur, A.M. and Granger, G.A., *Cell. Immunol. 24,* 277 (1976).
13. Walker, S.M., Lee, S.C. and Lucas, Z.J., *J. Immunol. 116,* 807 (1976).

DISCUSSION

LEONARD: Rocklin's findings are interesting, but there are reasons for concern when the separation and the preparative techniques devolve solely on isoelectric focussing. Relative to the issue of a small active peptide being attached to albumin and removed during isoelectric focussing, I recently had occasion to subject purified human albumin to flat bed electrofocussing. After an overnight run, a yellow band was seen on the gel, corresponding to a pH of about 4.5. During the next few hr, the yellow color disappeared. The OD 280 of fractions eluted from the bed showed 2 distinct peaks, one at pH 4.5, the other at about pH 5.5. It is known that treatment of albumin with activated charcoal removes albumin-bound fatty acids, and the isoelectric pH increases to about 5.5.It is thus likely that under certain conditions of isoelectric focussing, ligands attached to albumin may dissociate. The implications of this finding for the present work are self evident.

MOLECULAR BIOLOGY OF HUMAN LEUKOCYTE MIGRATION INHIBITORY FACTOR (LIF)
MODULATION OF LIF-INDUCED ESTEROLYSIS AND NEUTROPHIL MIGRATION INHIBITION BY cGMP

Klaus Bendtzen[1]

Department of Medicine TA
Rigshospitalet University Hospital
Copenhagen

Leukocyte migration inhibitory factor (LIF) produced in vitro by Con A-stimulated human mononuclear cells is a serine esterase and -protease by virtue of its susceptibility to the irreversible enzyme inhibitors phenylmethylsulfonyl fluoride (PMSF), diisopropylfluorophosphate (DFP) and physostigmine (1-4, 11). The PMSF-induced abrogation of LIF activity is concentration-, temperature- and time-dependent, and PMSF-inactivated LIF may be reactivated by the nucleophilic agent pralidoxime methansulfonate (2, 4).

Arginine esters and -amides selectively protect LIF against the blocking effect of PMSF (3, 4, 8). This protection is dependent upon the relative concentrations between the substrates and PMSF, suggesting that the substrates compete with the inhibitor for the enzymatically active site on the LIF molecule.

A similar protective effect of cGMP has also been demonstrated (5). The protection afforded by this nucleotide is highly specific, since noncyclic nucleotides and nucleosides as well as cyclic nucleotides differing from cGMP at the position of the diester bond (2',3'-cGMP), in the sugar residue (2'-deoxy-cGMP), or in the purine base (cAMP) were all ineffective.

[1]*Present address: Tufts-New England Medical Center, Boston, Massachusetts.*

ISBN 0-12-213950-X

Effect of cGMP on the Esterolytic Activity of Purified LIF

To demonstrate directly the enzyme property of LIF, i.e., that LIF not only binds arginine esters but also promotes a hydrolytic attack on these esters, we have recently attempted to purify LIF and to test the LIF-mediated esterolysis using a highly sensitive double-phase radioenzyme assay (6, 7). To follow the effects of the purification procedures, the supernatant serine esterases were labeled with ^{3}H-DFP. More than 95% of the labeled enzymes were removed by a three-step procedure: 1) irreversible blockade of contaminating histidine esterases by treatment with tosyl lysine chloromethyl ketone, 2) Sephadex G-100 chromatography for fractionation of the proteins as well as for removal of unreacted inhibitor and Con A, and 3) immunoadsorption of the eluted LIF-containing fractions with agarose-immobilized antibodies against protein contaminants of LIF-rich supernatants (7). This procedure eliminated all proteins detectable by crossed immunoelectrophoresis. The resulting esterase concentration was approximately 10^{-11}M (unconcentrated), and the esterolytic activity towards tosyl arginine (^{3}H) methyl ester (^{3}H-TAME) corresponded to that of 0.3 ng human thrombin per ml.

As shown in Table I, cGMP at concentrations as low as 10^{-7}M significantly reduced the esterolytic activity of purified LIF. Again, the inhibitory effect was highly specific, since GTP, 5'-GMP and cAMP did not modulate the rate of hydrolysis.

The kinetic behavior of LIF-induced esterolysis of ^{3}H-TAME is shown in Fig. 1. At relatively high (left) concentrations of the substrate Michaelis-Menten kinetics were obtained. As predicted from the results of cGMP/PMSF competition experiments (5), cGMP behaved kinetically as a competitive inhibitor, and a linear relationship in the double reciprocal plots was obtained. It is important to realize that the competitive nature of this inhibition indicates that even very low levels of cGMP may influence the enzyme activity of LIF, provided that the substrate concentration is low. Indeed, in most biological systems low and unsaturating levels of natural substrates are found.

TABLE I. Effect of cGMP and Other Nucleotides on LIF-induced Esterolysis of ^{3}H-TAME

Nucleotide		% loss of esterolytic activity[a]	
10^{-5}	cGMP	23 ± 12	($p<0.05$)
10^{-6}	cGMP	18 ± 6	($p<0.05$)
10^{-7}	cGMP	15 ± 8	($p<0.05$)
10^{-8}	cGMP	7 ± 6	(ns)
10^{-4}	GTP	3 ± 5	(ns)
10^{-4}	5'-GMP	-4 ± 7	(ns)
10^{-4}	cAMP	0 ± 6	(ns)

[a]Means of five different experiments. $P>0.05$ is considered not significant (ns); Mann-Whitney rank sum test.

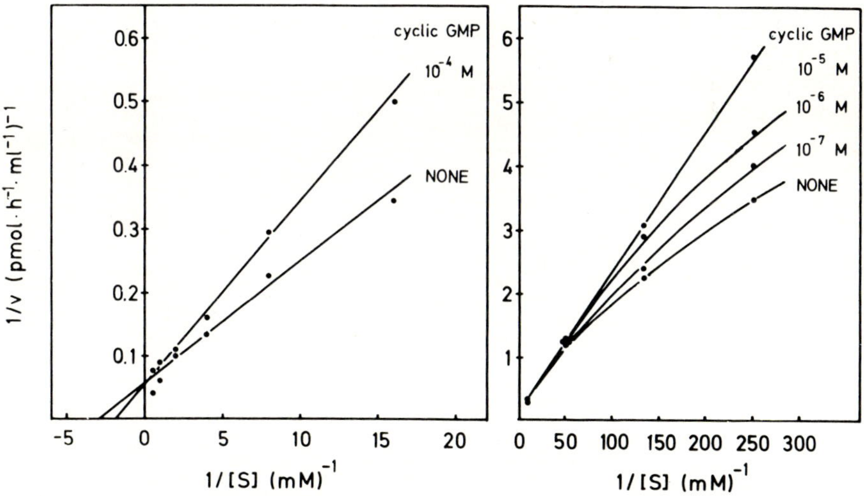

FIGURE 1. Lineweaver-Burk plots of LIF-induced initial reaction velocities (v) at high (left) and low (right) concentrations of ^{3}H-TAME. The influence of cGMP is also shown.
(Adapted from Ref. 6 with permission from Elsevier/North-Holland Biomedical Press).

Effect of cGMP on LIF-induced Inhibition of Neutrophil Motility

If cGMP inhibits PMSF-induced acylation of the catalytic centre of LIF and interferes with LIF-dependent esterolysis, the nucleotide would also be expected to inhibit the biological effect of the lymphokine. We have previously shown that exogenous cGMP and dibutyryl cGMP have little effect on LIF activity when tested after 22 hours of neutrophil migration (10). However, a slight but consistent reduction in LIF activity was observed after 3 hours of migration (10).

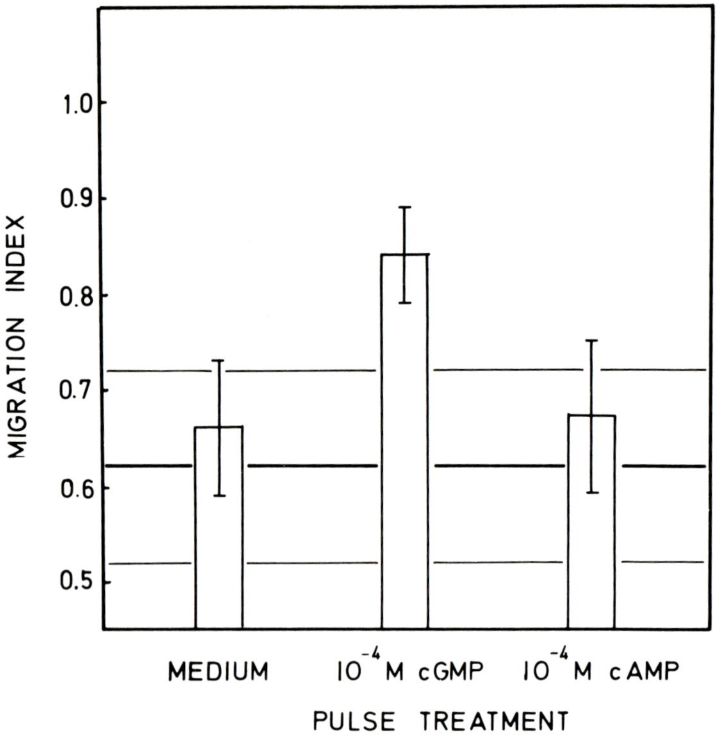

FIGURE 2. Ability of cGMP to prevent LIF-induced migration inhibition of neutrophils. Columns and bars are means ± 1 SD, n=6; horizontal lines are mean migration index ± 1 SD obtained when neutrophils were exposed to LIF and control supernatants throughout the entire migration period. The reduction in LIF activity caused by cGMP is significant (P<0.05; Mann-Whitney rank sum test).

Recently, the ability of cGMP to interfere with the LIF-neutrophil interaction has been further substantiated by the following experiment:

Neutrophils were pulse-treated at 37°C for 1 hour with LIF and control supernatants in the presence of cGMP, cAMP, or medium alone (Fig. 2). Then the cells were washed, resuspended in fresh medium without nucleotides and tested for migration inhibition. It can be seen that pulse treatment of neutrophils with LIF was as effective as continuous exposure of the cells to the lymphokine. The effect of LIF was not affected by cAMP, but when cells were pulsed with LIF in the presence of cGMP, little or no inhibition of migration was observed.

The natural substrate for LIF is unknown as is the biological significance of the cGMP-mediated modulation of LIF activity. The results of recent experiments indicate that LIF increases the intraneutrophil levels of cGMP (9). Whether cGMP is in fact an intracellular mediator of LIF - not necessarily acting alone - is not known. However, besides explaining the outcome of experiments where the effects of exogenous cGMP and cAMP have been investigated, such a model would provide an attractive regulatory mechanism by which LIF activity might be adjusted in vitro and, possibly, in vivo.

REFERENCES

1. Bendtzen, K., *Acta Path. Microbiol. Scand. Sect. C, 84,* 471 (1976).
2. Bendtzen, K., *Scand. J. Immunol. 6,* 125 (1977).
3. Bendtzen, K., *Scand. J. Immunol. 6,* 133 (1977).
4. Bendtzen, K., *Scand. J. Immunol. 6,* 1055 (1977).
5. Bendtzen, K., *Scand. J. Immunol. 8,* 53 (1978).
6. Bendtzen, K., *Biochim. Biophys. Acta 566,* 183 (1979).
7. Bendtzen, K., *J. Clin. Lab. Immunol. 2,* 37 (1979).
8. Bendtzen, K., *Scand. J. Immunol.* (1979)(In press).
9. Bendtzen, K., and Klysner, R., *Immunopharmacol.* (1979) (In press).
10. Bendtzen, K., and Palit, J., *Acta Path. Microbiol. Scand. Sect. C, 85,* 317 (1977).
11. Rocklin, R.E., and Rosenthal, A.S., *J. Immunol. 119,* 249 (1977).

DISCUSSION

MIZEL: (1) What is the turnover value for LIF? (2) Can Bendtzen rule out the possibility that the enzyme activity is associated with a protein which converts LIF to an active form?

BENDTZEN: (1) The Vmax of our purified LIF preparations was shown in the Lineweaver-Bürk plot. At saturating concentrations of the substrate, approximately 20 pmoles of TAME is converted in 1 hr at 32°C by the LIF material present in 1 ml of original supernatant. (2) The proposition posed by Mizel is theoretically possible but highly unlikely. In that case this protein and LIF should co-purify in various procedures including molecular/sieve chromatography and isoelectrofocussing. This possibility could be tested rather easily, for instance by preincubating LIF supernatants at 37°C for 1 hr. This would activate the putative LIF precursor, and addition at this stage of PMSF would not be able to block the LIF activity.

BRETZ: Since small molecular weight esters and amides are model substrates for proteinases and since proteinases are known to affect different types of cells, has Bendtzen sought to show proteolytic activity by LIF?

BENDTZEN: We have not been able to test for proteolytic activity of LIF, simply because LIF is found in very minute quantities, and conventional protease assays are not sensitive enough for this purpose. The fact that synthetic arginine amides protect LIF activity against the blocking effect of PMSF and that these amides seem to compete directly with the natural substrate for LIF in the agarose assay indicate that these amides have affinity for the catalytic site on the enzyme. There is reason to believe therefore, that LIF is a protease as well.

NEUTROPHIL MIGRATION INHIBITION FACTOR FROM T-LYMPHOCYTES (NIF-T): A NEW LYMPHOKINE*

Richard H. Weisbart
David W. Golde
Leonard Spolter
Peter Eggena
Heinrich Rinderknecht

Department of Medicine
UCLA San Fernando Valley Program
and UCLA
Los Angeles, California

I. BACKGROUND

We described a neutrophil migration inhibition factor produced by a T lymphoblast cell line (Mo) established from a patient with a T cell variant of hairy cell leukemia (1). In contrast, neutrophil migration inhibition activity was not detected in the supernatants from numerous other lymphoblast cell lines including T cell, B cell, Null cell, and myeloblast cell lines. We also studied a neutrophil migration inhibition factor produced by peripheral blood lymphocytes (PBL). T cells, B cells, or monocytes alone did not produce mediator activity in response to mitogenic stimulation, but assayable mediator was detected when T and B cells or T cells and monocytes were combined (2). The neutrophil migration inhibition factors from Mo cells and PBL have been isolated and compared. Both factors appear to be the same and are distinguishable from previously described neutrophil migration inhibition factors.

*Supported in part by Public Health Service Grant AI 13253.

ISBN 0-12-213950-X

II. METHODS

Neutrophil migration inhibition activity was produced by lymphoblast cells and PBL in serum free medium (3×10^6 cells/ml Medium 199). 8402, a T lymphoblast cell line that did not produce neutrophil migration inhibition activity was used as a control for studies involving Mo cells. PBL were isolated by Ficoll-Hypaque gradient centrifugation. Mediator activity was induced from PBL by Concanvalin A (Con A), and non-stimulated culture supernatants were reconstituted with the same concentration of Con A used in stimulated cultures. A microassay was used for neutrophil migration under agarose as previously described (3).

III. RESULTS

A summary of the results comparing the neutrophil migration inhibition factor from Mo cells and PBL is given in Table I. The migration inhibition factor from both Mo cells and PBL showed the same remarkable heat stability with activity persisting after heating to 80°C for 30 minutes. Neutrophil migration inhibition activity from both sources was abolished by treatment with pronase (1 mg/ml). Mediator activity from both sources showed the same elution pattern from DEAE Sephacel with activity eluted at 0.3M NaCl. Con A sepharose was cultured in the presence of PBL and incubated with supernatants from Mo cells. In both cases, assayable mediator activity was not eluted from Con A sepharose with 1M NaCl, but activity was specifically eluted with α-methyl-D-glucoside. Supernatants with neutrophil migration inhibition activity from PBL and Mo cells were electrophoresed for 4 hours at 300 volts in polyacrylamide gradient slab gels. Mediator activity from Mo cells and PBL was localized to a region corresponding to 35,000 to 45,000 daltons. Supernatants from Mo cells and PBL treated with diisopropylfluorophosphate (DFP)(10^{-3}M) for 30 minutes retained full activity. Trypsin added to the same supernatants was demonstrated to lose its activity after the same treatment with DFP. Neutrophils were incubated with supernatants from PBL and Mo cells, washed, and incubated for 2 and 20 hours before migrating them. In comparision to neutrophils incubated with control supernatants, the neutrophils incubated with active supernatants still showed inhibition of migration after 2 hours, but the inhibitory effect was absent by 20 hours. Culture supernatants did not contain chemotactic activity.

IV. DISCUSSION

The neutrophil migration inhibition factor from Mo cells and PBL are the same or remarkably similar. This mediator can be distinguished from other migration inhibition factors (MIF, NIF, and LIF) by its heat stability, selective production by T lymphocytes, resistance to inactivation by DFP, and molecular weight.

TABLE I. Neutrophil Migration Inhibition Factor[a]

	Source	
	Mo cells	PBL
Initial activity	42 ± 2	49 ± 5
Heat Stability 80° X 30 min.	28 ± 6	34 ± 4
Pronase Digestion	4 ± 4	-4 ± 6
Elution from Con A sepharose	45 ± 7	41 ± 5
MW by PAGE	35,000-45,000	35,000-45,000
Treatment with DFP (10^{-3}M)	42 ± 9	34 ± 5
Reversibility of inhibition of neutrophil migration		
2 hours	48 ± 4	42 ± 7
20 hours	0 ± 6	-1 ± 11

[a]% inhibition in the area of neutrophil migration ± S.E.M.

ACKNOWLEDGMENTS

We thank Amelia Kacena and Grace Chan for expert technical assistance, Renate Smart and Inga Anderson for preparation of the manuscript.

REFERENCES

1. Weisbart, R.H., Billing, R., and Golde, D., *J. Lab. and Clin. Med.* 93, 622 (1979).
2. Weisbart, R.H., Yu, D.T.Y., Billing, R., Fan, P.T., Clements, P.J., and Paulus, H.E., *Immunol.* 34, 815 (1978).
3. Weisbart, R.H., and Mickey, M.R., *J. Immunol. Methods*, 16, 269 (1977).

ASSESSMENT OF ACTIVITIES OF LEUKOCYTE MIGRATION INHIBITORY FACTOR (LIF), AND OF ANTIBODIES AGAINST LIF

F.C. den Hollander
J.I. van Lieshout
A.H.W.M. Schuurs

Organon Scientific Development Group
Oss, The Netherlands

I. PREPARATION OF LIF AND OF ANTI-LIF

Cells from human lymphoid cell lines RPMI 1788 and CCRF-SB were cultured to a density of 10^6 cells/ml in RPMI 1640 containing 10 ml/l human or 50 ml/l foetal calf serum (FCS) respectively. After centrifugation (2000 N/kg) the cells were resuspended in serum-free RPMI 1640 at 10^6 cells/ml, and incubated for another 48 h. The supernatant was harvested and β-propiolactone added (final concentration 1,0 g/l). After 24 h at 4^oC the pH was adjusted to 7,0.
The supernatant was ultrafiltrated through an Amicon hollow fiber cartridge with a molecular weight cut-off of 10^5 D. The filtrate was concentrated 20 times on a 5×10^3 D cartridge. The 10^5 - 5×10^3 D concentrate was dialysed against several changes of distilled water, and lyophilised.
This material (prep. 517.2, see table 1) was redissolved in 0,05 mol/l NH_4HCO_3 containing 9 g/l NaCl and fractionated on Sephadex G100. Fractions were collected and their absorbance at 280 nm was measured. The migration-inhibitory activity (test procedure see below) in each fraction was assessed. Three

ISBN 0-12-213950-X

activity peaks were obtained. The activity in only one of them (void volume peak) was found stable after pooling of the fractions. Activity could no longer be demonstrated in the other pooled fractions.
The void volume pool (prep. 527.2 table 1) was used for immunisation of rabbits. The material was injected in Freund's complete adjuvant into multiple sites on the back of the animal (Vaitukaitis, J. and Ross, G.T. in : Gonadotrophins. Eds. Saxena, B.B., Beling, C.G., and Gaudy, H.M. Wiley-Interscience, New York, 1971, pp. 435-443), followed by i.m. injections using equal volumes of Freund's incomplete adjuvant.

II. TEST PROCEDURE FOR LIF ACTIVITY AND STATISTICAL EVALUTION OF TEST DATA

Pig buffy coat cells, prepared by dextran sedimentation of erythrocytes, were washed with 0,155 mol/l NH_4Cl and suspended at a density of 6×10^8 viable cells/ml in MEMS containing 300 ml/l FCS. This was done right before use in the test. One such test accommodated 12 samples (8 unknowns, 1 medium control and the reference in triplicate). The samples were diluted in 4 different microtiter plates, using MEMS without serum. In each plate a different randomised order was used (four-block designed assay).
After addition of cells (final concentration 3×10^8 cells/ml) the microtiter plates were incubated for 1 h at 37°C. Samples of 5 μl of each of the wells were then transferred to a hole punched in an agarose layer (20 g/l medium 199 containing 150 ml FCS/ml) contained in a petri dish. This was done in duplicate from each microtiter plate. The agarose dishes were incubated for 20 h at 37°C. After a treatment with methanol and formalin, both for 30 min, the agarose was removed and the plates were washed and dried. The migration index was calculated using the formula (diameter sample/diameter medium control)^2 x 100.
The statistical analysis comprised checks on linearity and parallelism of the dose-response curves of standard and unknowns, and on block differences. This resulted in potencies with 95% confidence limits. Some of our results are presented in table 1. We arbitrarily defined our unit of migration inhibitory activity as that amount of standard which caused 30% migration inhibition. With our first standard 273.2 this level of inhibition was attained

with 50 μg of material and we therefore assigned to this preparation a potency of 20 U/mg. Subsequent standards such as 359.2 were assayed against the first one.

III. ASSESSMENT OF ANTI-LIF

The antisera were shown to contain anti-LIF activity by incubation with LIF (20 h, 4°C) and subsequent precipitation (at 4°C) of the immune complexes by 40% saturated ammonium sulphate. As control was used non-immune rabbit serum. Neutralisation of LIF is shown in fig. 1 for three different antisera in comparison with non-immune serum.

TABLE 1: Statistical evaluated LIF activities

Preparation	Origin	Potency in U/mg, including 95% confidence limits
273.2	CCRF-SB	20 (by definition)
359.2	CCRF-SB	7,4 (4,9-10,9)
488.2	RPMI 1788	117 (80-169)
517.2	RPMI 1788	29 (20-42)
527.2	RPMI 1788	3000*

* no confidence limits due to lack of parallelism with the standard

FIGURE 1: Comparison of non-immune serum and 3 immune sera with regard to their ability to neutralise LIF activity

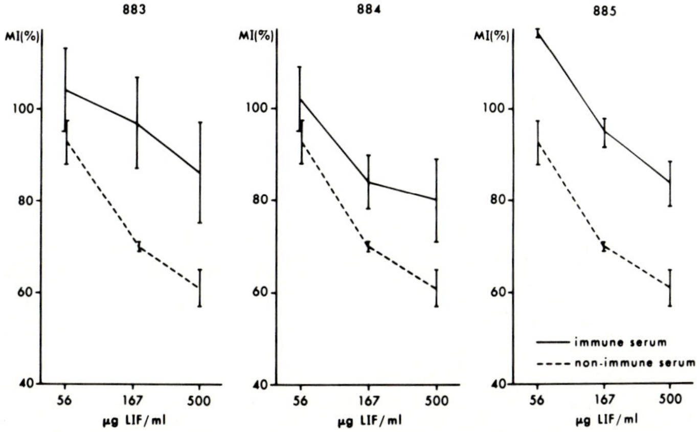

LYMPHOKINE MIMICRY BY PHORBOL MYRISTATE ACETATE (PMA) AND THE IONOPHORE A23187 - A NEW HYPOTHESIS FOR EXPLAINING THE ACTION MECHANISM OF MIGRATION INHIBITORY FACTOR (MIF)[1]

Yona Keisari
Edgar Pick[2]

Department of Human Microbiology
Sackler School of Medicine
Tel-Aviv University
Tel-Aviv, Israel

I. INTRODUCTION

Among all lymphokines, macrophage migration inhibitory factor (MIF) is the one having attracted a considerable part of the investigative effort. However, progress in the understanding of the intracellular mechanism of MIF action has been particularly slow. We have recently initiated a new approach to the study of the mechanism of MIF action, centered on the search for agents mimicking one or more of the biochemical events which are thought to occur in the macrophage subject to MIF action. In the present communication we summarize our studies with two such agents, phorbol myristate acetate (PMA) and the ionophore A23187, and offer a novel interpretation of the experimental results. We also suggest a new unified hypothesis to explain the action mechanism of MIF.

[1]*Supported by grant 1505 from the U.S. - Israel Binational Science Foundation and by a grant from F. Hoffmann-La Roche & Co. Ltd., Basle, Switzerland.*
[2]*To whom correspondence should be addressed.*

ISBN 0-12-213950-X

II. MATERIALS AND METHODS

PMA was obtained from Consolidated Midland Corporation, dissolved in dimethylsulfoxide (DMSO) to a concentration of 2mM and stored at -70°C. A23187 was a gift of E. Lilly & Co., and was stored as a 10mM stock solution in DMSO, at -70%, in the dark. Macrophage harvest, migration inhibition assays, chemiluminescence tests and superoxide anion release measurements were performed as previously described (1,2).

III. RESULTS

A. Effect of PMA and A23187 on Macrophage Migration

Guinea pig peritoneal exudate cells (PEC) were pulse-exposed to PMA (2nM-2μM) for intervals of 30 sec, 10 min and 60 min at 37°C, followed by washing of the cells and assessment of their migration from capillaries in culture medium. 0.2-2μM PMA caused pronounced inhibition of macrophage migration even when the length of the pulse was only 30 sec. When pulsing was prolonged to 10 min, as little as 20 nM PMA induced significant migration inhibition. Cell viability was not affected by incubation of macrophages for 1 h with up to 2 μM PMA. PMA did not stimulate lymphocytes to release MIF, indicating that inhibition of macrophage migration was the result of a direct effect of PMA on macrophages.

In another series of experiments, guinea pig PEC were allowed to migrate from capillaries in chambers containing the divalent cation ionophore A23187, dissolved in Eagle's MEM with varying concentrations of Ca^{2+}. We have recently shown that incubation of macrophages with 1-10 μM A23187 causes a marked influx of Ca^{2+}, as assayed by the uptake of ^{45}Ca by cells preequilibrated with ^{45}Ca in a medium containing 1.8 Ca^{2+} (2). A23187 was found to inhibit macrophage migration at concentrations in excess of 0.5 μM, in media containing 1.8 or 10 mM Ca^{2+} and 0.8 mM Mg^{2+}. When the migration assays were performed in Ca^{2+}-free medium, the inhibitory effect of A23187 was considerably reduced. Pulsing of macrophages with 10 μM A23187 for intervals of 5-60 min was sufficient to induce migration inhibition. However, at concentrations below 2.5 μM, A23187 was not effective in pulse exposure experiments. The migration inhibitory effect of A23187 was due to the direct interaction of the ionophore with macrophages since incubation of lymphocytes with the ionophore did not stimulate MIF production.

TABLE I. Induction of Chemiluminescence in Guinea Pig Peritoneal Macrophages by PMA and A23187

Stimulant	Concentration	Length of exposure of macrophages to stimulant	Stimulation ratio[a]
PMA	0.002 μM	1 min	1.0
	0.02 μM		12.5
	0.2 μM		47.6
	2 μM		69.4
A23187	10 μM	5 min	8.6
Opsonized zymozan	0.5 mg/ml	5 min	80.8

[a]Stimulation ratio = (counts per 30 sec in the presence of the stimulant) / (counts per 30 sec in the absence of the stimulant)

TABLE II. Superoxide Generation by Guinea Pig Peritoneal Macrophages Induced by PMA and A23187

Divalent cations in the medium[a]	nmol reduced cytochrome c per mg macrophage protein (90 min incubation)		
	-	PMA (2μM)	A23187 (10μM)
Ca^{2+}, Mg^{2+}	7.4	50.9	37.7
Ca^{2+}, -	4.8	48.1	31.9
- , Mg^{2+}	0	56.4	0.3
- , -	0	78.8	0.4

[a]The concentration of Ca^{2+} was 1.8 mM; that of Mg^{2+} was 0.8mM.

B. Induction by PMA and A23187 of Chemiluminescence and Superoxide Production

It has been reported that macrophages, like neutrophils, respond with a cyanide-insensitive respiratory burst to phagocytic and other membrane stimuli (3). In the course of this, oxygen is taken up and diverted from the oxidative phosphorylation pathway to a biochemical sequence, the essence of which is the formation of superoxide anions (O_2^-), H_2O_2, hydroxyl radicals ($OH\cdot$) and singlet oxygen (O_2^1). Chemiluminescence is the expression of the combined effects of these radicals; their relative contribution to the phenomenon is still uncertain.

We found that PMA induces rapid (within 1 min) chemiluminescence in oil-induced peritoneal macrophages in the same concentration range which also causes inhibition of migration (Table I). Chemiluminescence was also produced by incubation of macrophages with 10 µM A23187 but peak light emission was reached after 5-10 min of incubation. The intensity of luminescence was higher following stimulation with PMA, reaching levels close to those found with macrophages phagocytising opsonized zymosan. Results obtained in chemiluminescence assays were closely paralleled by the quantitation of O_2^- release. Both PMA and A23187 stimulated O_2^- production and the specificity of O_2^- - mediated cytochrome c reduction was confirmed by its total inhibition by superoxide dismutase (30 µg/ml). While PMA-induced O_2^- release was independent of divalent cations, A23187-stimulated O_2^- production only occurred in the presence of Ca^{2+} (Table II). Mg^{2+} was unable to replace Ca^{2+}, indicating that A23187 induces O_2^- production by a specific effect on Ca^{2+} transport.

IV. DISCUSSION AND WORKING HYPOTHESIS

We would like to suggest a novel hypothesis to explain the effects of MIF on macrophages. The essential points of this proposal are : a) MIF acts as a stimulant of the respiratory burst in macrophages; b) unstable products of oxygen reduction such as O_2^-, $OH\cdot$ and O_2^1 or the more stable H_2O_2, formed during the MIF-induced respiratory burst, are responsible for most, if not all the effects of MIF; c) inhibition of migration, the most common of all MIF effects, is the result of oxidative damage by oxygen by-products to membrane lipids or protein or to cytoplasmic elements, possibly belonging to the cytoskeleton, and d) MIF-mediated macrophage activation, as expressed by augmented bactericidal and cytotoxic capacity, is the functional expression of the enhanced ability of MIF-activated cells to produce H_2O_2 (and perhpas $OH\cdot$ and O_2^1) in response to phagocytic stimuli or other types of membrane perturbation. In this hypothesis we distinguish between two effects of MIF: a) an early effect, namely its ability to directly stimulate the respiratory burst, and b) a late effect, developing after the initial burst has burned out, and characterized by an enhanced capacity to produce potentially cytotoxic oxygen products in response to membrane stimulation.

There is a large body of evidence in support of this proposal: (1) Directed movement and phagocytosis by polymorphonuclear leukocytes (PMN) are decreased by exogenous H_2O_2 (4). Phagocytosis is also promoted in anaerobic conditions and the presence of the H_2O_2-catabolizing enzyme, catalase, promotes phagocytosis and cell movement (4); (2) PMN from humans treated with the antioxidant α-tocopherol demonstrate improved phagocytosis (4); (3) Incubation of PMN with the H_2O_2 scavenger 2,3-dihydroxybenzoic acid promotes phagocytosis and directed cell movement (5); (4) Three chemically unrelated agents - PMA, A23187 and Con A - which are potent inhibitors of macrophage migration are also active inducers of H_2O_2 formation in macrophages (6). The induction of O_2^- (the normal precursor of H_2O_2) formation by A23187 is Ca^{2+}-dependent. Sodium azide, which also blocks macrophage migration, induces O_2^- release by guinea pig macrophages (Keisari and Pick, in preparation) and OH· formation by human monocytes (7); (5) Ascorbic acid, acting as an oxidant, causes refractoriness of the adenylate cyclase of adrenal cells to stimulation by ACTH, provided that the cells are derived from rats deficient in α-tocopherol (8). Refracteriness was explained as being due to oxidative damage to the lipid environment of the enzyme. Such a mechanism could provide an alternative explanation for the MIF-induced adenylate cyclase refractoriness (9); (6) We have also found that D_2O promotes MIF action and have explained this by its stabilizing effect on microtubules (10). The same finding can, however, also be explained by the fact that D_2O prolongs the lifetime of O_2^1 in solution, which would promote oxidative damage (cited in Ref. 11); (7) Direct evidence for an oxidative process occurring in macrophages within 1 h of exposure to MIF is offered by the findings of Poulter and Turk (12) of increased oxidation of SH groups and a corresponding rise in SS groups. The same authors also described an increase in the oxidation of NADPH after 1 h contact of macrophages, with MIF; (8) Two recent reports indicate that macrophages (13) and PMN (14) incubated with lymphokine prepearations demonstrate increased O_2^- production, as assessed by the reduction of nitro-blue tetrazolium; (9) Resident peritoneal macrophages respond poorly to MIF, compared to oil-induced exudate cells (15). This is in good agreement with the increased ability of chemically-elicited peritoneal macrophages to produce O_2^- (16); (10) The stimulated hexose monophosphate shunt activity in macrophages exposed to MIF for 48 - 72 h (17) may be driven by the NADP resulting from the oxidation of NADPH, required for the reduction of O_2 to O_2^-; (11) Elevated prostaglandin production and release was described for MIF-treated (18), PMA-treated (19) and A23187-treated (20) macrophages. This could be the result of stimulated prostaglandin endoperoxide formation, as a side-effect of the respiratory burst (21); (12) A number of agents prevent MIF action but the biochemical mechanisms responsible for the effect are still unknown. These are: epinephrine, norepinephrine, prostaglandins of the E series, cysteine, antiproteases, hydrocortisone (see Ref. 22 for review). We suggest that all these agents act either as antioxidants or by inhibiting the respiratory burst. Epinephrine and norepinephrine scavenge O_2^- radicals (23); E type prostaglandins block macrophage chemiluminescence (24); cysteine could serve as a competitive substrate for oxidants; a number of protease inhibitors and synthetic serine protease substrates inhibit O_2^- formation in PMN (25), and hydrocortisone also inhibits O_2^- release by PMN (21); (13) SH binding reagents were found to impair PMN motility and adhesiveness, possibly by causing a decrease in the level of reduced glutathione, an important cellular buffer against H_2O_2 (26). Cysteine prevented the effect of SH-binding reagents on cell motility.

All these data provide firm support for the idea that MIF exerts its effects on macrophages by inducing the formation of potentially damaging oxidants, affecting the cell membrane and/or cytoplasmic components. The precise nature of the targets and the predominant damaging radical (O_2^-, H_2O_2, OH· or O_2^1) remain to be determined.

Finally, we would like to make the following predictions, all of which can be tested experimentally: a) MIF should not inhibit macrophage motility in the absence of oxygen. Since peritoneal macrophage migration persists under anaerobic conditions (15), this suggestion can be tested; b) MIF-treated macrophages should demonstrate increased production of oxygen reduction products such as O_2^- H_2O_2, OH· or O_2^1, an elevation in the ratio of oxidized/reduced glutathione and evidence of lipid peroxidation; c) The effects of MIF should be prevented by antioxidants, and OH· or O_2^1 scavengers. Inhibition of MIF action can also be expected by inhibiting the H_2O_2 generating enzyme, superoxide dismutase. Inhibition of catalase should enhance MIF effects; d) Macrophages of animals on a vitamin E-deficient diet should be more susceptible to MIF. Cells derived from subjects with a high level of superoxide dismutase should also be more responsive to MIF.

REFERENCES

1. Manheimer, S., and Pick, E. (1973). *Immunology 24*, 1027-1034.
2. Pick, E., Seger, M., Honig, S., and Griffel, B. (1979). *Ann. N.Y. Acad. Sci.* (in press).
3. Johnston, R.B. (1978). *Fed. Proc., Fed. Am. Soc. Exp. Biol. 37*, 2759-2764.
4. Baehner, R.L., Boxer, L.A., Allen, J.M., and Davis, J. (1977). *Blood 50*, 327-335.

5. Boxer, L.A., Allen, J.M., and Baehner, R.L. (1978). *J. Lab. Clin. Med. 92*, 730-736.
6. Nathan, C.F., and Root, R.K. (1977). *J. Exp. Med. 146*, 1648-1662.
7. Weiss, S.J., King, G.W., and LoBuglio, A.F. (1977). *J. Clin. Investig. 60*, 370-373.
8. Nathans, A.H., and Kitabchi, A.E. (1975). *Biochim. Biophys. Acta 399*, 244-253.
9. Pick, E. and Grunspan-Swirsky, A. (1977). *Cell. Immunol. 32*, 340-349.
10. Pick, E., Honig, S., and Griffel, B. (1979). *Int. Arch. Allergy Appl. Immunol. 58*, 149-159.
11. Klebanoff, S.J., and Rosen, H. (1978). *J. Exp. Med. 148*, 490-506.
12. Poulter, L.W., and Turk, J.L. (1975). *Cell. Immunol. 20*, 12-24.
13. Krueger, G.G., Ogden, B.E., and Weston, W.L. (1976). *Clin. Exp. Immunol. 23*, 517-524.
14. Salin, M.L., and McCord, J.M. (1977). *In* "Superoxide and Superoxide Dismutases" (A.M. Michelson, J.M. McCord and T. Fridovich, eds.), pp. 257-270. Academic Press, New York.
15. Pollock, E.M., Pegram, C.N., and Vazquez, J.J. (1971). *J. Reticuloendothel. Soc. 9*, 383-391.
16. Johnston, R.B., Godzik, C.A., and Cohn, Z.A. (1978). *J. Exp. Med. 148*, 115-127.
17. Nathan, C.F., Karnowsky, M.L., and David, J.R. (1971). *J. Exp. Med. 133*, 1356-1376.
18. Morley, J. (1974). *Prostaglandins 8*, 315-326.
19. Brune, K., Glatt, M., Kalin, H., and Peskar, B.A. (1978). *Nature (London) 274*, 261-263.
20. Gemsa, D., Seitz, M., Kramer, W., Grimm, W., Till, G., and Resch, K. (1979). *Exp. Cell Res. 118*, 55-62.
21. Goldstein, I.M., Malmsten, C.L., Kaplan, H.B., Jindahl, H., Samuelsson, B., and Weissmann, G. (1978). *Clin. Res. 26*, 518A (abstr.).
22. Pick, E. (1979). *In* "Biology of the Lymphokines" (S. Cohen, E. Pick, and J.J. Oppenheim, eds.). Academic Press, New York (in press).
23. McCord, J.M., and Fridovich, I. (1969). *J. Biol. Chem.* 244, 6049-6055.
24. Weidemann, M.J., Peskar, B.A., Wrogemann, K., Rietschel, E.T., Staudinger, H., and Fisher, H. (1978). *FEBS Letters 89*, 136-140.
25. Kitagawa, S., Takaku, F. and Sakamoto, S. (1979). *FEBS Letters 99*, 275-278.
26. Giordano, G.F., and Lichtman, M.A. (1973). *J. Cell. Physiol. 82*, 387-395.

DISCUSSION

EPSTEIN: The gene responsible for the action of the enzyme superoxide dismutase (SOD) has been localized to the human chromosome 21. Studies by Feaster and Epstein have demonstrated that the level of SOD is elevated in the polymorphonuclear leukocytes and monocytes of patients with trisomy 21, or Down syndrome. Thus Pick should be able to test his theory concerning MIF action via SOD by using the monocytes or polymorphonuclear leukocytes from patients with Down syndrome as target cells. If his theory is correct, the trisomic cells, containing more SOD, should be more sensitive to the action of MIF, and greater inhibition of migration should be observed, as compared with the migration of normal cells.

OPPENHEIM: If antioxidants interfere with the activity of MIF, one would predict that 2-mercaptoethanol, which is commonly used, and has scavenger activity mediated by its effect in generating reduced glutathione, also would interfere with MIF assays. Perhaps the use of 2-ME explains the difficulty that has been experienced in performing MIF assays with mouse macrophages.

PICK: There is little information on the effect of 2-mercaptoethanol on the biological effect of MIF. de Weck has been using 2-mercaptoethanol as a component of his culture medium for lymphokine production by human cells. It seems that under these conditions 2-mercaptoethanol does not interfere with activity. However, this may be a question of concentration; it is probable that in order to act as an antioxidant, one has to use a high concentration of 2-mercaptoethanol. I would remind you that both Bartfeld and Atoynaran and my colleague Keijari have found that cysteine and acetylcysteine block MIF action and this effect is probably identical to that of 2-mercaptoethanol. Perhaps de Weck could tell us whether the presence of 2-mercaptoethanol during the generation of MIF has any effect on the action of MIF produced in such cultures?

de WECK: I cannot give any meaningful statement on Pick's query for the reason that the population of macrophages used in the test is not pure and the effect of 2-ME could be due to various cellular interactions not limited to macrophages alone.

MAUEL: The following observation might support the hypothesis presented by Pick: mouse macrophages incubated with supernatants from Con A-stimulated lymphocytes tend to undergo degenerative changes after 72-96 hr in culture, which can be easily detected by microscopic observation. With respect to the effect of aminotrioxazole, our results, based on the monitoring of destruction of intracellular parasites by activated macrophages, suggest that this drug *decreases* killing of intracellular microorganisms, thus inhibits the effect of oxydative metabolism. We think that intracellular parasite killing in activated macrophages is mediated by H_2O_2 through endogenous peroxydatic activity. Aminotrioxazole is known to block peroxidase, thus presumably decreasing the toxic effect of H_2O_2.

OSTEOCLAST ACTIVATING FACTOR (OAF) PRODUCTION IS DEPENDENT ON PROSTAGLANDIN SYNTHESIS BY MONOCYTES[1]

Gregory R. Mundy[2]
Toshiyuki Yoneda[3]

Department of Medicine
University of Connecticut Health Center
Farmington, Connecticut

I. PROSTAGLANDIN SYNTHESIS IS NECESSARY FOR OAF PRODUCTION

The lymphokine osteoclast activating factor (OAF) is a powerful mediator of bone resorption (Horton et al., 1972). It is a likely pathogenetic factor in the localized bone destruction which occurs adjacent to collections of chronic inflammatory cells in patients with diseases such as rheumatoid arthritis, periodontal disease and tumor metastases in bone. It is the probable mediator of bone resorption in patients with myeloma (Mundy et al., 1974a) and malignant lymphomas (Mundy et al., 1974b; Mundy et al., 1978). Prostaglandins are also local mediators of bone resorption (Klein and Raisz, 1970; Raisz et al., 1975). As prostaglandins modulate the release of other lymphokines and both of these factors are likely to be produced in similar situations, we examined the effects of prostaglandins on OAF production.

Bone resorption was measured in vitro by the release of ^{45}Ca from fetal mouse long bones in organ culture (Yoneda and Mundy, 1979). Bone resorption was quantitated as the mean

[1]Supported by Grant AM-21584 from the National Institutes of Health and Grant CH-69B from the American Cancer Society.
[2]Recipient of Faculty Research Award FRA-148 from the American Cancer Society.
[3]On leave from the 2nd Department of Oral and Maxillofacial Surgery, Osaka University Dental School.

ISBN 0-12-213950-X

percent release of total ^{45}Ca from 4 individual bones and differences from bones cultured in control media were determined using Student's t-test for nonpaired samples. Human peripheral blood leukocytes comprising 85% lymphocytes and 15% monocytes were stimulated by PHA-M 1% for 24-72 hours. In some cultures drugs which block prostaglandin synthesis by inhibition of the enzyme prostaglandin cyclo-oxygenase were cultured with leukocytes. In these cultures OAF was not detected in the leukocyte culture supernatants (Yoneda and Mundy, 1979). Three inhibitors of prostaglandin synthesis were used--indomethacin, flufenamic acid and RO20-5720. The effects were the same for each inhibitor and were observed at concentrations of 10^{-5} and 10^{-6}M. Partial effects were seen at 10^{-7}M. These drugs inhibited OAF production at 24, 48 and 72 hours of culture, although they had no consistent effect on DNA synthesis as measured by ^{3}H-thymidine incorporation or protein synthesis as measured by ^{3}H-amino acid incorporation.

Since indomethacin, flufenamic acid and RO20-5720 are structurally unrelated inhibitors of prostaglandin synthesis, it is likely that their effects on inhibition of OAF production were secondary to inhibition of prostaglandin synthesis. To confirm this, we added exogenous PGE_1 (10^{-7}M) back to PHA-activated leukocytes cultured with indomethacin (Yoneda and Mundy, 1979). The exogenous prostaglandins had to be removed before assay for bone resorption by diafiltration. We found that exogenous prostaglandins restored OAF production in cultures treated with indomethacin. This data indicates that prostaglandin synthesis is required for OAF production by activated leukocytes.

II. ROLE OF MONOCYTE PROSTAGLANDINS IN OAF PRODUCTION

To determine which cells were responsible for OAF production and which were responsible for prostaglandin synthesis, we separated lymphocytes from monocytes by serial adherence to plastic petri dishes. More than 90% of the adherent cells were phagocytic and showed nonspecific esterase activity. Only the nonadherent cells obtained after three 24 hour periods of culture were used as enriched lymphocytes. When these latter cells were cultured with PHA they incorporated ^{3}H-thymidine but did not release OAF. However, when media harvested from adherent enriched monocytes were added to these activated lymphocytes, the lymphocytes released OAF. The monocyte-conditioned media did not contain OAF. When the monocytes were cultured with indomethacin, the harvested media did not cause the activated lymphocytes to release OAF.

When exogenous PGE_1 or PGE_2 were added to the activated lymphocytes, then OAF release also occurred. These results indicate that the activated lymphocyte is the cell of origin of OAF and the monocyte is the cell which produces prostaglandins. They also indicate that monocyte prostaglandins are necessary for OAF production and that the production of prostaglandins by monocytes may be a means of regulation of OAF production.

III. INCREASES IN CYCLIC AMP ARE REQUIRED FOR OAF PRODUCTION

It is likely that the effects of prostaglandins on OAF' production are mediated by cyclic AMP. When cAMP was measured in activated leukocytes, it was found that a peak in cyclic AMP always precedes OAF production. OAF production by activated leukocytes treated with indomethacin was restored by PGE_1, dibutyryl cyclic AMP, isobutylmethylxanthine (IBMX) and isoproterenol, all of which increase lymphocyte cyclic AMP content through different mechanisms. Similarly OAF release by activated lymphocytes was produced by adding dibutyryl cyclic AMP or IBMX to the cultures as well as PGE_1. This suggests that cyclic AMP accumulation in the lymphocytes is necessary for activated lymphocytes to release OAF and is in contrast to the widely held notion that cyclic AMP is a general inhibitor of immune cell functions (Bourne et al., 1974).

REFERENCES

Bourne, H.R., Lichtenstein, L.M., Melmon, K.L., Henney, C.S., Weinstein, Y., and Shearer, G.M. (1974). Science 184, 19.

Horton, J.E., Raisz, L.G., Simmons, H.A., Oppenheim, J.J., and Mergenhagen, S.E. (1972). Science 177, 793.

Klein, D.C., and Raisz, L.G. (1979). Endocrinol. 86, 1436.

Mundy, G.R., Raisz, L.G., Schecter, G.P., Cooper, R.A., and Salmon, S.E. (1974a). New Engl J Med. 291, 1041.

Mundy, G.R., Luben, R.A., Raisz, L.G., Oppenheim, J.J., and Buell, D.N. (1974b). New Engl J. Med. 290, 867.

Mundy, G.R., Rick, M.E., Turcotte, R., and Kowalski, M.A. (1978). Am. J. Med. 65, 600.

Raisz, L.G., Trummel, C.L., Mundy, G.R., and Luben, R.A. (1975). In "Calcium Regulating Hormones", p. 149. Excerpta Medica, Amsterdam.

Yoneda, T., and Mundy, G.R. (1979). J. Exp. Med. 149, 279.

DISCUSSION

WAKSMAN: We made a closely similar observation in studying the effect of IDS (inhibitor of DNA synthesis, produced by non-specific suppressor T cells) on lymphotoxin production by mitogen-stimulated T cells. IDS raises cyclic AMP in late G1 and arrests the stimulated cells in this phase of the cycle, i.e. prevents them from entering S and later mitosis. Lymphotoxin is produced in G1, and its production is greatly enhanced by IDS and the arrest of the stimulated cells in G1. Did Mundy look at the relation of his findings to the cell cycle?

MUNDY: I thank Waksman for his comments. We have not yet examined the events we described in relation to the cell cycle.

LITTMAN: We have just completed a series of experiments determining the effect of indomethacin on the production of two other monocyte dependent lymphokines, LIF and monocyte-complement stimulator (which stimulates C2 production by human monocytes). Indomethacin at 5 μg/ml did not inhibit the production of either of these lymphokines. Therefore, the effect Mundy has described regarding OAF dependence on monocyte PGE synthesis should not be generalized to other lymphokines.

MUNDY: I agree. There is no reason to believe that the regulatory mechanism for one lymphokine need be the same for all other lymphokines. Indeed there is good evidence that some other lymphokines are inhibited by exogenous prostaglandins. However, before concluding that the lymphokines Littman mentions are not prostaglandin dependent, it would be necessary to show that no prostaglandins were present in his cell cultures before he added indomethacin.

OPPENHEIM: Can Mundy overcome the inhibitory effect of indomethacin on the production of OAF by lymphocytes by adding PGE? This maneuver would presumably stimulate cAMP increases despite the presence of indomethacin.

MUNDY: Yes, we have indeed done the experiment suggested by Oppenheim. OAF production, inhibited by indomethacin, is restored by addition of exogenous prostaglandins of the E series. There is a simultaneous increase in measurable cyclic

AMP in the lymphocytes due to the prostaglandins. Incidentally we have found that indomethacin added to PHA-activated leukocytes inhibits cyclic AMP generation as well as OAF production.

DAVID: Do monocytes have to come from the same individual to help lymphocytes making OAF? Is there a genetic restriction? Did I understand Mundy to say that PGE_1 will substitute for monocytes added to pure lymphocytes?

MUNDY: We have worked only with human cells and both monocytes and lymphocytes have come from the same individual. Not only PGE_1 but other agents which increase lymphocyte cyclic AMP content such as dibutryryl cyclic AMP, IBMX and isoproterenol will substitute for monocytes in the production of OAF by activated lymphocytes.

WEBB: Our studies of a murine suppressor T cell also support the concept of PG induction of lymphokine production. This T cell is activated by PGE_2 to release a suppressor peptide. Thus it is possible to demonstrate both positive and negative effects of prostaglandins on mediator production and/or release.

MERGENHAGEN: Just as one cannot generalize on the influence of prostaglandins and cAMP on production of lymphokines, a parallel situation exists with regard to production of macrophage enzymes and monokines. While prostaglandin synthesis is obligatory for collagenase synthesis by the macrophage, the reverse holds for production of other mediators such as CSF and interferon by macrophages. That is, inhibition of prostaglandin synthesis increases the output by stimulated macrophages of both CSF and interferon. Furthermore, LAF production is not influenced by prostaglandins or elevated levels of cAMP.

OPTIMIZATION OF MIF-PRODUCTION IN HUMAN LYMPHOCYTE CULTURES STIMULATED BY CON A - SEPHAROSE

Udo Schwuléra
Hans H. Sonneborn[1]

BIOTEST-Serum-Institut GmbH
Flughafenstrasse 4
D-6000 Frankfurt - BRD

The production of MIF-active supernatants was carried out by incubating purified, human peripheral blood lymphocytes with insoluble mitogen, Concanavalin A (Con A), in serum free medium. These supernatants were assayed for their ability to inhibit the migration of lymphocytes and macrophages from packed capillary tubes. We investigated the influence of various parameters of the standard protocol (i.e. Con A concentration, incubation period and cell density), in order to obtain the optimal conditions for the release of MIF into the culture supernatant.

The presence of higher concentrations of insoluble Con A led to an increase in free, soluble Con A in the supernatants which nonspecifically inhibited cell migration (Fig. 1).

An increase in the time of incubation produced a higher MIF-activity in the medium, however, viable cell recovery decreased markedly (Fig. 2).

[1]present address: BIOTEST GmbH, Geleitsstrasse 103, D-6050 Offenbach - BRD

ISBN 0-12-213950-X

When the cell density of the cultures was increased, the MIF activity of the supernatant was also enhanced. Again cell viability is the limiting factor and at 3 - 4 x 10^7 cells/ml optimal conditions are reached (Fig. 3).

A combination of these parameters, limited by cell viability, led us to employ the following conditions for optimal MIF production:

2,5 - 3 x 10^7 lymphocytes/ml

20 µg insoluble Con A / ml

45 - 60 hr incubation

2 x 10^{-5} M 2 - mercaptoethanol
in RPMI - 1640 with L-glutamine.

Under these conditions lymphocyte viability is $>$ 80 % following incubation and the MIF activity in the supernatants is markedly increased.

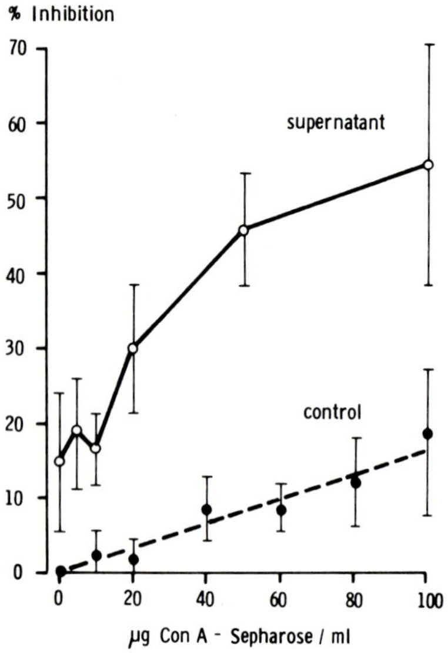

FIGURE 1. Stimulation of human peripheral blood lymphocytes by varying concentrations of Concanavalin A and its influence on MIF production. MIF activity in the supernatants was assayed on human peripheral blood lymphocytes admixed with guinea pig, peritoneal macrophages as indicator cells using the capillary technique.

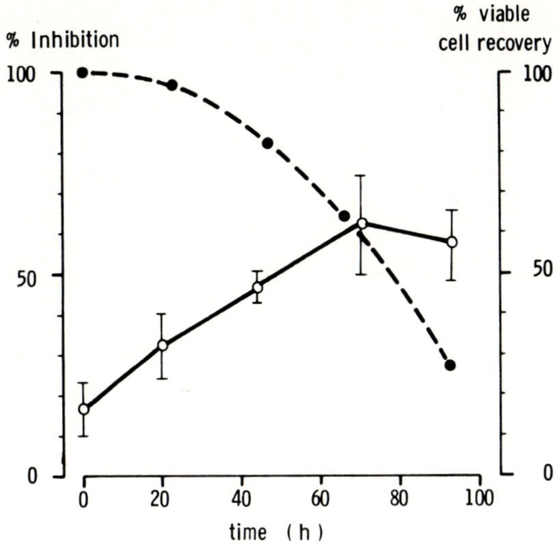

FIGURE 2. Effect of prolonged incubation on MIF production.

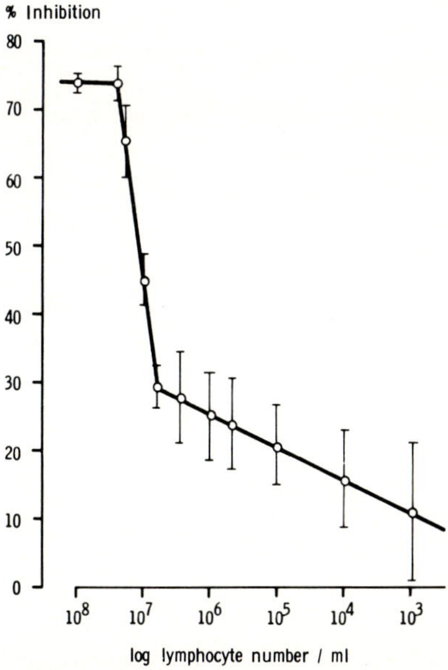

FIGURE 3. MIF activity of supernatants generated by cultures of increasing cell concentration.

PRODUCTION OF COSTIMULATOR AND VARIOUS CYTOKINE ACTIVITIES (CSF,MIF,TRF) IN MOUSE LYMPHOID CELL CULTURES. USE OF A SMALL REACTOR VESSEL

B.Bödeker
J.Lehmann
P.F.Mühlradt

Gesellschaft für Biotechnologische Forschung mbH
Braunschweig

Many groups are investigating the various cytokine activities appearing in cultures of mitogen- or otherwise stimulated lymphoid cells. Conditions for production of these activities vary between different groups and are not always well defined.

We made use of a small reactor vessel in which culture conditions such as pH or partial oxygen pressure (pO_2) could be monitored as well as regulated to study the effects of various parameters on cell survival and the production of several lymphokines in Con A stimulated lymphocyte cultures. Our interest focussed on the costimulator activity (1).

Methods. The reactor vessel consists of a glass dish,i.d. 10 cm, height 3.5 cm, carrying a stainless steel cover equipped with inlets and outlets for gases, pH and pO_2 electrodes, a hanging magnetic stirrer, and a rubber septum for aseptically taking or introducing samples. Splenocytes from CBA/J mice were cultivated at pH 7.3 in 250 ml of serum-free RPMI 1640 at a concentration of 1×10^7 cells/ml in the presence of 1μg Con A/ml.Costimulator (CS) activity was tested by thymidine incorporation in thymocytes at a concentration of 5×10^5 cells/well in microtiter plates. Cultivation was done in RPMI with 5% NCS. Con A (6 μg/ml) and CS were present from the beginning, 1μCi ^{3}H-thymidine (final concentration 5 μM) was added 6 h before harvesting at 72 h. TRF was tested by A. Schimpl (2), CSF was tested by H. Laukel (3), MIF by H. Sorg (4) as described.

Results and Discussion. A study of the influence of pO_2 and speed of stirring at constant pH and constant cell concentration on the liberation of several cytokine activities is

ISBN 0-12-213950-X

summarized in Table 1. The pO_2 drops very sharply as soon as the cells are added to the reactor and stays low unless the culture is stirred. pO2 can be regulated by the speed of stirring, the composition and the flow rate of the gas mixture with which the medium is equilibrated. The latter was kept constant in these experiments.

TABLE 1. Influence of pO2 and Stirring on the Production of Cytokine Activity in the Bioreactor

Exp.	pO_2 1[a]	pO_2 2[b]	stirring speed	cell survival	cytokine activity CS[c]	MIF[d]	TRF[e]	CSF[f]
	(Torr)		(RPM)	(%)	(% of maximal act.)			
1	151	77	30	24	100	0	30	55
2	151	22	--	41	83	30	45	35
3	56	13	30	48	43	100	100	70
4	48	19	150	44	80	0	15	100

Samples were taken after 26 h. [a] pO_2 at the beginning, [b] 6 h later. 100 % activity corresponds to:

[c] 150 µl SN giving 23500 cpm/culture (control 100 cpm)
[d] 400 µl SN yielding 3500 PFC (control 25)
[e] 1:6 diluted SN inducing >40% inhibition
[f] 1:1 diluted SN giving rise to 40 colonies

There was an inverse relationship between cell survival and pO2 , high oxygen content being cytotoxic. The influence of pO2 on cytokine production is more complex. The production of MIF and TRF is favored by anaerobic conditions. Liberation of CSF is beneficially influenced by stirring while pO2 has no pronounced influence. CS liberation is not influenced by stirring *per se* but is limited by oxygen supply. Thus, anaerobic conditions such as are prevalent at the bottom of petri dish cultures lead to slow liberation and low yields of CS (see Fig. 1). The results show that the activities of individual cytokines which are all produced in mitogen-stimulated spleen cell cultures can vary with seemingly trivial changes of the culture conditions, and that it is possible to select conditions favorable for the formation of each particular cytokine.

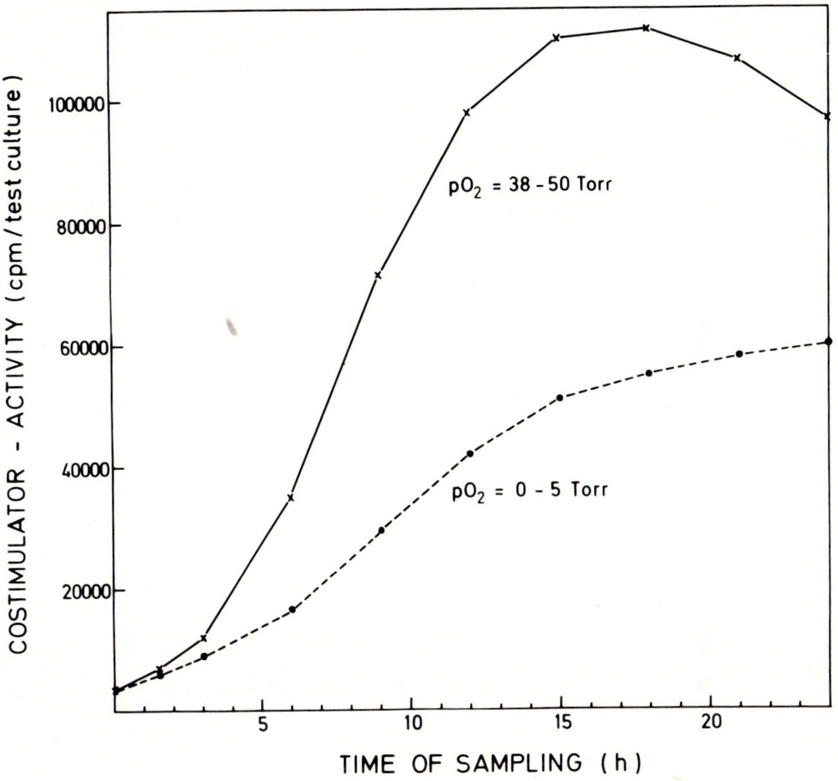

Fig. 1. Kinetics of release of CS activity at low and high pO_2

References

1. Paetkau, V., Mills, G., Gerhart, S., and Monticone, V. *J. Immunol. 117, 1320 (1976)*
2. Müller, G., Hübner, L., Schimpl, A., and Wecker, E. *Immunochemistry 15, 27 (1978)*
3. Bradley, T.R., and Metcalf, D., *Austr. J. Exp. Biol. and Med. Scie. 44, 287 (1966)*
4. Neumann, Ch., and Sorg, C., *Eur. J. Immunol. 8, 582 (1978)*

MACROPHAGE ACTIVATING FACTOR (MAF) INDUCED MACROPHAGE CYTOTOXICITY: SIMILARITIES IN MAN AND GUINEA PIG

W. Hallowell Churchill
Deborah Cameron

Department of Medicine
Harvard Medical School
Peter B. Brigham Hospital
Robert B. Brigham Hospital
Boston, Massachusetts

In vivo evidence suggesting that macrophages influencing tumor growth come from several sources. First, animals treated with adjuvants such as BCG are more resistant to tumor growth (1). Macrophages from these animals kill the tumor cells in vitro (2). Second, morphologic studies have shown that there is a correlation between the number of macrophages and the tumors tendency to metastasize or regress (3,4). Moreover, macrophages found at the site of tumor rejection have the morphologic findings on light and electron microscopic study of activated macrophages (5). Third, macrophages teased from these tumors and then tested for their capacity to kill the same tumors in vitro are effective killer cells (6). In attempting to answer how macrophages acquire enhanced resistance to tumors in vivo, we and others have used in vitro systems to show that lymphocytes release a factor, macrophage activating factor (MAF), which modifies many macrophage functions among which is enhancement of cytotoxicity for tumor cells (7-10).

In our previous studies with the guinea pig hepatoma system, we have shown that guinea pig MAF and another mediator guinea pig migration inhibitory factor (MIF) share many properties. These two mediators have not yet been separated by fractionation procedures. Removal of cell surface fucose or sialic acid renders macrophages unresponsive to these mediators (11,12). Finally, cell surface proteinases modify macrophage responsiveness to both mediators (13-15).

ISBN 0-12-213950-X

More recently we have developed a method which, for the first time, permits the study of MAF induced macrophage cytotoxicity in man and find that human MAF is similar to guinea pig MAF both in the physical properties and in the mechanism of interaction with macrophages.

Our assay for MAF induced cytotoxic macrophages has been described in detail (16). Briefly, Ficoll-Hypaque mononuclear cells are plated in microtiter wells, washed after one hour, and allowed to incubate for 5 days during which time they acquire the capacity to respond to MAF. At the end of the 5 day incubation, the macrophage monolayers are washed and antigen induced MAF is added for 24 hours. The macrophages are then washed to remove the mediator and tritiated target cells are added for a period of 24 hr co-cultivation. Cytotoxicity is then determined by measuring the tumor cells remaining after incubation with macrophages. This method has been shown to be a valid measure of cellular cytotoxicity. The results from experiment to experiment are compared at a standard attacker:ratio of 20:1. Maximum cytotoxicity is induced after 24 hr incubation with MAF. The target cells used for these studies include several long-term malignant cell lines and also cultures of normal cells.

Studies of the specificity of mediator induced cytotoxic macrophages have yielded results which are in agreement with results of similar studies in other species (17,18,19). In our initial studies, the effect of cytotoxic macrophages on six malignant targets and five normal targets were determined. These results, shown in Table I, indicate that the normal targets are resistant to the effects of cytotoxic macrophages, whereas the activated macrophages were cytotoxic to five of the six tumor targets (16).

These studies were subsequently extended to targets originating from the same genetic pool. Pairs of osteosarcoma and fibroblast lines from 5 patients were supplied to us by Dr. Steve Rosenberg. These 5 pairs of malignant and normal target cells were then tested for susceptibility to mediator induced cytotoxic macrophages. In two of the matched pairs, the malignant target was killed, whereas the normal target was resistant to the effect of macrophages. In two other pairs, both the malignant and normal targets were resistant and in the remaining pair both malignant and normal targets were sensitive to the effects of activated macrophages.

These results indicate that some but not all of the pairs of malignant and normal targets showed a pattern of susceptibility similar to that described in other systems with the normal targets being resistant and the malignant targets susceptible to the effects of activated macrophages.

TABLE I. *Effect of in Vitro Activated Macrophages on Malignant and Normal Target Cells*

	Percent cytotoxicity										
	Malignant target cells						Nonmalignant target cells				
Exp #	SK-BR-3	HT-29	Caki-1	Calu-1	SK-Mes-1	MA-160	WI-38	MRC-5	M-7	MA-112	MA-349
1	35	33	23	-	25	-	-	-	-	-	-
2	48	-	30[a]	-	-4	-	-	-	-	-	-
3	16	-	5[b]	-	13	-	-	-	-	-	-
4	-	26	18	-	-22	-	-	-	-	-	-
5	13	-20	6[b]	-	23	33	-	-	-	-	-
6	-	32	5[b]	4[b]	11	50	-	-	-	-	-
7	-	-	-	13[a]	-	16	-	-	-	-	-
8	-	-	-	6[b]	13	21	-	-	-	-	-
9	30[a]	-	-	-	-	-	-8[b]	-	-	-	-
10	23	-	-	-	-	-	-5[b]	-	-	-	-
11	28	-	-	-	-	-	0[b]	-	-	-	-
12	13	-	-	-	-		0[b]	-	-	-	-
13	-	-	-	-	-		-	-7[b]	4[b]	0[b]	0[b]
14	-	-	-	-	-		-	-8[b]	-12[b]	2[b]	5[b]

All results significant at $p < 0.05$ except as noted.

[a] $P \leq 0.10$

[b] Not significant.

Data from Cameron and Churchill (16).

In order to better understand the variation from target to target of sensitivity to activated macrophages, two other variables were examined. Keller has previously reported that target cell growth rates can be related to sensitivity to cytotoxic macrophages (20). In our studies, however, we were unable to make any such correlation between growth rate and susceptibility. Indeed, in the case of the two matched pairs studied, the doubling time of the resistant fibroblasts and the sensitive tumors were identical. This finding confirms our previous studies with allogeneic malignant and normal target cells (16).

Malignant cell membranes differ in many respects from normal cell membranes. These differences include increased Con A receptors (21,22), increased surface sialic acid (23), decreased fibronectin (24) and changes in glycosyl transferases (25). It is possible that some of these differences might permit preferential adherence of activated macrophages to malignant targets rather than to normal targets. Because an increase in surface sialic acid is one of the more consistent differences between malignant and normal cell membranes, we compared the sialic acid content of resistant and sensitive targets using the method described by Warren (26). Among the matched pairs the sensitive tumor targets had about twice as much sialic acid as the resistant targets did. Of special interest was the finding that one of the resistant tumors had a sialic acid content in the range of that found on resistant normal targets. The only exception was that the fibroblast target, which was killed by the macrophages, had a sialic acid content in the lower range of that found with other resistant normal targets. These preliminary findings suggest that sialic acid content may correlate with susceptibility to macrophage cytotoxicity, but further studies will be required to settle this issue.

Guinea pig macrophages acquire enhanced responsiveness to MAF after treatment with either the cell surface reactant diazotized sulfanilic acid or with an inhibitor of surface proteinases such as antithrombin III (15). We therefore carried out experiments to determine if the response of human macrophages to human MAF might be regulated by a similar mechanism. Monocyte derived macrophages were pretreated with either 50 to 100 μg/ml of AT III or of soybean trypsin inhibitor after which the macrophages were tested for responsiveness to MAF. Similar experiments were carried out after pretreatment with 10^{-3} 10^{-4}M DSA. The response of macrophages to subthreshold amounts of MAF was consistently enhanced by these treatments. After soybean trypsin inhibitor, treatment, the extent of kill was increased up to three times the cytotoxicity of macrophages exposed only to the subthreshold amounts of MAF. A similar enhancement was seen after AT III or DSA treatment.

The mechanism of this enhancement is not yet defined. However, it is known that macrophage surface proteinases destroy guinea pig MIF (27). We, therefore, have examined the possibility that differences in inactivation of MAF by treated or control macrophages could account for the observed enhanced response to MAF. Aliquots of MAF were exposed to either treated or normal macrophages for 1 hr at 37°C. After this incubation, the cells were removed by centrifugation and the MAF tested for activity on normal macrophages. In these experiments MAF activity was depleted to a much greater extent by normal macrophages than it was by incubation with macrophages pretreated with DSA or AT III. These results are consistent with the view that decreased inactivation of MAF by the treated macrophages might account for the enhanced response to MAF because the dose of MAF is known to be related to the extent of cytotoxicity induced. Thus, it would appear that the mechanisms regulating the effect of MAF at the cell surface, are very similar to what has been previously described for guinea pig MIF.

Our preliminary studies of the physical properties of human MAF indicate that it is also similar to human MIF in terms of size and distribution of activity after isoelectric focussing. Weiser *et al.* have fractionated MIF by isoelectric focussing using techniques similar to those described by Remold *et al.* (28). The MIF was prepared from Con A stimulated human lymphocytes. The fractions were then tested both for MIF and MAF activity. After isoelectric focussing, the activity of both mediators appears to be distributed in parallel fashion with maximum activity in two peaks. Further studies are required to settle whether these two peaks of activity are analogous in properties to pH 3 and pH 5 MIF described for guinea pig MIF by Remold *et al.* (28). In our own previous studies with guinea pig MIF, we have demonstrated that MAF activity exists in both the pH 3, pH 5 MIF fractions (Churchill and Remold, unpublished observations) so this preliminary evidence in man indicates that an analogous situation may well exist. Further kinetic studies and physical characterization of human MAF are needed to determine what properties human MAF shares with human MIF.

Thus, it would appear from the initial studies of human MAF, that it is similar in many respects to guinea pig MAF. Fractionation procedures have not yet separated MAF from MIF in either species. The specificity of the MAF induced macrophages is similar for both. Finally, the response of guinea pig and human MAF appears to be regulated by similar mechanisms on the macrophage cell surface. Hopefully, further study of the MAF macrophage interaction in man will elucidate the role of cytotoxic macrophages in health and in disease.

REFERENCES

1. Old, L. J., Clarke, D. A., and Benacerraf, B., *Nature 184*, 291 (1959).
2. Hibbs, J. R., Jr., Lambert, L. H., Jr., and Remington, J. S., *Proc. Soc. Exp. Biol. Med. 139*, 1049 (1972).
3. Evans, R., *In* "The Macrophage in Neoplasia" (M.A. Fink, ed) p. 27, Academic Press, New York (1976).
4. Russell, S. W., Doe, W. F., and Cochrane, C. G., *J. Immunol. 116*, 164 (1976).
5. Dvorak, H. F., Dvorak, A. M., and Churchill, W. H., Jr., *J. Exp. Med. 137*, 751 (1973).
6. Van Loveren, H., and den Otter, W., *J. Nat. Cancer Inst. 53*, 1057 (1974).
7. Piessens, W. F., Churchill, W. H., and David, J. R., *J. Immunol. 114*, 293 (1975).
8. Churchill, W. H., Piessens, W. F., Sulis, C. A., and David, J. R., *J. Immunol. 115*, 781 (1975).
9. Rucco, L. P., and Meltzer, M. S., *J. Immunol. 119*, 889, (1977).
10. Fidler, I. J., *J. Natl. Cancer Inst. 55*, 1159 (1975).
11. Churchill, W.H., and Wong, C., submitted for publication.
12. Liu, D. Y., Higgins, T. J., Petschek, K. D., Remold, H. G., and David, J. R., *Fed. Proc. 37*, 1400 (1978).
13. Remold, H. G., and Rosenberg, R. D., *J. Biol. Chem. 250*, 6608 (1975).
14. Remold, H. G., *J. Immunol. 118*, 1 (1977).
15. Piessens, W. F., Remold, H. G., and David, J. R., *J. Immunol. 118*, 2078 (1977).
16. Cameron, D. J., and Churchill, W. H., *J. Clin. Investigation 83*, 977 (1979).
17. Piessens, W. F., Churchill, W. H., and David, J. R., *J. Immunol. 114*, 293 (1975).
18. Cleveland, R. P., Meltzer, M. S., and Zbar, M., *J. Nat. Canc. Inst. 52*, 1887 (1974).
19. Meltzer, M. S., Tucker, R. W., Sanford, K. K., and Leonard, E. J., *J. Nat. Cancer Inst. 54*, 1177 (1975).
20. Keller, R., *J. Natl. Cancer Inst. 56*, 369 (1976).

21. Aub, J. C., Sanford, B. H., and Wang, Li-Hsia, *Proc. Nat. Acad. Sci. 54*, 400 (1965).
22. Burger, M. M., *Fed. Proc. 32*, 91 (1973).
23. Beek, W. P. van, Smets, L. A., and Emmelot P., *Cancer Res. 33*, 2913 (1973).
24. Beek, W. P. van, Emmelot, P., and Homburg, C., *Br. J. Cancer 36*, 157 (1977).
25. Buck, C. A., Glick, M. C., and Warren, L., *Biochemistry 9*, 4567 (1970).
26. Warren, L., *J. Biol. Chem. 234*, 1971 (1959).
27. Remold, H. G., and Mednis, A. D., *J. Immunol. 122*, 1920 (1979).
28. Remold, H. G., and Mednis, A. D., *J. Immunol. 118*, 2015 (1977).

CHARACTERISTICS OF HUMAN MACROPHAGE ACTIVATION FACTOR[1]

Mildred C. McDaniel

College of Medicine
East Tennessee State University
Johnson City, Tennessee

This preliminary report characterizes the lymphokine, macrophage activation factor(s) (MAF) as to molecular weights and aggregation. MAF is defined by a bioassay based on the cytotoxicity of mouse macrophages toward a syngeneic tumor line. The source of MAF is the supernatant from a human Burkitt's lymphoma cell line, Namalwa, which produces MAF as a constitutive product.

I. EXPERIMENTAL

A. Cytotoxic Assay (MAF)

C57Bl/6 mice are used as the source of peritoneal exudate cells. The B16 melanoma line, F10, was provided by Dr. I.J. Fidler, Frederick Cancer Research Center. The macroassay of Fidler[2] has been adapted to a microassay. C57Bl/6 mice are injected intraperitoneally with 2 ml of thioglycollate five days before the harvest of the peritoneal exudate cells. The cells are plated in 96 well plates at a concentration of 50,000 cells/well in 0.1 ml of RPMI 1640-10% FCS. After 30 minutes incubation at 37°C the media and nonadherent cells are removed and 0.1 ml of medium is added back. MAF containing fractions in 0.1 ml volumes are added to the wells and

[1]*This research was supported by NCI Contract NO1-CO-75380 and VA 2A (74) III-43-0100-02*

[2]*Norbury, K., and Fidler, I, (1975) J. Immun. Methods, 7, 109.*

ISBN 0-12-213950-X

the plates are incubated 48 hours. All fractions are assayed in quadruplicate at each dilution.

F10 cells are labelled with ^{125}I-iododeoxyuridine (IUdr) overnight. The tumor cells are washed twice and harvested with trypsin. The medium is removed from the macrophages and the F10 cells in 0.1 ml medium are added at a concentration of 5,000 cells/well (10:1 ratio of macrophages to tumor cells). After one day in culture all media and nonadherent tumor cells are removed and replaced with new medium. Medium is replaced on the third day also. After five days incubation, the cultures are washed with saline twice and lysed with 0.1N NaOH. The residual ^{125}I-IUdr is determined on a gamma counter. % Cytotoxicity is determined by:

$$\% \text{ Cytotoxicity} = \left[1 - \frac{\text{cpm target cells with activated macrophages}}{\text{cpm target cells with normal macrophages}} \right] \times 100$$

B. Chromatography

Supernatant from cells is harvested, desalted on a Sephadex G25 column and lyophilized. The lyophilized powder is stored at -20°C or -70°C. A column of Sepharose 6B-Cl equilibrated with 6M guanidine-HCl pH 8.0 solvent is loaded with 20-50 mg protein from lyophilized cell supernatant dissolved in 1 ml of guanidine without reduction or alkylation the day before the column is run. Fractions are collected and the protein concentration is determined by absorbance readings at 235 nm. Every three or four fractions are pooled and dialyzed twice against water and a third time against normal saline. The fractions are collected, filtered through a 0.2 μ filter and assayed immediately and/or stored at -20°C.

II. RESULTS

Namalwa grown in 2% FCS produces MAF activity in three molecular weight ranges: 70-90,000, 25-40,000 and 12,500 and below. Virtually the same ranges of MAF activities were found in trypsin digests of Namalwa cell surfaces grown in 2% FCS. When the cells are incubated in 10% FCS, activity is only recovered at molecular weights of 12,500 and below *(TABLE I)*. FCS alone has no MAF activity throughout the continuum of column fractions. To compare the MAF produced by a lymphoma cell line with human lymphocytes, supernatants from tonsil

TABLE I. MAF Fractions from Guanidine Chromatography

	Incubation conditions	Molecular weight	Cytotoxicity ± 95% confidence limits
Namalwa[a]	10% FCS, 24 hours	12,500 to <10,000	33 ± 9% 47 ± 13%
Namalwa[a]	2% FCS, 24 hours	70,000 ± 7,000 25,000 ± 2,500 12,500 ± 1,250 <10,000	12 ± 2% 32 ± 14% 25 ± 5% 26 ± 10%
Namalwa[a]	2% FCS, 24 hours trypsin[b] treated	85,000 ± 8,500 to 75,000 ± 7,500 23,000 ± 2,300 <10,000	22 ± 4% 20 ± 6% 17 ± 3% 25 ± 15%

[a] $2X10^6$ cells/ml in RPMI 1640 at 37°C.
[b] Washed cells treated with 0.05% trypsin for 5 min at 37°C.

lymphocytes incubated in zero FCS for 48 hours had MAF activity in the void volume peak (greater than 100,000 daltons) and a single additional MAF fraction below 10,000.

From cells grown in 10% FCS the low M.W. region containing MAF (12,000 and below) was dialyzed and concentrated then divided: one sample (control) was stored at -20°C; the second sample was incubated in 6M guanidine-HCl at 37°C for 24 hours, and the third was placed in 10% FCS for 24 hours at 37°C, then in 6M guanidine-HCl. Samples 2 and 3 were chromatographed on a guanidine column and fractions assayed for MAF along with the control. Sample 2 displayed MAF activity only in the void volume and at 70,000 daltons, while sample 3 had MAF activity from 70,000 to ca. 10,000 daltons. In addition when Namalwa cells in 2% FCS were treated with levamisole and Sepharose ConA, MAF activity was restricted to 45,000 and 90,000 daltons but when this supernatant was heated at 37°C overnight in 6M guanidine-HCl, all activity appeared at 90,000.

Human MAF appears to be a monomer of less than 10,000 M.W. which associates at 37°C to larger aggregates of ca. 12,000 - 25,000, 70,000 - 90,000, and greater. The monomer appears to be stabilized by higher concentrations of FCS and should have only a transient existence in zero FCS.

MACROPHAGE CYTOTOXICITY FACTOR PURIFICATION AND SEPARATION FROM MIF

Eva Maria Kniep
Botho Kickhöfen
Herbert Fischer

Max-Planck-Institut für Immunbiologie
Freiburg, FRG

I. PREPARATION

Mouse spleen cells (10^7/ml) are stimulated with 2 ug/ml ConA. After 24 hours the MCF-containing supernatant is collected.

II. PURIFICATION PROCEDURES

MCF can be adsorbed onto the anion exchanger QAE-Sephadex at pH 8 and eluted with a salt gradient. It can further be adsorbed onto the cation exchanger SE-Sephadex at pH 4. Elution is achieved with high salt concentrations at pH 7.5. Other possibilities to obtain a partial purification are binding to hydroxyapatite (elution with 0.5 M phosphate) and to Blue-Sepharose (elution with high salt concentrations).
The drawback of all these procedures is the necessity to concentrate and desalt the crude supernatant prior to its application; both steps lead to a considerable loss of activity. Attempts to perform two of these purification steps consecutively inevitably led to a loss of 90-99% of activitiy. Therefore we looked for a material which would adsorb MCF in the presence of salt and the other components of Eagle's medium. Such materials are phenylalanine-Sepharose and phenyl-Sepharose.

ISBN 0-12-213950-X

III. COMBINED PURIFICATION STEPS

A. Salt-Mediated Hydrophobic Chromatography on Phenylalanine-Sepharose

Solid ammonium sulfate is added to the MCF-containing supernatant to yield a concentration of 2 M. The solution is passed over a column of phenylalanine-Sepharose. Ten ml phenylalanine-Sepharose are sufficient to adsorb the activity out of 1 l supernatant. Elution is performed stepwise with decreasing ionic strength. MCF activity is eluted with buffer containing 1 M ammonium sulfate. A 5-fold purification is achieved with this step; in addition, the solution is concentrated 20-fold (Fig. 1).

B. Salt-Mediated Hydrophobic Chromatography on Phenyl-Sepharose

The active fraction eluted from phenylalanine-Sepharose is applied directly on a phenyl-Sepharose column. Activity is eluted at pH 10.5 with the aid of ethylene glycol. With this step, a further 5-fold purification and a 3-fold concentration is obtained (Fig. 2).

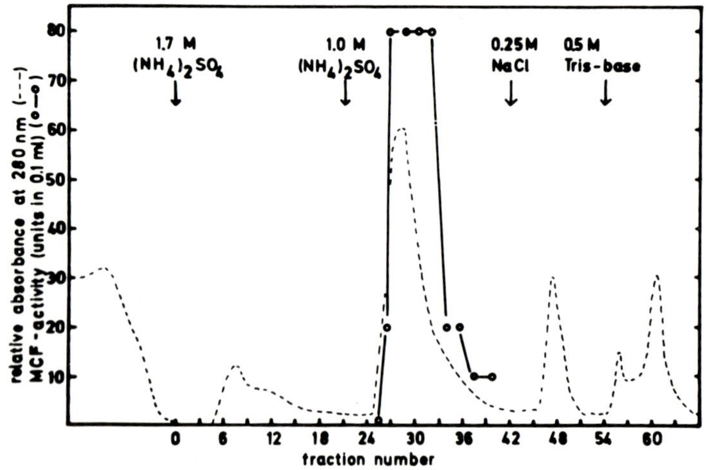

FIGURE 1. Chromatography on phenylalanine-Sepharose. Ammonium sulfate (880 g) was dissolved in 2750 ml supernatant and the solution passed over a column (1.5 x 24 cm) of phenylalanine-Sepharose equilibrated with 0.04 M Tris acetate buffer, pH 7.6, containing 2 M ammonium sulfate. Elution was performed with the indicated salt concentrations in the same buffer. Remaining proteins were washed off with 0.5 M Tris, pH 10.5 plus 10% ethylene glycol.

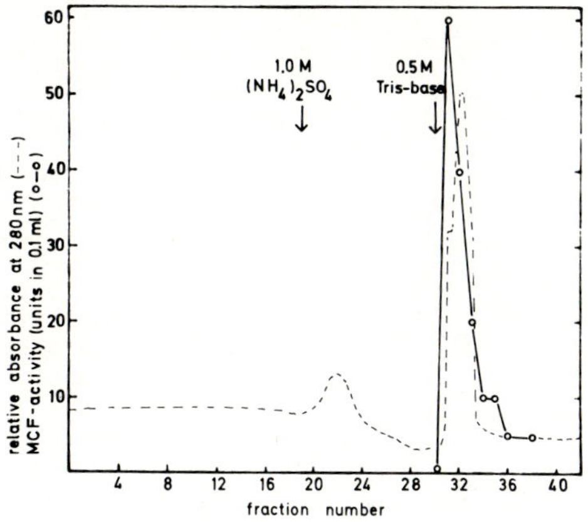

FIGURE 2. Chromatography on phenyl-Sepharose. The active fraction (see Fig. 1) was passed over 10 ml phenyl-Sepharose (syringe) equilibrated with the buffer described in the legend to Fig. 1 containing 1 M ammonium sulfate. Activity was eluted with 0.5 M Tris plus 10% ethylene glycol.

C. Gel Filtration on Ultrogel AcA44

The MCF-containing material purified by two hydrophobic chromatographies is concentrated to 10 ml by ultrafiltration and passed over an Ultrogel AcA44 column. The active peak corresponds to a molecular weight of 20 000 - 30 000 (Fig. 3). This is in contrast to the molecular weight of 45 000 which was estimated from Sephadex G-100 chromatography (data not shown). Possibly, the factor is retained through unspecific adsorption to the gel material. With the combination of purification methods described here, the loss of activity is minimized by avoiding dialysis between the single steps and limiting ultrafiltration to one 5-fold concentration step (Table 1).

TABLE 1. Purification of MCF

Purification step	Volume (ml)	Activity (units)	Protein (mg)	Recovery (%)
Supernatant	2750	55 000	182	100
Phenylalanine-Sepharose	160	53 000	35	96
Phenyl-Sepharose	56	11 200	7	20
Ultrogel	70	16 000	1	30

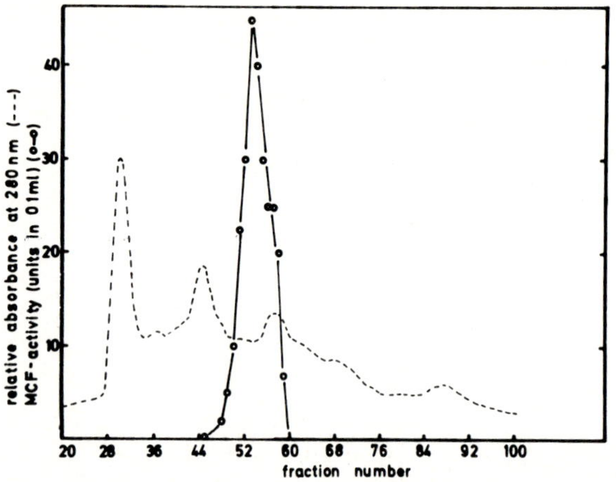

FIGURE 3. Gel filtration on Ultrogel AcA44. The active fraction (see Fig. 2) was concentrated to 10 ml using Amicon PM10 membranes and applied to a 2 x 150 cm Ultrogel AcA44 column in 0.1 M Tris acetate buffer, pH 7.0 plus 1 M NaCl. Flow rate: 5 drops per minute. Marker: BSA: fr. 36; Ovalbumin: fr. 44; Chymotrypsinogen A: fr. 52; Myoglobin: fr. 63.

IV. PROPERTIES

A. Heat Inactivation

Partially purified MCF looses half of its activity when heated at 50°C for 30 minutes, whereas the crude supernatant is more stable. Half of its activity is lost by heating at 60°C for 1 hour.

B. pH-Stability

MCF is fully stable in a pH range between 5.5 and 11.

C. Glycoprotein Nature of MCF

All attempts to adsorb MCF onto Con A-Sepharose resulted in a partial adsorption of 25 - 50% of activity which could be eluted with 0.1 M α-D-methylmannoside. Rechromatography of the unadsorbed material led to the same distribution of activity. Thus, adsorption seems to be a rather unspecific effect. Spleen cells stimulated with Con A in the presence of 1 mM 2-desoxy-D-glucose which inhibits the glycosilation of proteins produce normal amounts of MCF activity. Therefore, if MCF is a glycoprotein, the sugar part is not essential for its activity.

D. Isoelectric Focusing

Preparative isoelectric focusing was performed in flat bed gels. In the absence of urea, activity was found to be widely distributed between pH 4.5 and 7.5. Isoelectric focusing in the presence of 8 M urea, however, results in two sharp peaks of activity at pH 7.6 and 8.6 (Fig. 4).

V. SEPARATION FROM MIF

Migration Inhibition Factor (MIF) which also acts on macrophages was sometimes proclaimed to be the same protein as MCF because these two activities could so far not be separated. After isoelectric focusing in the presence of 8 M urea, however, MIF is found at about pH 4.5 with a minor activity at pH 6.0 (Fig. 4). Thus, MCF and MIF can be clearly separated.

Chromatography on Ultrogel AcA44 has proved to be a second means for the separation of MCF from MIF activity. Whereas MCF is retarded by the gel material, MIF is found in a peak corresponding to its molecular weight of 45 000 (data not shown).

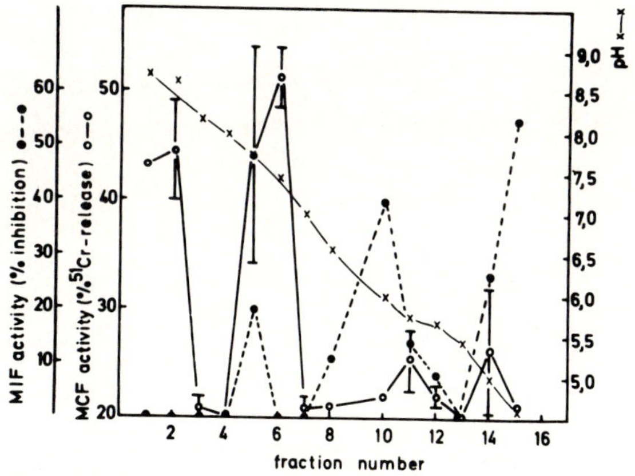

FIGURE 4. Isoelectric focusing of the partially purified MCF and MIF-containing sample.A 10-ml sample was supplemented with 0.25 ml of each Servalyte pH 4-6 and 6-8 and 3.6 g urea and applied half way to the anode on an Ultraphor chamber. Gel bed: 5 g Pheragel in 70 ml H_2O with 5.5 M urea and 2.5 ml Servalyte as above. After partial drying, the urea concentration was about 8 M.
Electrophoresis: 7 h, 8 W, max. 1200 V. Fifteen fractions were collected, washed by centrifugation in syringes equipped with a porous sheet and dialyzed against Eagle's medium prior to testing.

DISCUSSION

1. Purification Procedures

PICK: Would McDaniel explain the reason behind her use of levamisole to stimulate MAF production in Namalwa cells? Why does she believe that the molecular weight of levamisole-induced MAF is different? Is this difference in any way related to the different molecular weight pattern described by David for supernatants of 24-48 hr cultures as compared to 0-24 hr cultures?

McDANIEL: Whitcomb reported that human peripheral lymphocytes increase protein production and MIF production when stimulated with both Con A and levamisole. At the Frederick Cancer Research Center Fidler and I sought to increase MAF production by Namalwa cells (a B cell line) so we added Sepharose-Con A and levamisole. MAF produced in 24 hr had molecular weights of 45,000 and 90,000 and in 48 hr manifested a molecular weight of 90,000 only. I do not know why this difference in molecular weight appeared consequent to the addition of Sepharose-Con A and levamisole. One change I did observe is a reduction in protein synthesis by stimulated Namalwa cells. The heterogeneity of human MAF that David finds in 48 hr supernatants may be due to the same association phenomena I encountered in Namalwa MAF on heating at 37°C. As the incubation period is increased, larger molecular forms of MAF appear in the supernatant. This can occur also in 6 M guanidine, thus ruling out hydrophilic or hydrophobic interactions. Therefore I feel that human MAF polymerizes by some enzymatic reaction on the cell surface or by active sulfhydryl groups on the "monomer" of human MAF.

PICK: I would appreciate Kniep giving us more detail on the methodics used in purifying mouse MCF, particularly the reasoning behind the use of phenyl-sepharose and blue sepharose. Do others have experience in the use of phenyl-sepharose for lymphokine purification?

KNIEP: The advantage of hydrophobic chromatography is that supernatants can be applied directly without prior desalting or concentration. Blue sepharose does not have this advantage and therefore I do not use it anymore.

DAVID: Heinz Remold has successfully used phenyl-sepharose to isolate guinea pig MIF.

ISBN 0-12-213950-X

SCHIMPL: Phenyl-sepharose has been used to bind several lymphokines contained in murine Con A-induced supernates (in 2M $(NH_4)_2SO_4$). Colony stimulating factor (Havemann, Marburg) can be eluted by 0,6 M $(NH_4)_2SO_4$/24 mM Tris- acetate while TRF, MCF and MIF are eluted by 0,25 M Tris-base, 35% ethylene glycol.

WIETZERBIN: Immune interferon type II binds very well to phenyl-sepharose and blue sepharose. Phenyl-sepharose retains interferon (type II) under physiological conditions (PBS). We can recover IF activity with a specific activity of 10^4 U/mg from phenyl-sepharose and with a specific activity of 10^5 U/mg from blue sepharose.

2. *Identity of MAF/MCF with other Lymphokines*

MELTZER: Is there really evidence that some supernatants manifest MAF activity without parallel MIF activity?

ROCKLIN: There is evidence that human MIF and MAF are similar based on the use of human monocytes as indicator cells. David and I showed that human lymphokines generated by SK-SD and filtered over Sephadex G 100 columns contained a fraction (MW 25,000) which possessed both MIF activity and a principle that caused enhanced cell adherence and glucose oxidation through the HMPS pathway by human monocytes.

de WECK: The fact that the MCF activity (induction of cytotoxicity in mouse macrophages) does not always correlate with MIF activity in human cell lines can be taken to indicate that the two activities are different.

SORG: We too have tested the supernatants of the same lymphoblastoid lines for MIF. We found some deviations from results of de Weck's group. However, I would not be inclined to take this as evidence for *or* against MIF and MAF being identical.

PICK: Would it then be appropriate to conclude that MIF can *not* be dissociated from monophage cytotoxicity factor (MCF) and macrophage activation factor (MAF).

KNIEP: In our hands MCF and MIF *could* be separated by two methods: (1) Isoelectric focussing in the presence of 8 M urea (2) Gel filtration on Ultrogel.

HADDEN: In the guinea pig system we have observed that MAF induction of bactericidal capacity for Listeria monocytogenes *can* be dissociated from MIF by vacuum dialysis prior to Sephadex chromatography or isoelectric focussing. In Sephadex column fractions of MW 40-70,000 and isoelectric focussing fractions of pH 3.5-4.5 and 8.0 we found MAF activity. In these fractions, MIF activity was negligible at a 1x concentration relative to starting supernatant while MAF activity was expressed as low as a further 1:10 dilution. Tentatively these data suggest that MAF can be dissociated from MIF activity.

LOHMANN-MATTHES: Murine MCF and MAF are raised under identical conditions. The macrophage cytotoxicity factor (1972) was designated MCF, because we tested exclusively for cytotoxic effects. Probably some of the characteristics of MAF may be secondary to activation with MCF: for instance spreading occurs by incubating macrophages with PGE^1 which is secreted upon activation by MCF.

SALVIN: Both MIF and MAF have been produced in sensitized mice *in vivo* by intravenous challenge with specific antigen. The peak of MIF release into the circulation occurs at 2-4 hr after challenge, whereas the peaks of MAF release are at 1 or 24 hr (possibly indicating more than one substance that is different from MIF). The MAF is measured by the NBT assay. Also, some strains of mice release MAF *in vivo*, but not MIF, and vice versa.

WAKSMAN: Could David tell us about SIRS (soluble immune response suppressor), which I understand is another incarnation of MIF and MAF?

DAVID: Studies with Pierce and Kühner showed that the activity of mouse SIRS and MIF were not separable by Sephadex chromatography cesium chloride, or enzyme susceptibility (both SIRS and MIF act on macrophages).

MAYER: I would like to return to the issue of dose-response assays in the present context. Does anyone have dose-response curves for MAF and MIF on the same cell supernatant?

MELTZER: In collaboration with Kühner we have compared murine MAF and MIF over a wide range of dose-response. The dose-response curves were identical.

CHURCHILL: MAF and MIF in guinea pigs and MAN have many similarities as shown by the following table:

Comparison of MAF and MIF attributes

	MAF		MIF	
	GP	MAN	GP	MAN
Receptors				
Fucose	+		+	+
Sialic Acid	+	ND	+	
Enhancement of mediator by treatment with				
AT III	+	+	+	?+
STI	ND	+	+	
DSA	+	+	+	
Fractionation				
pH3	+	+*	+	+
pH5	+	+	+	+

* preliminary data

Thus far we have not separated MIF from MAF in guinea pig or in man. Other data presented at this workshop suggest however that *mouse* MIF and MAF are separable.

MELTZER: What are the relationships of MIF/MAF/MCF to interferons?

KNIEP: We have a hint that MCF is different from interferon. Interferon is reported to bind to poly-I-Sepharose whereas MCF does not.

SORG: Neumann has data indicating that MIF and IF are not the same: (1) MIF and IF are produced by different cells. (2) An antiinterferon (IF) serum prepared by Gresser reacts only with IF. (3) Preliminary chemical characterization suggests that MIF and IF are different.

McDANIEL: The cell line Namalwa is used both as a source of interferon and of MAF. However, the active MAF fractions from 2% FCS supernatants have no interferon activity. Namalwa interferon is leukocyte interferon, MW 18,000 and stable in guanidine and urea.

KIRCHNER: Interferon has been clearly shown to have the same effects as SIRS and MAF. Interferon shortly will be available in a highly purified form. If it then still holds up that interferon has all these effects, it remains possible that MAF and SIRS are different molecules that exert the very same effects as interferon.

HADDEN: In comparing lymphokines and interferon (provided by W.E. Stewart II) in the Schultz and Chirigos tumoricidal system we find that interferon will activate peritoneal macrophages *to kill* tumor targets (i.e. with a net loss of cells) at a macrophage-target ratio of 10:1. On the other hand, lymphokine MAF (both supernatants and Sephadex fractions) induces only mild effects seen as *growth inhibition* (reduction in increase in cell number) at ratios of 50:1. Based upon this and other comparisons, we are far more impressed by interferon as an activation mechanism than by so-called lymphokine MAF.

MACROPHAGE ACTIVATION BY LYMPHOKINES: CHARACTERIZATION OF LYMPHOKINE SIGNALS FOR TUMORICIDAL AND MICROBICIDAL ACTIVITIES AND FOR PROSTAGLANDIN SYNTHESIS

Monte S. Meltzer
Larry M. Wahl
Edward J. Leonard

National Institutes of Health
Bethesda, Maryland

Carol A. Nacy

Walter Reed Army Institute of Research
Washington, District of Columbia

Macrophages recovered from peritoneal cavities of mice can be activated for tumor cytotoxicity by any one of several in vitro treatments. Two such treatments are supernatants from antigen or mitogen-stimulated spleen cell cultures (lymphokines) and endotoxic lipopolysaccharides from gram-negative bacteria (LPS) (1). In our system, macrophages treated with as little as a 1/30 dilution of lymphokines for 4-8 hours prior to addition of prelabeled tumor cells were significantly tumoricidal. Tumor cytotoxicity was estimated by measurement of radiolabel released into culture supernatants after 48 hours. LPS was much less effective than lymphokines as an in vitro activation stimulus. Tumor cytotoxicity by macrophages pretreated with up to 1 ug/ml LPS was minimal (Fig.1a). Although LPS had only a slight direct effect on macrophage tumoricidal activity, as little as 1 ng/ml LPS significantly increased the cytotoxicity of lymphokine-activated macrophages (Fig.1b). The interaction of LPS and lymphokines on macrophage tumoricidal activity was synergistic: if the slight direct effect of LPS is subtracted from the combined activity of LPS and lymphokines throughout the lymphokine dose-response curve, significant increases in cytotoxic activity persist (shaded area in Fig.1b). This synergistic interaction was critically dependent upon treatment sequence (Fig.1c). With suboptimal concentrations of LPS (1

ISBN 0-12-213950-X

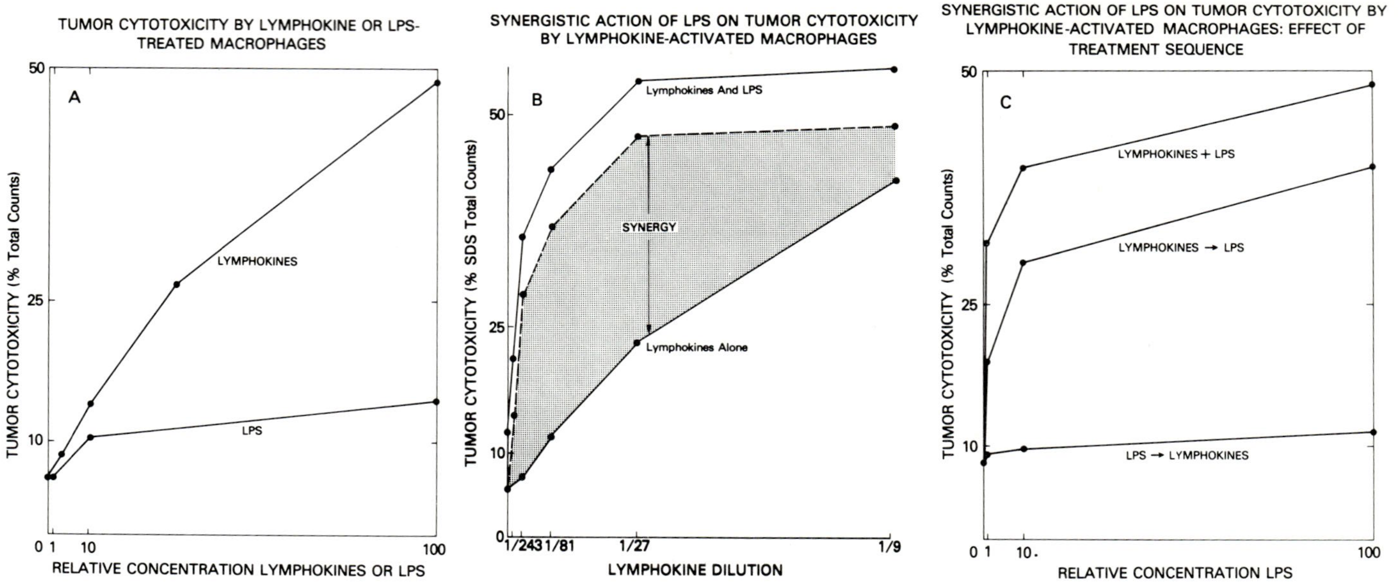

FIGURE 1. Synergistic action of LPS on tumor cytotoxicity by lymphokine-activated macrophages: (a) effect of treatment with LPS or lymphokines alone, (b) synergistic effects of combined treatment and (c) effects of treatment sequence.

ng/ml) and lymphokines (1/300 dilution), which by themselves were ineffective, strong tumoricidal activity was evident with macrophages treated simultaneously with LPS and lymphokines for 6 hours or with macrophages treated first with lymphokines for 5 hours followed by a LPS pulse of 1 hour. In contrast, macrophages treated first with LPS for 1 hour and then with lymphokines for 5 hours were not cytotoxic.

The interaction of lymphokines and LPS for alterations in macrophage function was also evident with prostaglandin (PGE) synthesis. In contrast to tumoricidal activity, the more effective stimulus for PGE secretion was LPS, not lymphokines (Fig.2a). Macrophages treated with lymphokines for 4-12 hours released little or no PGE over a subsequent 16-20 hour incubation. Over the same time span, macrophages treated with up to 1 ug/ml LPS synthesized significant levels of PGE. PGE release by macrophages treated with both LPS and lymphokines, however, was markedly increased over that by cells treated with LPS alone (Fig.2b). As with macrophage tumoricidal activity, effects of both stimuli on PGE synthesis were synergistic: subtraction of the slight direct effect of lymphokine treatment from the combined activity of LPS and lymphokines resulted in a persistent increase in PGE synthesis throughout the LPS dose-response curve (shaded area in Fig.2b). This synergistic interaction was also dependent upon treatment sequence (Fig.2c). With suboptimnal concentrations of LPS (1 ng/ml) and lymphokines (1/300 dilution), which were ineffective by themselves, significant PGE synthesis was evident with macrophages treated for 6 hours with both stimuli. In contrast to tumor cytotoxicity, however, the most efficient treatment was not the concurrent mixture but rather treatment with lymphokines first for 6 hours followed by a LPS pulse for 1 hour. Macrophages treated with LPS first for 1 hour followed by a lymphokine pulse of 6 hours released little or no PGE. It should be emphasized that initial treatment of macrophages with LPS did not preclude further response to lymphokines. Macrophages treated with LPS first could develop tumoricidal activity or increased PGE synthesis after lymphokine treatment when, and only when, these lymphokine-treated cells were pulsed again with LPS (Fig.3).

Thus, for both macrophage cytotoxic activity and for PGE synthesis multiple signals were required, each given in precise sequence: macrophages must be primed with certain factors in lymphokine supernatants first and then treated with LPS for full expression of functional activity. Fractionation of lymphokine supernatants by Sephadex G-200 gel chromatography revealed that priming activities for macrophage tumoricidal activity and for PGE synthesis were similar: both eluted in the 50,000 MW region (Fig.4a) (2). Macrophage tumoricidal activity and PGE synthesis appear then to be regulated by common mechanisms. The relationship between these two macrophage functions, however, was not through cause and effect. Macrophage cytotoxicity by lymphokines and LPS was not affected by indomethacin (0.05 mM) or by aspirin (1.0 mM), yet these treatments effectively inhibited PGE synthesis.

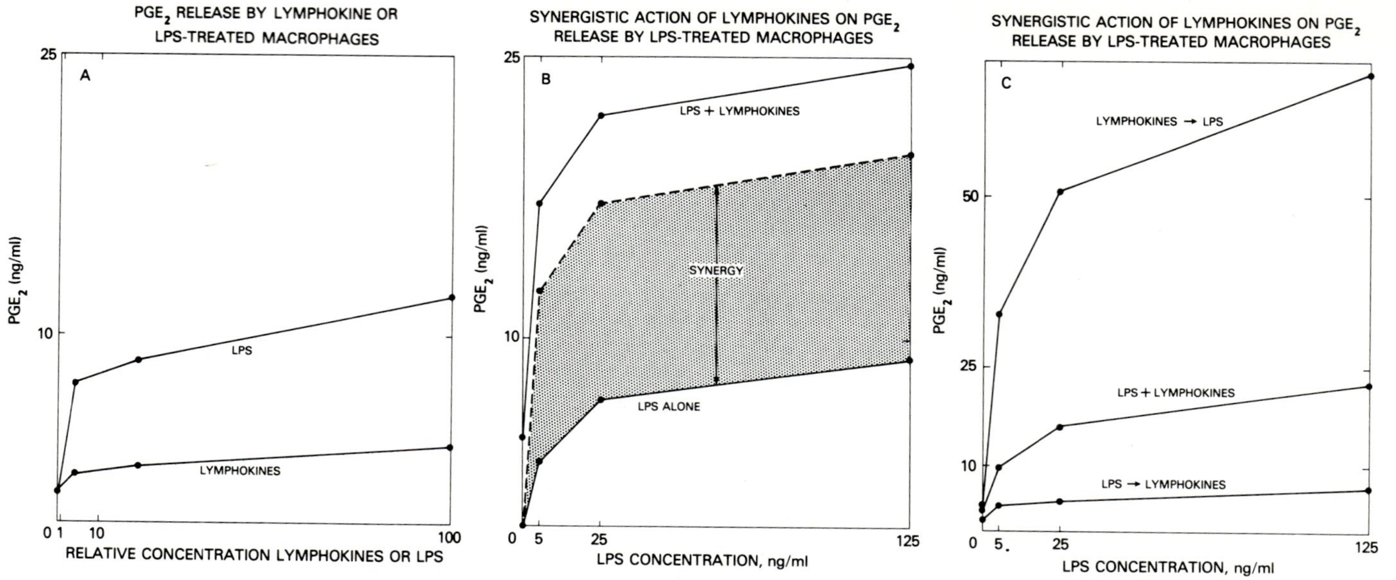

FIGURE 2. Synergistic action of lymphokines on PGE synthesis by LPS-treated macrophages: (a) effect of treatment with LPS or lymphokines alone, (b) synergistic effects of combined treatment and (c) effects of treatment sequence.

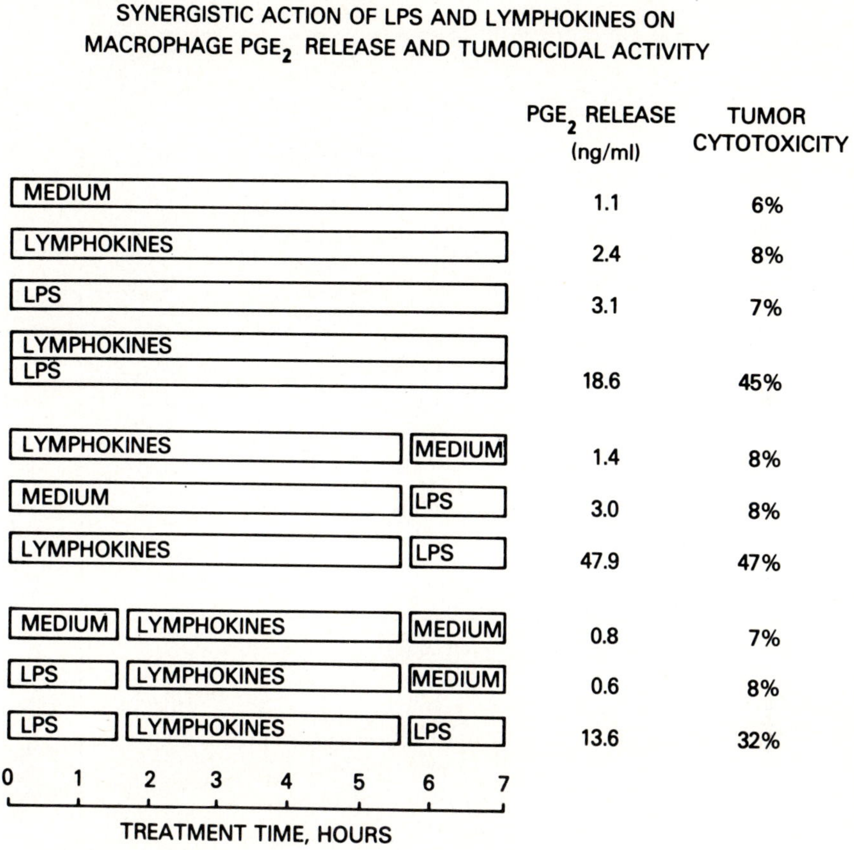

FIGURE 3. Synergistic interaction of lymphokines and LPS for macrophage tumoricidal activity and PGE synthesis: effects of treatment sequence.

The preceding results document instances in which different and probably unrelated functions of activated macrophages were regulated by common signals in lymphokine supernatants. These are not, however, the only lymphokine signals which regulate macrophage activation. We have previously shown a strict correlation throughout a wide range of in vivo and in vitro treatments between development of macrophage tumoricidal and microbicidal activities. The test organism for macrophage microbicidal activity was Rickettsia tsutsugamushi, an obligate intracellular parasite (3). Macrophages from (a) in vivo immune responses or chronic infection but not from sterile inflammatory exudates and (b) macrophages treated in vitro with lymphokines but not control supernatants showed strong tumoricidal activity. These macrophages also had strong rickettsiacidal activity: macrophages treated with lymphokines after rickettsial infection developed

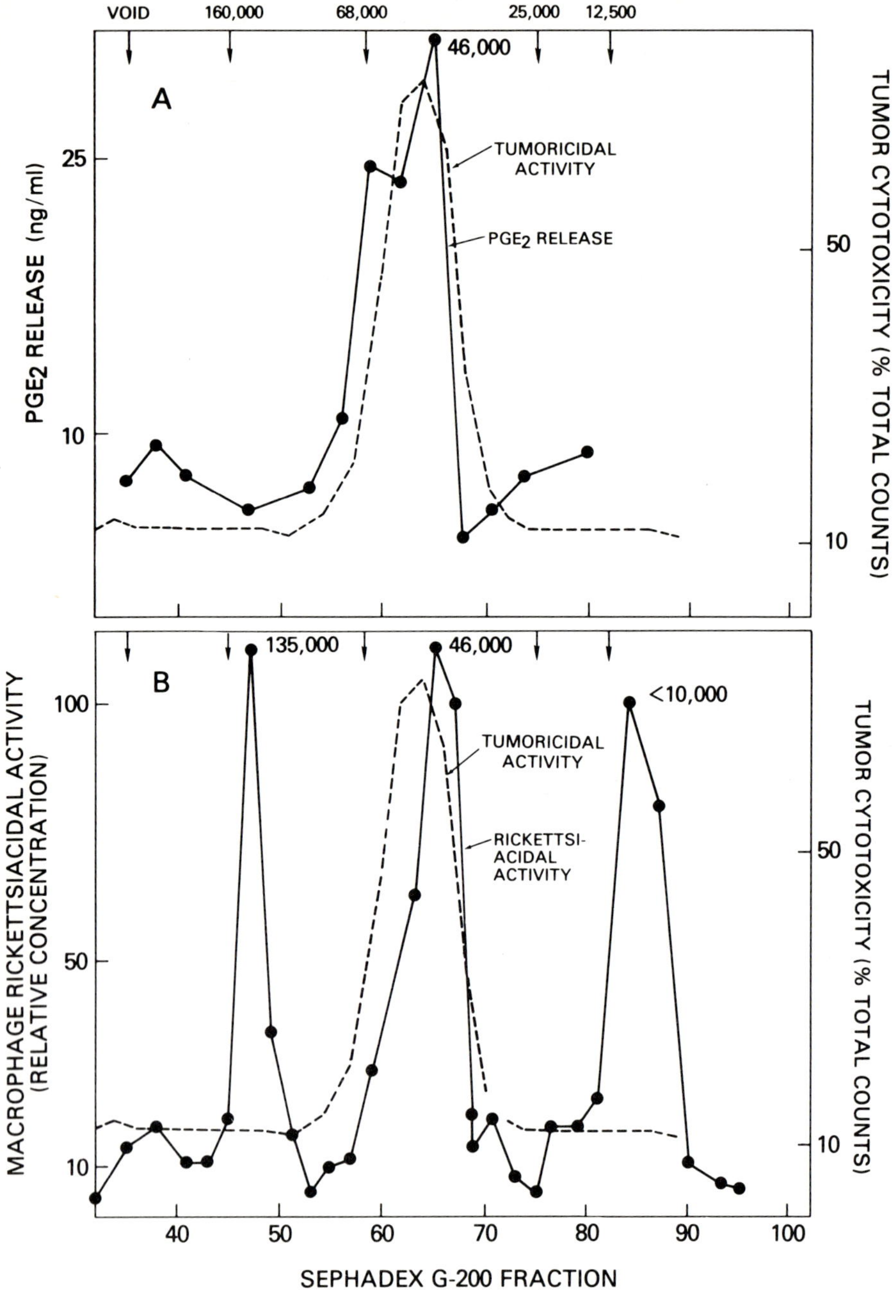

FIGURE 4. Chromatography of lymphokine supernatants on Sephadex G-200: activity of eluted fractions for (a) macrophage tumor cytotoxicity and PGE synthesis and (b) macrophage tumor cytotoxicity and rickettsiacidal function.

capacity to kill the intracytoplasmic parasite; control cells, however, suffered progressive rickettsial growth and cytolysis. Fractionation of lymphokine supernatants by Sephadex G 200 again revealed that activities for activated macrophage function, induction of both tumoricidal and rickettsiacidal capacity, eluted in the 50,000 MW region (Fig.4b). It was of considerable interest to note, however, that lymphokine activities for microbicidal but not for tumoricidal activity also eluted in two other regions: 135,000 and less than 10,000 daltons. Thus, we could document, for the first time, that tumoricidal and microbicidal functions of activated macrophages could be dissociated and that these activities appear to be regulated by completely different lymphokine signals.

REFERENCES

1. Ruco, L.P. and Meltzer, M.S. J. Immunol. 121,2035,1978.
2. Leonard, E.J., Ruco, L.P. and Meltzer, M.S. Cell. Immunol. 41,347,1978.
3. Nacy, C.A., Meltzer, M.S., Russell, P.K. and Osterman, J V. Fed. Proc. 38,1078,1979.

DIFFERENT PATHWAYS OF MACROPHAGE ACTIVATION TO CYTOTOXICITY

M.-L.Lohmann-Matthes, H.Lang and W.Domzig

Max-Planck-Institut für Immunbiologie,Freiburg,FRG

INTRODUCTION

Besides the nonspecific cytotoxicity, which is induced by activation with the lymphokine macrophage cytotoxicity factor (MCF) cells of the macrophage lineage possess two other mechanisms to kill tumor targets, the K cell-like cytotoxicity against antibody coated tumor cells and the NK-like cytotoxicity against NK-susceptible tumors. Data on cooperative effects of the different mechanisms are presented.

MATERIAL AND METHODS

Bone-marrow cultures, preparation of promonocytes and the cytotoxic assays are done as described (Lohmann et al. 1979; Domzig et al. 1979)

RESULTS

1. Three Different Mechanisms of Macrophage-mediated Cytotoxicity

a. Lymphokine induced macrophage mediated cytotoxicity-macrophages are incubated for 24 h with the lymphokine MCF (see Kniep et al. in this volume). Figure 1 shows a dose response curve for 3 different mouse strains. This type of macrophage mediated cytotoxicity is nonspecific and is directed against all tumors tested.

ISBN 0-12-213950-X

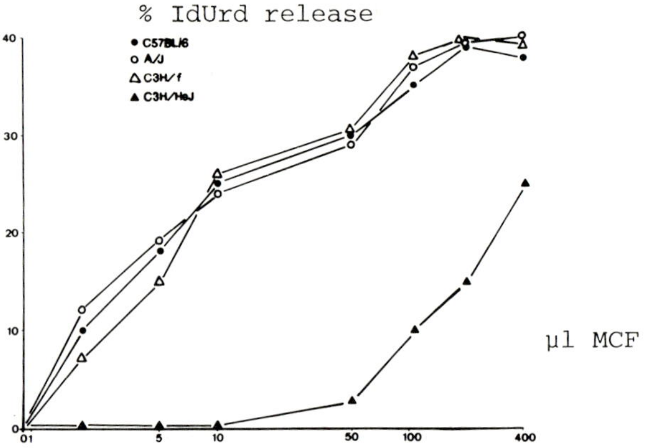

Fig. 1. MCF-induced macrophage cytotoxicity

b. Antibody-dependent macrophage mediated cytotoxicity against tumor cells. Young macrophages and macrophage precursor cells (promonocytes) have the capacity to kill antibody coated tumor targets. Table I shows that only macrophage precursor cells and young macrophages but not the resident peritoneal macrophage are active in this system.

Table 1. *Antibody-dependent cytotoxicity by various macrophages*

Effector cells	% spec. ^{125}IdUrd release of AB-coated P815
Promonocytes	42
Young macrophages from a 8 day bone-marrow culture	46
Thioglycollate induced macrophages	35
Normal wash out peritoneal macrophages	0

Ratio 8:1 18 h Assay

Fig. 2 compares the kinetics of antibody dependent and lymphokine induced killing. The lag phase in the latter system represents the time which is needed for activation.

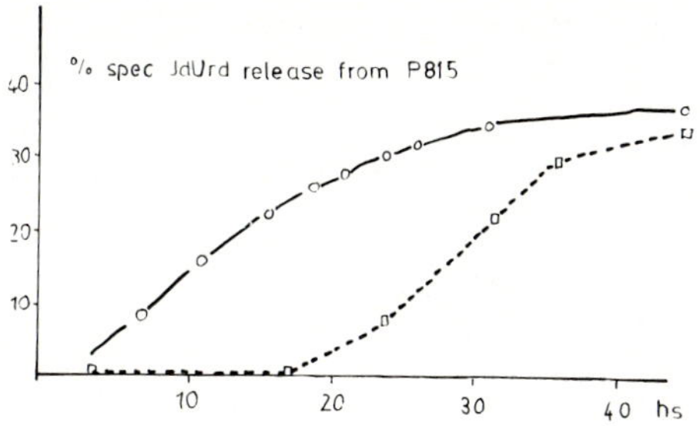

Fig. 2. Kinetics of antibody-dependent and lymphokine-induced killing

c. NK-cell activity performed by promonocytes. Table 2 demonstrates that the nonadherent, nonphagocytic, esterase negative macrophage precursor cell promonocyte kills very effectively tumors, which are susceptible for natural killing. The promonocyte is likely to be identical with the NK-cell. Its killing capacity is enhanced by interferon preparations.

Table 2. *Natural killing by promonocytes*

Effector cells	% spec. ^{125}IdUrd release YAC	P815
C57B1/6 Promonocytes	60	4
Ratio 50:1		6 h Assay

2. Cooperative Effects Between the Different Cytotoxicity Mechanisms.

a. NK-killing is enhanced, when the target cells are coated with antibody.

b. Figure 3 shows cooperative effects between activation by MCF and antibody dependent cytotoxicity. Macrophages are preactivated for 24 h with MCF over a large dose range. Antibody-dependent cytotoxicity is enhanced by preactivation with MCF at dosages, which fail to induce nonspecific lymphokine-cytotoxicity. The experiment shown in Figure 3 was done with bone-marrow macrophages from C3H/HeJ mice. Identical cooperative effects are obtained with other mouse strains. The deficiency of C3H/HeJ mice to respond to lymphokines is completely compensated in this cooperative system.

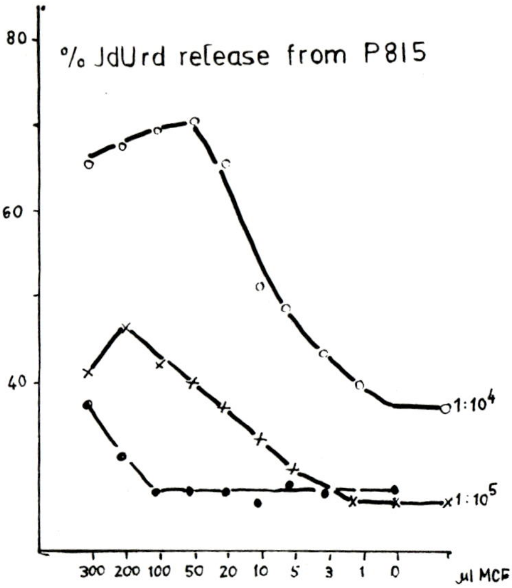

Fig. 3. Cooperative effects between MCF-induced and antibody-dependent cytotoxicity.

All macrophages were preactivated with MCF for 24 h.

●—●—●—●	MCF activated macrophages
o—o—o—o	MCF activated macrophages + rabbit anti 5178Y antiserum $1{:}10^4$
x—x—x—x	MCF activated macrophages + rabbit antiserum $1{:}10^5$

The enhanced cytotoxicity, which is obtained in the described cooperative system, is specific and the specificity corresponds to the specificity of the antisera used for coating the tumor targets.

COMMENTS

Macrophages possess three different mechanisms by which they can kill tumor targets. These mechanisms can cooperate and produce additive effects. In the case of cooperation between antibody and MCF-induced cytotoxicity preactivation with

MCF is already highly significant at MCF dosages, which are far below the dosage, which induces nonspecific MCF-induced cytotoxicity. CeH/HeJ mice are low responder for the activation with MCF to cytotoxicity (Ruco et al. 1978). However, this deficiency is fully compensated in the described cooperative situation. Since under most in vivo conditions antibody is produced at the same time as lymphokines, these data on the cooperative effect of the two mechanisms allow to understand, why C3H/HeJ mice do not suffer from increased incidence of infections and tumors.

Our experiments show, that in the cooperative situation of antibody-dependent and lymphokine-induced cytotoxicity, the specificity of the reaction corresponds to the specificity of the antisera used. The nonspecific effect of the lymphokine activation does not come up at these small dosages, which are used for the cooperative preactivation. These data explain our earlier findings on specific macrophage mediated cytotoxicity. At that time MCF was prepared from allogeneically sensitized spleen cells, which were reexposed to the sensitizing antigen in vitro (Lohmann-Matthes et al. 1973). The supernatant produced by these allogeneic cultures contained small amounts of MCF (compared to supernatants of Con A stimulated spleen cells) and certainly also small amounts of antibody were present. The effect, which we measured at that time, was most likely a cooperative effect similar to the one described here. As soon as chemical characterization started, the lymphokine preparations were concentrated 10 to 100-fold. The resultant preparation contained a much higher amount of the nonspecific lymphokine. Therefore, the effects observed with these concentrated preparations showed the nonspecific nature of lymphokine-induced macrophage mediated cytotoxicity. The described cooperative effects are likely to play an important role under in vivo conditions.

REFERENCES

1. Lohmann-Matthes, M.-L., Domzig, W. (1979). *Eur. J. Immunol. 9,* 261
2. Domzig, W., Lohmann-Matthes, M.-L. (1979). *Eur. J. Immunol. 9,* 267
3. Ruco, L. P., Meltzer, M. S. (1978). *J. Immunol. 120,* 1054
4. Lohmann-Matthes, M.-L., Ziegler, F. G. and Fischer, H. (1973). *Eur. J. Immunol. 3,* 56

DETERMINATION AND CHARACTERIZATION OF MACROPHAGE-CYTOTOXICITY-FACTOR (MCF) BY MEASURING CHEMILUMINESCENCE (CL) OF MACROPHAGES

Herbert Fischer
Eva-Maria Kniep
Martin Ernst

Max-Planck-Institut
für Immunbiologie
Freiburg i.Br.

Bernhard Peskar

Pharmakologisches Institut
Freiburg i.Br.

Granulocytes, macrophages and also lymphocytes (1) respond to external signals with a burst of chemiluminescence (CL) which can be measured - either directly or with the aid of luminol - in tissue culture medium at 37°C, in a scintillation counter (2). The burst of light is due to the generation and reaction of oxygen species (O_2^-; $^1O_2$; H_2O_2; $\cdot OH$) which in the case of granulocytes have been proven to be highly important for the microbicidal activity of these cells (3). In macrophages, CL and generation of reactive oxygen species is much less and can only be compared to granulocyte CL, when highly activated macrophages are tested. In this case, hydrogen peroxide in sufficient amounts to lyse target cells can be generated (4). The obvious correlation between free radical formation and CL suggested a closer analysis of MCF induced macrophage activation and cytotoxicity with the help of CL.

We have studied the effect of purified macrophage cytotoxicity factor (MCF) on 5-6 day cultured bone marrow macrophages from C57Bl mice. Experimental details of macrophage cultivation and measurement of CL have been described elsewhere (1). MCF was purified by Kniep et al. (this conference).

As is shown in Fig. 1 preincubation with a low dose of MCF leads to an enhanced CL response to Con A; with higher doses this effect is levelled out or even decreased, an effect which is neither due to increased PGE release nor to cell damage.

We have also studied the zymosan induced CL response of MCF activated macrophages, which seems not to be significantly

ISBN 0-12-213950-X

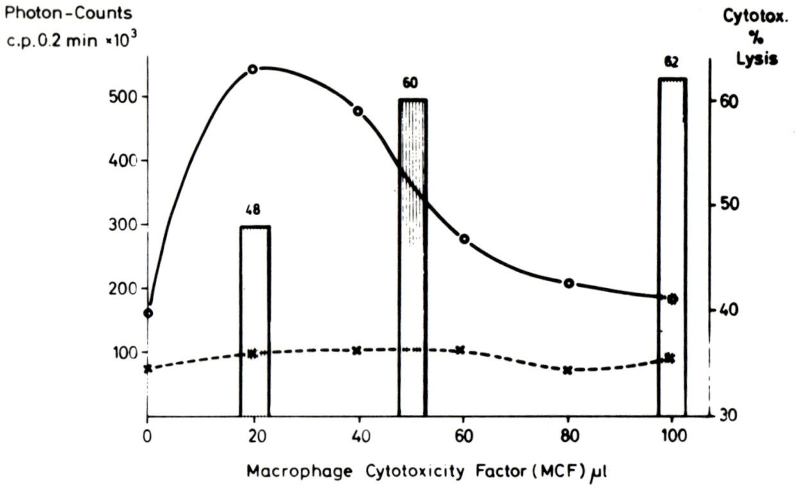

FIGURE 1. Con-A induced Chemiluminescence after 20 h pre-incubation with MCF.
5 day cultivated C57Bl macrophages were incubated for 2o hours with increasing amounts of MCF ($1o^6$ mac/2.5 ml Eagle's Hepes) 15 min prior to Con A (8o µg/ml) luminol (4o µg/ml) was added. Circles indicate net photon counts per 5 min after Con A addition to MCF treated macrophages. Crosses indicate net photon counts per 5 min after Con A addition to macrophages treated with heat inactivated MCF. Bars indicate the percentage of cytotoxic lysis depending on the amount of MCF.

altered(data not shown). Recently, an improved photon counting machine has enabled us to measure the CL of various samples during the 8-12 hours required for macrophage cytotoxicity.

The results shown in Fig. 2 seem to us especially meaningful since direct interaction between activated macrophages and target cells is monitored. Clearly, antibody-coated target cells evoke a much higher metabolic response which occurs mostly during the first 3 hours of co-cultivation. However, it is also clear (see lower graph) that MCF-activated macrophages have a consistently higher output of CL during the whole course of the cytotoxicity assay compared to non-preactivated macrophages.

The obvious correlation with short term killing in antibody-mediated cytotoxicity and the long term MCF induced cytotoxicity suggests, that improved measurements of CL can be used to analyse both macrophage activation and macrophage cytotoxicity.

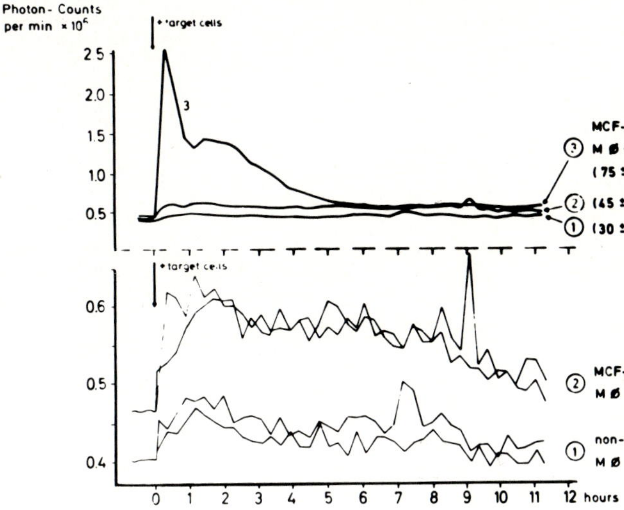

FIGURE 2. Macrophage CL induced by addition of P815 target cells.

Integral CL represents net photon counts per 11 hours. Cytotoxicity means the percentage of cytotoxic target cell lysis after 15 hours. Curves (1) CL of non-activated macrophages. Integral CL: 24 x 10^6; curves (2) CL of MCF (200 µl) activated macrophages. Integral CL: 71 x 10^6; curve (3) CL of MCF (200 µl) activated macrophages induced by antibody coated target cells. Integral CL: 439 x 10^6.

REFERENCES

1. Wrogemann, K., Weidemann, M.J., Peskar, B.A., Staudinger, H. Rietschel, E.T. and Fischer, H., Eur. J. Immunol. 8, 749 (1978).
2. Allen, R.C., Stjemholm, R.L. and Steele, R.H., Biochem.Biophys. Res. Commun. 47, 679 (1972).
3. Johnston, R.B., Fed. Proc. 37, 2759 (1979).
4. Nathan, C.F., Silverstein, S.C., Brukner, L.H. and Cohn, Z.A., J.exp. Med. 149, 100 (1979).

DISCUSSION

3. Mechanisms of Macrophage Activation: Lymphokine Signals and Macrophage Heterogeneity

MELTZER: There is evidence from several laboratories that lymphokine responsiveness of macrophages varies with the state of maturation. For example, resident peritoneal macrophages respond very poorly to lymphokines as regards this activation for tumor cytotoxicity. Inflammatory macrophages, less mature peroxidase-positive cells are about 10-fold more responsive to the same concentration of lymphokine. Peripheral blood monocytes, the putative precursor of inflammatory cells, however, do not respond at all. Is there evidence from other groups that lymphokine response varies with maturation?

CHURCHILL: Human peripheral blood monocytes will not respond to MAF until they have been in culture for 5 days. This response begins after 3 days in culture. Thus we believe that the capacity to respond to MAF is acquired during the maturation of monocytes into macrophages. In the guinea pig the effector cell is an oil-induced or casein-induced peritoneal exudate cell.

ALTMAN: What is the available information on the expression of Ia antigens on macrophages during their differentiation stages?

LOHMANN-MATTHES: Studies by Gisler and Müller-Stern show that 60-80% of the macrophages cultured from the bone-marrow express Ia antigens. In contrast only 15-20% of the resident peritoneal macrophages are Ia positive. A correlate of these findings is that bone-marrow macrophages are particularly efficient in antigen presentation. Up to now it is not known whether the expression of Ia reflects a macrophage subpopulation or whether the expression of Ia is correlated with maturation processes.

BELLER: We have found that Ia antigen (as detected by hybridoma anti Ia and fluorescent Fab_2 RAMG), is present on only 5-10% of uninduced or peptone-elicited murine PEC, but is found on 60-70% of splenic and thymic macrophages. Antigen presentation to macrophage-depleted *Listeria*-immune T cells is similarly about 10-fold better in thymic and splenic macrophages than in PEC. Of interest is the finding made with Chris

ISBN 0-12-213950-X

Lu, that thymic macrophages are capable of presenting antigen much earlier in ontogeny than the splenic macrophages. Thymic macrophages can already present optimally on day 8 (the earliest day so far tested) while spleen macrophages demonstrate no antigen presentation function on day 8 and about 50% of maximal adult activity on day 18. Thinking that Ia might be increased in an antigen-presenting population, we injected mice with *Listeria* i.p. The PEC harvested from these animals were 50-75% Ia positive.

LEON: Could the differential response to lymphokines of monocytes and macrophages of different age be due, in part, to the presence of other cell types in the preparations? I am referring to cell types which could either exert direct suppressive effects or secrete suppressive factors.

LOHMANN-MATTHES: Promonocytes (macrophage precursor cells) are active in K-cell killing of tumor targets and in NK-killing. In addition, they can be activated to cytotoxicity by MCF; however, during the 24 hr activation process by MCF, they also mature to adherent macrophages. The only suppressive effect which is known so far is the suppression of NK-activity. There is evidence (see Holden in these proceedings), that prostaglandin E_1 suppresses NK-activity. Since prostaglandin E_1 is produced by macrophages, the NK-activity of promonocytes is suppressed and perhaps regulated by mature macrophages.

MELTZER: Is there any further information on synergistic effects between lymphokines and other agents with respect to action on macrophages?

LOHMANN-MATTHES: We have done experiments with young bone-marrow macrophages as effector cells. These macrophages were preactivated with subthreshold dosages of our lymphokine MCF (MAF), which failed to induce non-specific cytotoxicity. However, addition of antibody, which had also been diluted to a concentration where no antibody-dependent cytotoxicity occurred, resulted in a strong synergistic cytotoxicity for target cells, dependent on the specificity of the antisera used. This finding explains our earlier data on "specific macrophage-mediated cytotoxicity", since these early experiments (1972) were done in an allogeneic system, where both MCF and antibody, were secreted into the supernatants in subthreshold amounts, and thus acted in a synergistic way on macrophages.

CHURCHILL: With human and guinea pig macrophages, cytotoxic macrophages can be induced by endotoxin or by MAF. However, in preliminary experiments, we have not observed a synergistic interaction between MAF and endotoxin such as Meltzer has described in the mouse system.

MAUEL: We have results which appear to be similar to the effect reported by Meltzer. Using an assay based on intracellular killing of Leishmania parasites by lymphokine-activated mouse peritoneal macrophages, we observe that when our lymphokine preparation is diluted to such an extent that induction of intracellular parasite killing is no longer observed, full activity is restored by addition of nanogram amounts of LPS.

WAKSMAN: I would like to make a purely theoretical point: "Activation" can involve a variety of cell changes (1) stimulation of cell to move through cell cycle, i.e. synthesize DNA and undergo mitosis; (2) simple activation of membrane (movement, phagocytosis, other?); (3) reversible activation, in sense of increased organelles, increased lysosomal hydrolases; (4) differentiation (irreversible) to new phenotype. As an example of this last kind of change consider David's demonstration, 10 years ago, that LK-activated macrophages develop over 3 days into a type of cell containing decreased lysosomal hydrolases (epithelioid cell transformation?). These four types of change are not necessarily consequences of the same signals. Accordingly, it is really unlikely that all macrophage-activating factors will be the same or have the same effect.

EPSTEIN: I would like to affirm Waksman's admonition. We must be more circumspect in our use of the term "activation of macrophages". For example, Lee and I (Cell. Immunol. in press, 1979) have shown that interferon can inhibit the maturation of human monocytes to macrophages. Yet interferon treated cells are more phagocytic in terms of the proportion of cells that phagocytize zymosan and the number of particles phagocytized. Thus although the interferon treated cells have more of the attributes of monocytes than macrophages (in terms of morphologic appearance and the specific activity of intracellular lysosomal enzymes) they function more like macrophages (with regard to increased phagocytic capacity).

DIENER: I can offer still another example emphasizing the ambiguity one is confronted with when trying to understand the physiological significance of MAF activity. Brown, in my laboratory, has shown that allogeneic restriction, as well as genetically determined macrophage-dependent non-responsiveness to certain antigens, may be overcome in the presence of MAF and free antigen when using the T cell proliferation assay. However, when the same assay is carried out with macrophage-bound antigen, restriction of responsiveness is observed (J. Immunogenetics, in press).

4. Mechanisms of Killing by Activated Macrophages

McDANIEL: There was a report in JNCI, 1977 by Hanna and collaborators on an extensive study of the killing of guinea pig hepatoma cells by preconditioned macrophages. Over a period of 9 hr the macrophages injected a small dense particle the size of a lysosome into tumor cells. The tumor cell then came apart and disintegrated. While the particle could not be shown directly to be a lysosome, because of the fixing techniques used, there are reasons for suspecting that it is a lysosome.

GRANGER: Levey in our laboratory and Redding in Nicholson's laboratory have shown that murine peritoneal macrophages from tumor alloimmune mice, or from thioglycolate-induced mice can release in vitro a 140,000 MW protease which is quite unstable in solution, binds rapidly to target cells and causes growth inhibition and cell lysis.

KIRCHNER: Among the most potent mechanisms for inducing cytostatic macrophages in mice, is the administration of *C.parvum*. A variety of substances are produced by the spleen of these animals 7-10 days later such as PGE and interferon. Nevertheless, in each case it has to be proven that these substances are actually involved in cytostasis/cytotoxicity. It now seems likely that in most cases the production of these substances is only associated with cytotoxicity but they are not involved in the cytotoxic mechanism itself.

OPPENHEIM: It is noteworthy that there are now reports that PGs can generate some H_2O_2. This is affirmed by the fact that indomethacin counteracting PGs indirectly decreases H_2O_2 production. Then too, there is the recent work by Cohn and associates in which it was shown that H_2O_2 is the agent responsible for macrophage killing and that MAF is the only signal that is capable of stimulating macrophages to produce peroxide.

PICK: I rather dispute Oppenheim's interpretation. Prostaglandins of the E series were found by Fischer's group to block chemiluminescence by macrophages, which is an expression of respiratory activity. I do not consider that there is evidence for prostaglandin-stimulated H_2O_2 formation.

HADDEN: I would point out that we can dissociate PG production and activation of guinea pig peritoneal macrophages for killing Listeria monocytogenes. First measuring PGE_2 and $PGF_{1\alpha}$ secretion at 1,3 and 5 days of culture, we found constitutive production but no greater production by antigen-preincubated supernatants and fractions than by antigen-reconstitution. Introduction of indomethacin and cyclo-oxygenase inhibitors did not prevent activation.

MELTZER: We have obtained data showing that tumor cytotoxicity and PGE_2 synthesis by LK-treated macrophages are controlled by the same signals but there is no cause and effect relationship: one can completely inhibit PGE_2 synthesis with indomethacin or aspirin without affecting tumor cytotoxicity.

LYMPHOKINE STIMULATION OF COMPLEMENT COMPONENT SYNTHESIS BY HUMAN MONOCYTES[1]

Bruce H. Littman

Medical College of Virginia
Virginia Commonwealth University
Richmond, Virginia

INTRODUCTION

Monocytes and macrophages produce many complement components (1). We have recently demonstrated that the synthesis of the second complement component (C2) can be stimulated by lymphokine-rich lymphocyte culture supernate (2). The purpose of the present investigation was to characterize this lymphokine called Monocyte Complement Stimulator (MCS) and to compare it to macrophage Migration Inhibitory Factor (MIF), another lymphocyte product affecting numerous macrophage functions (3). The results indicate that MCS and MIF are different lympnokines.

MATERIALS AND METHODS

Cell populations and cultures

Mononuclear cells are obtained by differential density centrifugation of heparinized blood on a Ficoll-Hypaque gradient and resuspended at 10^7/ml in medium 199 supplemented with HEPES buffer, penicillin and streptomycin (2).

Adherent monocytes are isolated from the mononuclear cell population by incubation in the presence of 10 % heat-inactiv-

[1]*Supported by NIH Grants AM 20317 and AM 18976 and the Charles W. Thomas Research Fund from the Medical College of Virginia*

[2]*Recipient of a Research Career Development Award #KO4 AM-00336, National Institute of Arthritis and Metabolic Diseases, National Institutes of Health*

ISBN 0-12-213950-X

ated AB+ serum for 90 minutes and repetitive washing. The number of adherent cells is quantitated by fluorometric determination of DNA. Purified lymphocyte subpopulations are added to adherent monocytes in cultures producing MCS or lymphokine-rich supernates are added to stimulate C2 production (2).

Lymphocyte subpopulations are prepared by rosetting mononuclear cells with neuraminidase treated sheep erythrocytes (E_{VCN}) followed by Ficoll-Hypaque centrifugation (4). Purity was examined by re-rosetting with SRBC, determing surface immunoglobulin positive cells by immunofluorescence, and identifying cells phagocytic for polystyrene beads (4).

MCS containing supernates

5×10^6 mononuclear cells/ml of 15 % heat-inactivated AB+ serum in supplemented medium 199 were cultured 48 hours with the streptokinase-streptodornase (SK-SD) (active supernate). Control and active supernates are dialyzed against fresh medium 199 and millipore filtered prior to testing for MCS.

Assay for MCS activity

Supernates are diluted with supplemented medium 199 and made to contain a final concentration of 15 % inactivated AB+ serum, added to adherent monocytes and cultured for five days. Duplicate 0.1 ml aliquots of these culture supernates are tested in a standard assay for hemolytically active C2 (2, 5).

Sephadex G100 gel chromatography

Control and active supernates are concentrated by dialysis and lyophilization. They are fractionated on a calibrated sephadex G100 columns. Fractions are pooled, lyophilized, and reconstituted with distilled H_2O, dialyzed against distilled H_2O for 24 hours, HBSS for 24 hours and finally medium 199. They are millipore filtered and stored at - 20° C.

Isoelectric focusing

Concentrated supernates or fractions are subjected to isoelectric focusing using pH 3.5 - 10 ampholines and sucrose density liquid chromatography. Fractions are pooled, dialyzed against water and lyophilized. They are reconstituted with medium 199, dialyzed against medium 199 and millipore filtered prior to testing fro lymphokine activities.

Protease treatment

Insoluble chymotrypsin (on carboxy-methylcellulose) and insoluble trypsin (on polyacrylamide beads) are washed extensively with medium 199, incubated with control and active supernate for 18 hours at 30° C at pH 8.6 or 7.2. The MCS activity of enzyme-treated and control supernates is compared. Treated supernate did not abolish MCS activity, showing that inhibition was not due to detached protease affecting responding monocytes.

RESULTS

Cells producing MCS

In seven experiments MCS was produced by SK-SD stimulated T-lymphocytes and monocytes but not by antigen-stimulated rosette negative B-lymphocytes, monocytes and "Null" cells. The result of such an experiment is given in Fig. 1

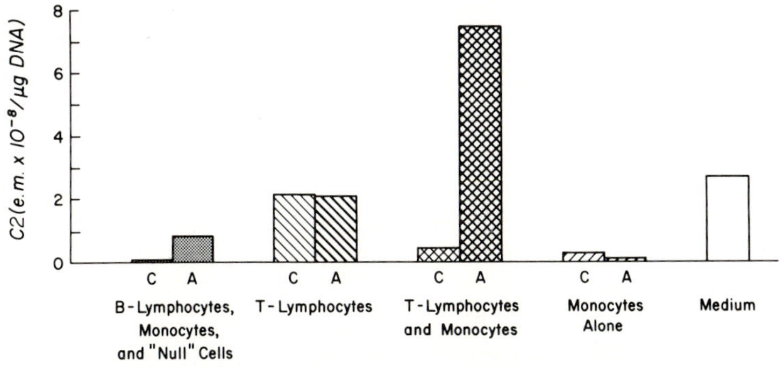

Fig. 1. Production of MCS by different cell types. "C" refers to control supernate and "A" refers to active supernate produced by the various cells.

Only rosette positive T-lymphocytes produced MCS while the monocyte containing rosette negative population did not. This result was obtained in three experiments and indicates that to obtain MCS production by T-lymphocytes, they must be co-cultured with monocytes and antigen initially. T-lymphocytes are then able to produce MCS independent of monocytes.

In another series of experiments, monocytes and T-lymphocytes were treated with pactamycin, an irreversible inhibitor of protein synthesis, and washed. Untreated monocytes were cultured with treated T-lymphocytes and untreated T-lymphocytes with treated monocytes. The resultant cultured mixtures of cells were stimulated with antigen and MCS production was determined. The results are given in Table 1.

Tab. 1. Pactamycin Treatment of Monocytes and T-lymphocytes: Effect on MCS Production

Treatment of cells			*Percent*
		Net	*Inhibition*
Monocytes	*T-cells*	*MCS*[a]	*MCS Production*
Medium	*Medium*	*24.26*	*0*
Pactamycin	*Pactamycin*	*0.64*	*97*
Medium	*Pactamycin*	*6.73*	*72*
Pactamycin	*Medium*	*7.62*	*69*

[a] *C2 e.m. x* 10^{-8}*/μg DNA*

Treatment of MCS with insolubilized chymotrypsin or with insolubilized trypsin resulted in destruction of MCS activity. This, together with the pactamycin inhibition experiment indicates that MCS activity depends on a protein moiety and that its production requires intact protein synthesis.

Comparison with MIF

Supernates derived from lymphocyte subpopulations were tested for both MCS and MIF; only monocytes and T-lymphocytes produced MCS. MIF was found in this supernate but was also produced by rosette negative cells. Thus a supernate is produced which has MIF and no MCS activity (Fig. 2).

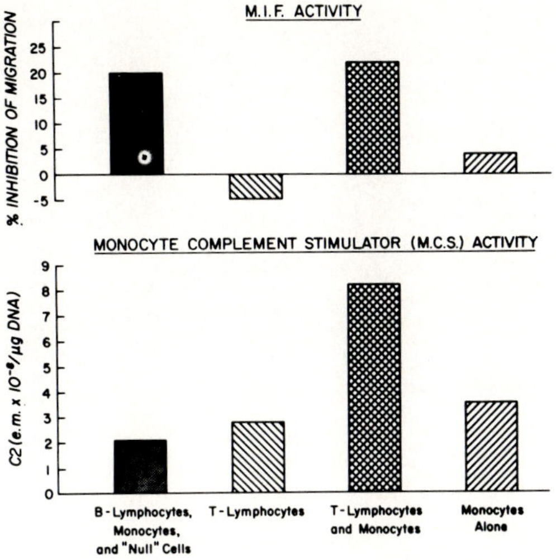

Fig. 2. MCS and MIF activities produced by various lymphocyte subpopulations.

The heat stability of MIF and MCS was compared by incubating supernates at 56° C for 30 minutes and testing heated and unheated aliquots MCS and MIF activities. The results (not shown) indicate that MCS is heat labile while MIF activity is retained after heating.

Sephadex G100 chromatography

Sephadex G100 chromatographic separation of active and control supernates is shown in Fig. 3. Peak MCS activity elutes with molecules of 25,000 daltons, the reported size of human MIF (3). MIF is also found with molecules of this size as indicated in Fig. 4A. However MCS activity is present to a lesser extent in fractions corresponding to a higher molecular weight with significant activity eluting with molecules of 20 - 50,000 daltons.

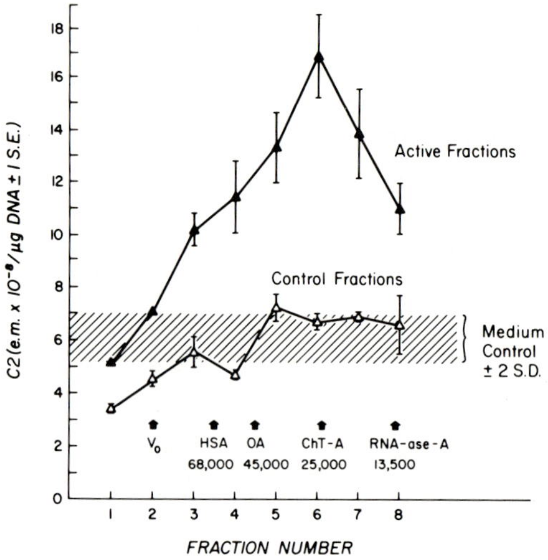

Fig. 3. Sephadex G100 chromatography of MCS-related control supernates.

Isoelectric focusing

MCS was found in fractions corresponding to an isoelectric point of 6.5 - 7.5.

A. SEPHADEX G100 SEPARATION

FRACTION	M.W.	NET MCS e.m. C2 x 10^{-8}/µg DNA	MIF % INHIBITION	
1	80,000-100,000	2.4	-18	6
2	56,000-80,000	-0.3	4	-3
3	40,000-56,000	3.8	-9	-7
4	28,000-40,000	3.1	1	-11
5	20,000-28,000	14.7	51	36
6	14,000-20,000	1.5	-22	-20
7	10,000-14,000	4.5	1	3

B. ISOELECTRIC FOCUSING OF SEPHADEX FRACTION 5

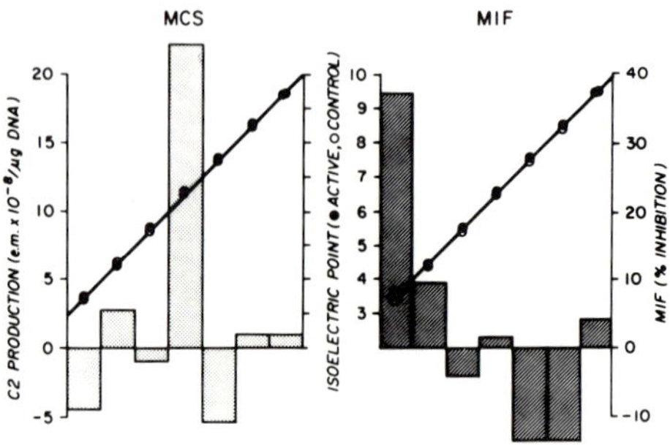

Fig. 4. Sequential sephadex G100 chromatography and isoelectric focusing of MIF and MCS.

Sequential sephadex G100 chromatography and isoelectric focusing were performed and fractions were tested for both activities as shown in Fig. 4. MIF and MCS are both present in sephadex fraction 5, corresponding to a MW of 25,000, isoelectric focusing of this fraction separated MIF from MCS. MIF activity was present at isoelectric point of pH 3.5 - 4.0 while MCS was found at pH 6 - 7.

DISCUSSION

This study has shown that MCS is a lymphocyte product stimulating C2 production by human monocytes. Its production requires intact protein synthesis by monocytes and T-lymphocytes. During the first 24 hours of antigenic stimulation these cells cooperate in MCS production by T-lymphocytes. Susceptibility to trypsin and chymotrypsin digestion affirm MCS as protein.

Like MIF, MCS has a molecular size of 25,000 daltons but it differs in heat lability and is not produced by monocytes and B-lymphocytes. Moreover, MCS can be separated from MIF by isoelectric focusing. MCS has an isoelectric point of 6.5 - 7.5 whereas MIF was 3.5 - 4.0. Accordingly MCS differs from MIF in several respects.

REFERENCES

1. Colten, H. R., *Progr. Immunol. 1,* 183, 1974
2. Littman, B. H. and Ruddy, S., *J. Exp. Med. 145,* 1344, 1977
3. David, J. R., *Fed. Proc. 34,* 1730, 1975
4. Littman, B. H., David, J. R. and Rocklin, R. E., *Cell. Immunol. 24,* 241, 1976
5. Ruddy, S., Klemperer, M. R., Rosen, F. S., Austen, K. F. and Kumate, J., *Immunology 18,* 943, 1970
6. Bhuyan, B. K., Dietz, A. and Smith C. G., *Antimicrob. Agents Chemother. 184,* May, 1961
7. Block, L. H., Jaksche, H., Bamberger, S. and Ruhenstroth-Bauer, G., *J. Exp. Med. 147,* 541, 1978
8. Littman, B. H. and Ruddy, S., *Clin. Res. 25,* 485A, 1977

DISCUSSION

EPSTEIN: In interferon research, we have studied the stability to low pH and heat for many years. Now I see that many investigators working with other lymphokines are likewise routinely ascertaining stability to low pH and heat. But I fail to see what information concerning their molecular configuration will be derived in this manner.

LACHMAN: If factors which are generated in cultures containing endotoxin lose activity when heated this at least implies that the factor is not residual endotoxin.

LITTMAN: Aside from increasing C_2 production in monocytes, MCS appears to promote monocyte differentiation. Monocytes produce C_2 when incubated for more than 2 - 3 days without MCS but they produce C_3 and C_4 immediately upon isolation. MCS seems to act by speeding up the differentiation of monocytes into C_2 producing macrophages. It does not increase the synthesis of C_3 and C_4, perhaps because as monocytes these cells have already differentiated to the stage where they produce these complement components. The differentiation of monocytes into C_2 producing cells is irreversible as removing MCS will not turn off C_2 production. This favors the view that monocytes have differentiated into macrophages, a one-way phenomenon. This process differs from other forms of macrophage cultivation such as tumor cell killing, which is a reversible phenomenon. The relationship of MCS to MAF is unknown, but it clearly is different from MIF.

OPPENHEIM: Perhaps as suggested by Littman, MCS is really a colony stimulating factor (CSF). As will be discussed in greater detail subsequently, CSF is a class of lymphokines which also activates macrophages to produce plasminogen activator, LAF, and increased phagocytosis. Thus it can mimic some of the biological effects of MAF.

MERGENHAGEN: Has Littman determined whether activated B cells produce factors which influence complement synthesis by monocytes?

LITTMAN: Supernates of antigen-stimulated sheep erythrocyte rosette-negative cells, mainly B cells and monocytes, do not produce MCS. On the other hand, T lymphocytes and monocytes do produce MCS under the same conditions and using cells from the same donor.

CHARACTERIZATION OF LYMPHOTOXIN AND TUMOR INHIBITION PROPERTIES IN A LYMPHOKINE PREPARATION DERIVED FROM THE CULTURED MOUSE L1210 LYMPHOMA[a]

B. W. Papermaster, J. E. McEntire, C. D. Gilliland
S. J. Buchok

Cancer Research Center
Columbia, Missouri

M. E. Smith

National Institutes of Health
Bethesda, Maryland

Lymphokine properties are detectable in the supernatant fluids of the mouse L1210 lymphoma which can be propagated in continuous culture in RPMI 1640 medium containing 10 percent FCS. The supernatant fluids can be concentrated by ultra filtration and lyophilization and contain MIF, lymphotoxin, chemotactic factor, macrophage activation factor, among other lymphokines. Such supernatants are capable of inducing regression, not only of the homologous (synergeneic) L1210 lymphoma, but also the allogenic B-16 melanomas. Preliminary purification and characterization of lymphotoxin is described. We conclude that malignant lymphoid cell lines may produce lymphokine molecules constitutively in a manner analogous to myeloma cells synthesizing immunoglobulins. As such, cultured lymphoid cell lines of mouse and human origin become useful tools for both production and genetic analysis of immunoregulatory molecules and their mechanisms of action.

[a]*These studies were supported in part by DHEW grant No. 1-RO1-25740-01.*

ISBN 0-12-213950-X

INTRODUCTION

Mediators of cellular immunity have been termed lymphokines by Dumonde and his associates (1). These have been reviewed extensively in recent symposia and review articles, and consist of a family of horomonal secretory products produced by both T and B lymphocytes involved in regulation of immune functions (2,3).

During the last decade, numerous long term cultured lymphoblast cell lines of both malignant and non-malignant origin have been shown to be sources of various lymphokines (4). Recently, de Weck et al. have studied a number of cultured human lymphoblastoid cell lines for their ability to produce different mediators and have reported these in a preliminary study*. We here report the use of the cultured mouse lymphoma L1210 cell line as a source of various lymphokine activities. Thus, L1210 is an excellent production source of mouse lymphokine molecules for molecular characterization and ultimate study of lymphokine regulation by molecular genetic techniques.

METHODOLOGY AND RESULTS

The L1210 cell line is propagated in RPMI 1640 medium containing 10 percent fetal calf serum and can routinely be grown from small inocula of 10^5 cells or less and has been cloned repeatedly (5). Alternation of *in vivo* and *in vitro* propagation tends to maintain the cell line's stability and malignancy and insures its histocompatibility and uniformity. The cultured cell line can be grown in concentrations up to 2 X 10^6 cells ml. These properties enable a high concentration of cells to be produced along with a cell line culture (5). Log phase growth is achieved in one or two days after inoculation and large volumes of 12 liters or more are maintained in spinner flasks of approximately 2 to 3 liters capacity. Cultures are pooled, the cells are removed by sedimentation at 800 X G and the supernatants are concentrated as described in methods. Conditions for cell growth are optimal between the pH range of 6.8 and 7.3, with supplementation by glutamine every 48 hours. A study of L1210 growth conditions by Dr. C. Stahli in our laboratories (personal communication) has indicated that glucose levels and key amino acids, phenylalanine and arginine, are critical for growth control of this

**Presented at annual meeting, FASEB, Dallas, Texas, April 10, 1979.*

cell line. Additional metabolic studies are underway regarding lymphokine production conditions. Methodology for the preparation of supernatant lymphokines has been described (4). More recent preparation steps include desalting and removal of dye over Sephadex G-25 and further separation on agarose A-5m and Sephadex G-200, electrophoresis on polyacrylamide and sodium dodecyl sulface (SDS) gels and affinity chromatography. Additional monitoring during preparation and purification can be obtained by exogenous labeling of proteins with ^{125}I or biosynthetically with ^{3}H-amino acids (6). Control materials are treated in an identical manner as active supernates and include 1) unfractionated starting material and 2) fractions from fresh culture medium (not incubated with cells) in order to rule out artifacts acquired during preparation or concentration. Starting materials, which have been partially separated on Sephadex G-200, and polyacrylamide gels have shown biologic activities associated with a large molecular weight fraction excluded from the G-200 gel filtration column and another fraction associated with albumin, as well as smaller molecular weight fractions. The active protein in the G-200 excluded peak was identified as alpha-2 macroglobulin, (α-2M). Both α-2M and albumin from the G-200 retained peak have been shown to act as carrier proteins for dissociable, smaller molecular weight-labeled fractions. Using an antialbumin affinity column and SDS gel electrophoresis, Smith, et al. have shown that biologically active lymphotoxin containing material could be separated from carrier protein in SDS gels and 6M guanidine-HCl columns (6).

A more detailed characterization of these fractions was obtained using biosynthetic labeling of cell secretory products with high specific activity (>40 ci/mmole) ^{3}H-aminoacids and exogenous labeling of the culture medium proteins with ^{125}I which allowed us to separate carrier and/or culture medium peptides from those synthesized by the cell. *In vitro* assays for lymphokine properties of tumor active supernatants have been described previously (4).

Two transplantable mouse tumors have provided preliminary quantitative information on the ability of lymphokine containing supernatants to induce tumor regression: 1) the L1210 lymphoma in DBA/2 mice propagated both as a subcutaneous and acites tumor and 2) the B-16 melanoma propagated subcutaneous tumor in C57/Bl mice. These tumors have been used extensively by the National Cancer Institute drug screening program for the determination of anticancer activity (7). In our studies up to the present time, comprising some 400 DBA mice and over

200 C57 mice, we have used the crude, partially fractionated supernatant material prepared as described above. We are presently utilizing more purified materials in our current studies obtained by acid or detergent extraction and chromatography or electrophoresis in dissociating solvents.

Lymphotoxin activity from L1210 cell lines was measured in concentrated lyophilized supernatants by trypan blue staining, measuring cell uptake of ^{3}H-thymidine, or release of Cytosol lactic dehydrogenase (LDH) by direct cell lysis as described by Smith et al. (6). Quantative measurements of specific activity could be made by dilution studies using the 50 percent killing level as an index of biologic activity and basis for calculation of specific activity measurements. Lymphotoxin activity has been partially purified from the albumin peak on Sephadex G-200 gel filtration columns and by elution from an anti-BSA affinity column (Fig. 1A) and elution by mannose from a Con A affinity column (6). The resulting material showed dissociation of ^{3}H counts from albumin in SDS gels and biologically active lymphotoxin with peaks at 12,500 and 25,000 daltons (Fig. 1B).

Tumor response curves were calculated by mean diameter of tumor size and median survival times. Tumors of 2 mm diameter could be recognized seven days after inoculation of L1210 tumor cells in a shaved area of the ventral surface of the abdominal subcutaneous tissue in DBA/2 mice. Inoculations of lymphokine containing materials or control substances began on the seventh day, intralesionally, and, in some groups, interperitoneally. Inoculations were continued either daily or three times a week, depending on the series and thereafter up to 20 to 25 days. The survival times of control and treated animals are indicated in Table I and the study of tumor growth as a measurement of tumor size is indicated in a similar study of tumor growth in C57 black mice bearing the B-16 melanoma. The result of these tumor studies clearly has shown that the administration of lymphokine containing supernatants alone will act to produce regression of subcutaneous tumors in several different ways: 1) tumor fails to grow at the same rate as control tumors; 2) the tumor undergoes a regression that essentially is complete, resulting in total slough of the tumor, scar formation, and healing of the original site of tumor growth; 3) the tumor undergoes partial regression, but eventually grows out, metastasizes and kills the animal in a delayed fashion. With fast growing tumors such as L1210, in the ascites form or even for complete eradication of B-16 melanoma, a combination of L1210 lymphokine containing prepar-

FIG. 1A. AFFINITY CHROMATOGRAPHY ON SEPHAROSE ANTI-BSA PROVIDES PARTIAL PURIFICATION OF L1210 LYMPHOTOXIN BOUND TO ALBUMIN. 10 MG OF PARTIALLY PURIFIED ALBUMIN CARRYING ^3H LABELLED SECRETED PRODUCTS WAS ADDED TO A COLUMN OF SEPHAROSE ANTI-BSA AND THE NON ADSORBED PROTEIN AND LABEL WAS ELUTED AT pH 7.4 IN 0.01M PO_4 AND 0.9% NaCL. THE ARROW INDICATES ADDITION OF ELUTION BUFFER, pH 2.2, 0.1M CH_3COONa, 0.5M NaCL WHICH RESULTED IN ELUTION OF THE FRACTION IN FIG. 1B.

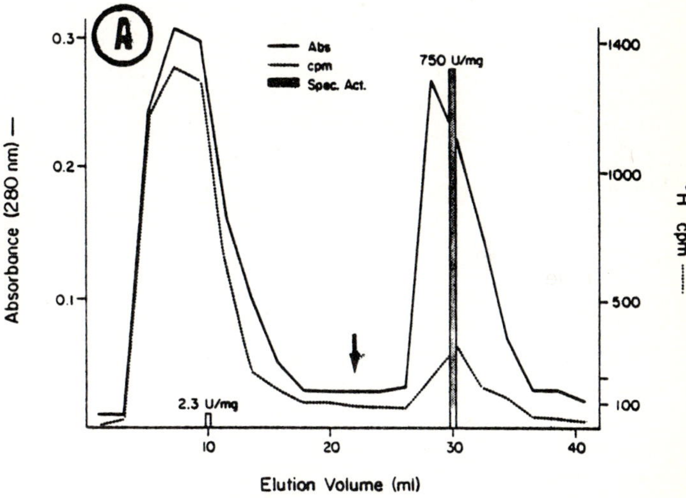

FIG. 1B. SDS-GEL ELECTROPHORESIS OF ALBUMIN BOUND LYMPHOTOXIN. THE FRACTION ELUTED AT pH 2.2 ABOVE WAS BOILED FOR 2 MINUTES IN 1% SDS CONTAINING 5% 2-MERCAPTOETHANOL. THIS MATERIAL WAS THEN SUBJECTED TO ELECTROPHORESIS IN 5.6% POLYACRYLAMIDE GELS IN 1% SDS, pH 7.4. THE MATERIAL WAS LABELLED WITH ^{125}I BEFORE REDUCTION AND DISSOCIATION. NOTE THAT ALL THE ^{125}I COUNTS FORM A SYMMETRICAL PEAK AT THE MIGRATION DISTANCE FOUND FOR BSA. THE ARROWS REFER TO M.W. CALIBRATION MARKERS. ALL OF THE ^3H LABELLED MATERIAL HAS DISSOCIATED FROM BSA.

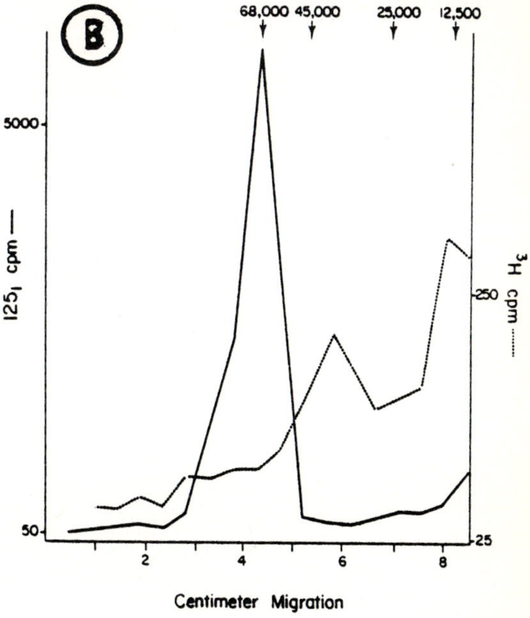

ations with MeCCNU** proved to be highly efficacious and produced prolongation of survival time. A particularly beneficial aspect of this chemoimmunotherapeutic combination was the excellent condition of the animals during drug treatment. The treated animals appeared to be healthier, lost less weight, and were more active than controls receiving the drug only, prompting us to begin some analogous Phase I chemoimmunotherapy trials in patients.

Table 1. Chemoimmunotherapy with MeCCNU and Lymphokines in L1210 Tumor Bearing Mice

Group	n	MST (in days)	100% kill
LK only	60	17	22
Tumor cells only	60	17	20
Medium control only	10	18	22
MeCCNU only (20-40 mg)	60	25	60 ($p<.01$)
Medium control + MeCCNU	10	21	22
LK + MeCCNU (20 mg)	50	25	35 ($p<.05$)
LK + MeCCNU (40 mg)	10	>75	(cured)

MeCCNU dose in mg/kg, LK = Lymphokine prep. as above was injected q 48 hr. for 21 days, n = sample size.

REFERENCES

1. Dumonde, D.C., Wolstencroft, R.A., Panayi, G.S., Matthew, M., Morley, J., and Howson, W.T. (1969). Nature, 224, 38
2. Cohen, S., David, J., Feldman, M., Glade, P.R., Mayer, M., Oppenheim, J.J., Papermaster, B.W., Pick, E., Pierce C.W., Rosenstreich, D.L., and Waksman, B.H. (1977). Cell. Immunol. 33, 233.
3. Yoshida, T., and Cohen, S. (1977). In "Mechanisms of Tumor Immunity" (I. Green, S.Cohen, and R.T. McClusky,eds.). p. 87, John Wiley and Sons, Inc., New York
4. Papermaster, B.W., Holtermann, O.A., Klein, E., Parmett, S., Dobkin, D., Laudico, R., and Djerassi, I. (1977). Clin. Immunol. Immunopathol. 5, 48.
5. Moore, G.E. and Ulrich, K. (1965). J. Surg. Res. 5,70.
6. Smith, M.E. and Papermaster, B.W. (1979). Purification of mouse lymphotoxins. Submitted for publication.

***Methyl 1-(2 chloroethyl)-3-(4 methylcyclohexyl)-1-nitrosourea (NSC 95441).*

LYMPHOTACTIN - A CHEMOTACTIC LYMPHOKINE FOR T CELLS

John C. Houck
Catherine M. Chang

Virginia Mason Research Center
Seattle, Washington

The lymphocyte population found in cutaneous delayed-type hypersensitivity has been shown to consist largely of cells not reactive to the immunologic stimulants which brought about the response (McCluskey, 1963). Approximately 95% of these lymphocytes were felt to be in the reactive area because of chemotaxis produced by the release, from a small number of sensitive lymphocytes, of an appropriate mediator. Recently Ward has shown that the supernatants from transformed, but not non-transformed, lymphocytes contain a material which can be shown to be chemotactic for lymphocytes in the Boyden Chamber assay (Ward, 1971). In the same paper it was pointed out that factors normally chemotactic for both polymorphonuclear leukocytes and macrophages had no effect chemotactically on lymphocytes. Finally, we have shown that thymus extracts contain a material which is specifically chemotactic for lymphocytes and which is not species-specific (Houck, 1976, 1977). This paper describes the purification of this lymphotactic material which we call "lymphotactin".

MATERIALS AND METHODS

Two batches of thymus from six-month-old vaccinated calves were pooled, representing three animals each and were extracted at $4^{o}C$ with 10 ml of 0.05 M tris buffer pH 7.4 per gm. After mincing and sonicating, the extract was allowed to stand at $4^{o}C$ overnight. After centrifugation, the clear supernatant was removed and passed through a 30,000 dalton Amicon ultrafilter and concentrated and dialyzed over a 10,000 dalton

ISBN 0-12-213950-X

Amicon ultrafilter. This fraction was centrifuged and lyophilized.

The thymus from three male Hartley strain guinea pigs (250 to 400 grams) were pooled and extracted in a similar fashion as was the thymus of two other groups of similar sized guinea pigs which had received four daily intraperitoneal injections of 5.4 μg/0.2 ml PPD_2 or PPD_2 and glycogen as has been described previously (Houck, 1973). Previous studies have indicated that only the immunologically stimulated guinea pig thymus extracts demonstrated significant amounts of lymphokine (i.e. Macrophage Inhibitory Factor activity); the immunologically unstimulated animals' thymus did not contain any MIF (Houck, 1973). Assays of lymphocyte chemotaxis were performed using the Boyden chamber assay as modified for lymphocytes by Ward (Ward, 1971) by using Millipore filters containing 5 μm holes. These chambers were obtained from Bellco Glass, Inc. (Bethesda, MD) and into one side of these chambers was introduced 5×10^6 lymphocytes obtained from Ficoll-Hypaque gradient purification (Boyum, 1968) from the peripheral blood of rabbits in a medium composed of Medium 199 supplemented with 20% calf serum in the appropriate amounts of Penn Strep and glutamine. These Boyden chambers were incubated with a test material on the other side of the Millipore filter for 17 hrs in a CO_2 incubator as has been described previously (Houck, 1976; Boyum, 1968). The lymphotactic activity of the various extracts was expressed as the mean number of lymphocytes per 5 microscopic fields (100 x) which had passed through the 5 μm Millipore filter and the ratio of these mean cell numbers to those demonstrated using only medium without the added fraction being tested, was calculated.

EXPERIMENTAL RESULTS

Crude isotonic saline extracts of the thymus from pools of guinea pig which had received PPD or PPD plus glycogen or merely IP injections of isotonic saline to serve as control, were, after dialysis and lyophilization, assayed for their chemotactic attraction for rabbit lymphocytes in the Boyden chamber system. The ratio of the number of cells that crawl through these filters when exposed to the test sample vs the saline control, are indicated in Table 1 and indicate that while normal, untreated guinea pig thymus apparently contains no chemotactic principle for these lymphocytes, after immunologic stimulation by PPD, a significant amount of such activity could be demonstrated. The addition of glycogen to serum to permit the release of the various products of the activation of complement which are known to be chemotactic for both polymorphonuclear leukocytes and macrophages (Ward, 1971) did not demonstrate any chemotactic activity toward lymphocytes under this assay system. It is clear from data of Table 1 that PPD and IP oyster glycogen treatment in vivo resulted in thymus tissue which contained considerably larger amounts of lymphotactic activity than did the PPD alone. Extracts of fetal or newborn calf thymus, however, demonstrated no lymphotactic and no MIF activity (Houck, 1973). Extracts of four-month-old calf lung, kidney and liver also contained no lymphotactic activity at any concentration in this assay system. Extracts of spleen were lymphotactic, however, at concentrations similar to that of thymus extracts.

TABLE 1

Chemotactic Effects of Various Amounts of Crude Lymphotactin Preparation in Vitro (Boyden chambers) and in Vivo (I.P., three guinea pigs after 18 h at 37°C)

Fraction (mg/ml)	in Vitro chemotactic ratio: Preparation I	in Vitro chemotactic ratio: Preparation II	in Vivo lymphocytes/peritoneal washout: Preparation II
0 (control)	—	—	0.5×10^6
1.0	1.5	2.0	42.0×10^6 [a]
5.0	1.6	2.3[a]	—
10.0	1.9[a]	2.7[a]	30.0×10^6 [a]
12.5	3.3[a]	4.1[a]	—
25.0	2.6[a]	3.5[a]	—

[a] Significantly different from 0 control ($P < .05$).

Three hundred grams of wet weight calf thymus was subjected to extraction, ethanol fractionation (30%) and Amicon ultrafiltration (10,000-30,000 D). This preparation was injected IP into three groups of 3 male 400 g Hartley guinea pigs each. One group received control isotonic saline IP; another group received 1 μg IP of ultrafiltered lymphotactin activity in 10 ml of saline which had been heated to 56° for 30 min and then cooled and the third group received unheated lymphotactin. After centrifugation and dilution, differential cell counts were performed in the usual fashion and the results are presented for each animal in Table 2. These data indicate that thermally inactivated or medium control IP injections produced no significant increases in the number of lymphocytes removed from 25 ml of peritoneal wash. Active lymphotactin increased the lymphocyte count IP by three to five fold, however.

TABLE 2

Effects of 1 μg of Crude Lymphotactin on the Differential Count of I.P. Cells 4 h after Injection

	Mean differential count			
Fraction	Monocytes ($\times 10^6$ cell)	Lymphocytes ($\times 10^6$ cell)	PMN ($\times 10^6$ cell)	Eosinophiles ($\times 10^6$ cell)
Control				
Animal 1	5.25	2.25	0	0
Animal 2	8.55	0.75	0	0
Animal 3	6.88	2.95	0	0
Inactive (56°C)				
Animal 4	5.90	3.88	0.35	2.56[a]
Animal 5	4.86	1.80	0	2.25[a]
Animal 6	6.67	2.26	0	2.37[a]
Active				
Animal 7	5.75	13.11[a]	4.14[a]	0
Animal 8	6.01	15.16[a]	0	1.43[a]
Animal 9	8.51	7.94[a]	0	1.52[a]

[a] Significantly higher than mean of controls ($P < .05$).

This ultrafiltered fraction which demonstrated both in vitro and in vivo chemotactic effects on lymphocytes, was subjected to isoelectric focussing over a pH gradient of 5-8 (Vesterberg, 1966). With a 1% Ampholine sucrose gradient, 206 mg were introduced into the isoelectric focusing device at 4°C and exposed to 600 volts for 48 hours. The results are presented in Fig. 1 with the fractions pooled as indicated. After extensive dialysis over a 10,000 dalton Amicon ultrafilter to remove sucrose and Ampholine, fraction 1 (with an isoelectric point ranging from pH 5.68 to 6.04) was the only peak demonstrating lymphotactic activity in the Boyden chamber system.

It was noticed that a large amount of lymphotactic activity had been lost after isoelectric focusing, probably during the dialysis required to remove sucrose. The isoelectric focusing procedure was repeated in the 5-8 pH range and sucrose and Ampholine were removed using a 1000 dalton Amicon ultrafilter (UM-2). A great deal more material remained when this membrane was used to accomplish dialysis. This material in turn was subjected at a concentration of 200 μg/gel to analytical acrylamide gel electrophoresis at 4°C at pH 9.5, 8 and 2.5 using 7.5% gels (Davis, 1964). Only 1 dense protein staining band could be demonstrated just behind the front; the position approximately equivalent to that of pre-albumin.

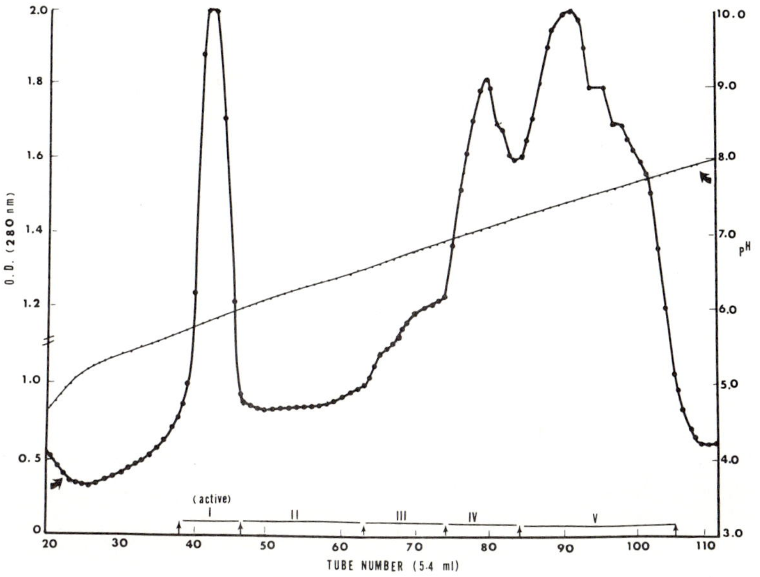

Fig. 1. Isoelectric focusing of 206 mg of ultrafiltered thymus extract in 1% Ampholine (pH 5.0-8.0) at 600 V for 48 h at 4°C. Fractions were collected at 5.4 ml/tube and pooled as indicated by roman numerals.

Concentrations of as little as 0.5 μg/ml of the eluted portions of the gel extracts demonstrated significant lymphotactin activity in the Boyden Chamber assay system (i.e. a chemotactic ratio of 3.4). The extracts of the non-staining areas of the unstained gels demonstrated no lymphotactic activity at all (i.e. the ratio was 0.9 to 1.1).

The molecular weight of the purified activity was determined using SDS gel electrophoresis (Weber, 1969) and G-75 exclusion chromatography. Both methods gave a molecular weight of 10,500 D. No evidence of any chemotactic activity by the purified lymphotactin towards either of polymorphonuclear leukocytes or macrophages could be demonstrated in this system. Purified lymphotactin from calf thymus was demonstrated to be equally chemotactic quantitatively toward both human and rabbit lymphocytes.

Preliminary studies utilizing fluorescent stains for immunoglobulins suggested that all of the lymphocytes which were found to migrate through the pores of the Millipore filter were in fact, T cells rather than B cell lymphocytes.

CONCLUSIONS

Thymus from immunologically experienced animals (calf and guinea pig) contains a specific chemotactic factor for T cell lymphocytes from either rabbit or man. This lymphotactic factor (or lymphotactin) is a sialoprotein weighing 10,500 D with an isoelectric point of approximately 5.9. It is thermolabile and destroyed by trypsin and sialidase digestion. It is not chemotactic for macrophages or polymorphonuclear leukocytes or B cell lymphocytes *in vitro*. It is also chemotactic for lymphocytes *in vivo* in guinea pigs. This non species-specific, but apparently T-cell specific, chemotactic substance cannot be found in tissue extracts other than thymus or spleen. We propose that this lymphotactin serves as a chemotactic signal when released by a small number of lymphocytes sensitive to a given antigen which will thereby amplify the immune response by recruiting inexperienced cells into contact with the antigen.

REFERENCES

Boyum, A. (1968). Scand. J. Clin. Lab. Invest., Suppl. 77.

Davis, B. (1964). Ann. N. Y. Acad. Sci. 121, 404.

Houck, J., and Chang, C. (1976) Inflammation 1, 217.

Houck, J., and Chang, C. (1977) Inflammation 2, 105.

Houck, J., Chang, C. and Platt, M. (1973) Proc. Soc. Exptl. Biol. Med. 143, 858.

McCluskey, R., Benacerrof, B., and McCluskey, J. (1963). J. Immunol. 90, 466.

Vesterberg, O., and Svenson, H. (1966). Acta Chem. Scand. 20, 820.

Ward, P., Offen, C., and Montgomery, J. (1971). Fed. Proc. 30, 21.

Weber, K., and Osborne, M. (1969). J. Biol. Chem. 244, 4406.

LYMPHOCYTE MEDIATOR MODULATION OF BASOPHIL MOTILE STRUCTURES[1]

Ann M. Dvorak
Stephen J. Galli
Anne Galli
M. Elizabeth Hammond
Harold F. Dvorak

Department of Pathology
Massachusetts General Hospital
Boston, Massachusetts

Basophils may participate in either immediate or delayed-type hypersensitivity reactions (A. Dvorak, 1978). Chemotaxis experiments suggest that the participation of basophils in delayed hypersensitivity reactions may be due to the generation of lymphokines by the sensitized lymphocytes present in such reactions (Ward, et al. 1975).

The present study was done to assess whether lymphokine-containing lymphocyte culture supernatants produce morphological alterations in guinea pig basophils that could be correlated with their behavior in chemotaxis experiments, and to compare such morphological alterations to those observed in other motile leukocytes. Because a preliminary report suggests that a factor(s) in the supernatant of mononuclear cell cultures releases histamine from human basophils (Theuson et al. 1977), we also looked for morphological or biochemical evidence of lymphokine-induced degranulation of guinea pig basophils.

[1]Supported by USPHS grant no. CA19141

ISBN 0-12-213950-X

Guinea pig basophils were incubated with lymphokine-containing lymphocyte culture supernatants or control supernatants dialyzed against culture medium, or culture medium alone for 1 to 72 hrs. Cell cultures were prepared by a variety of techniques for viewing by light microscopy, electron microscopy, for quantitation of basophil motile forms, and for determination of both cell-associated and released histamine.

Motile basophils were identified in all cultures and at all culture intervals examined. At 24 hrs. motile basophils were most abundant in cultures supplemented with MIF-containing lymphocyte supernatants, where they accounted for up to 64% of all viable basophils ($p < 0.05$ compared to cultures containing control lymphocyte culture supernatants (up to 58% motile) and $p < 0.0005$ compared to basophils cultured in medium alone (up to 45% motile), chi-square test).

Nonactivated basophils (Fig. 1A) were round with a variable surface composed of uniformly distributed villi and folds. Motile basophils, present either in control medium (Fig.1B), in control supernatants or in lymphokine-containing lymphocyte culture supernatants (Fig. 2), had a narrow, villi-covered cytoplasmic projection rich in glycogen and microfilaments, a

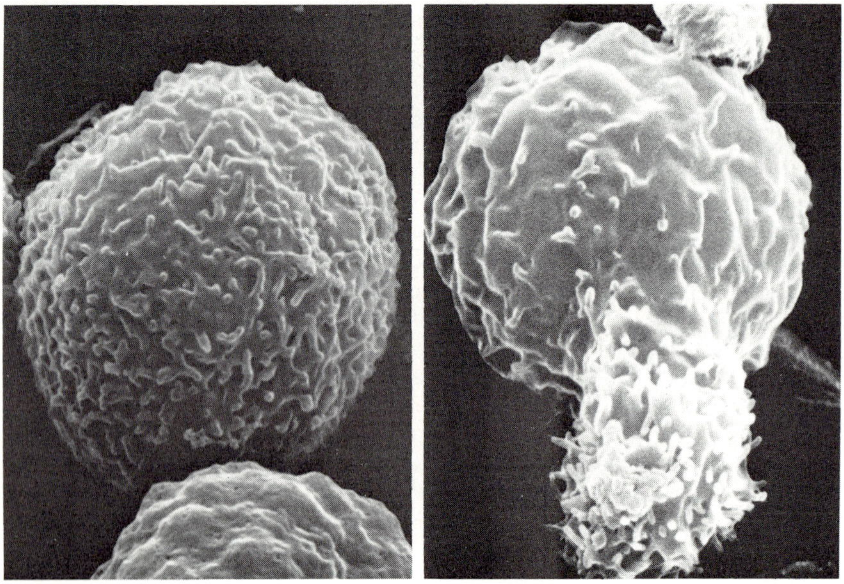

FIGURE 1. A round control basophil shows surface villi, ridges, and folds in A. The motile basophil in B, present in a complete medium control (MEM with 10% guinea pig serum), shows an elongated villi-covered motile structure. A&B, 11,000x.

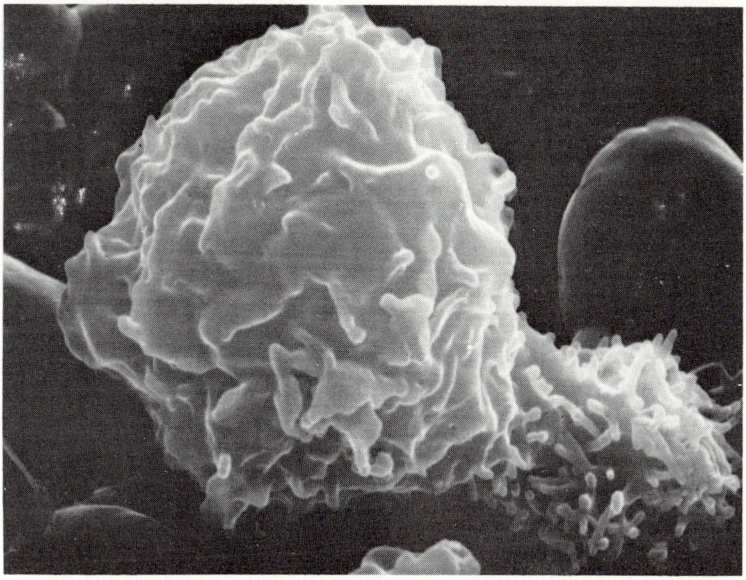

FIGURE 2. Activated basophil in the presence of lymphokine-containing lymphocyte culture supernatant shows an elongated motile structure and prominent smooth folds at the opposite cellular pole. 15,000x.

structure much like that previously described for lymphocytes. At the opposite (anterior)pole, motile basophils frequently exhibited a prominent complex of smooth-surfaced folds and ruffles which was both devoid of villi and relatively free of associated cytoplasmic organelles. There was neither morphological evidence of degranulation nor increased histamine release by motile basophils.

The increased numbers of motile basophils observed in cultures supplemented with lymphokine-containing lymphocyte supernatants could be due to the presence of basophil chemotactic factor(s), although other factors may also contribute to this phenomenon.

REFERENCES

Dvorak, A.M. (1978). In "Immediate Hypersensitivity: Modern Concepts & Developments" (M. Bach, ed.), Immunology Series, Vol. 7, p. 369, Marcel Dekker, Inc., New York.

Theuson, D.O., Speck, L., and Grant, J.A. (1977). Fed. Proc. 36,1300.

Ward, P.A., Dvorak, H.F., Cohen, S., Yoshida, T., Data, R., and Selvaggio, S.S. (1975). J. Immunol. 114, 1523.

COLONY STIMULATING ACTIVITIES (CSA) IN SUPERNATANTS OF DIFFERENT LEUKOCYTE CULTURES

Wulf-Diether Gassel
Herbert Laukel
Klaus Havemann

Medizinische Poliklinik und Klinik
Universität Marburg
Marburg, W. Germany

Human leukocyte cultures are known to produce colony stimulating activity (CSA) inducing granulocyte/macrophage progenitor cells (CFU-C) to form colonies in semisolid media (1). Human CFU-C inducing activity (CSAh) can be separated from an activity inducing mouse CFU-C (CSAm). Cultures were either performed with human bone marrow according to Robinson and Pike plating 200,000 non adherent cells (2) or with mouse marrow according to Bradley and Metcalf (3).

Cultures of Concanavalin A (ConA) stimulated spleen cells and peripheral mononuclear leukocytes, acute monocytic leukaemia (AMoL) cells as well as mixed lymphocyte cultures (MLC) were investigated for release of CSA. Appropriate unstimulated controls were studied in parallel. An example of the results obtained from a spleen cell culture demonstrating the release of CSAh is given in Fig. 1. Optimal conditions for release of CSAh were $1x10^7$ cells/ml and ConA concentrations of 5 µg/ml or more. Similar results were obtained with mononuclear leukocytes from peripheral blood. However, employing these conditions in the different culture systems the yield of CSAh showed great differences (Fig. 2). Except AMoL cells which already exhibited high spontaneous release without further augmentation after stimulation, stimulated cultures revealed a marked increase of CSAh as compared to control cultures. Stimulated spleen cells showed a more significant increase than cultures from other sources.

ISBN 0-12-213950-X

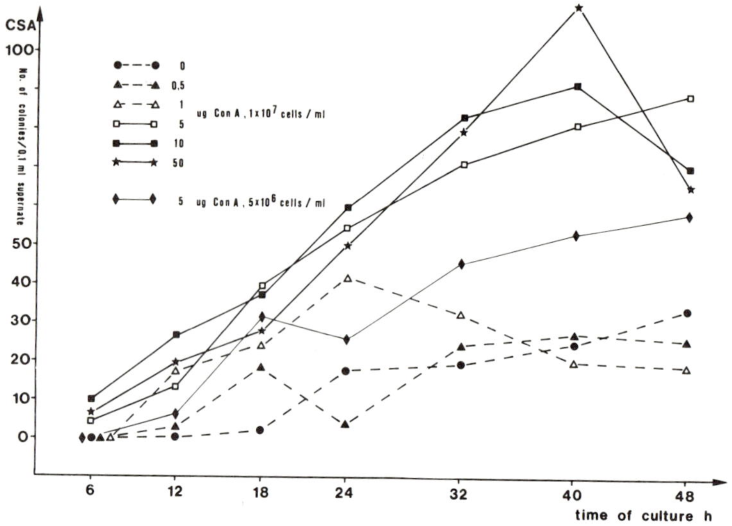

FIGURE 1. Kinetic of CSAh production in spleen cell culture: the activity of the supernatants depending on cell and Concanavalin A concentration per ml is demonstrated.

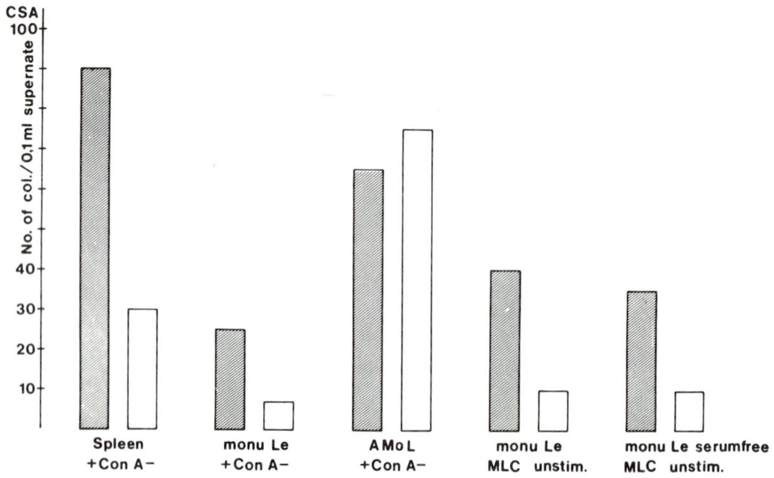

FIGURE 2. Yield of CSAh from different human stimulated (filled columns) and unstimulated (open columns) leukocyte cultures: MonuLe - peripheral mononuclear leukocytes, AMoL - acute monocytic leukaemia cells, ConA, MLC-mixed lymphocyte culture.

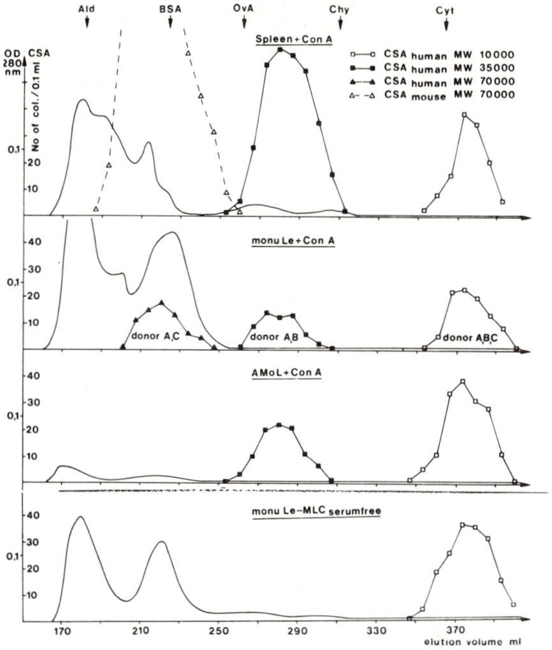

FIGURE 3. Elution profile of different leukocyte culture supernatants from Sephadex G 100 (OD 280 nm ——); the marker proteins are indicated on top.

Concentrated supernatants of the different stimulated cells were subjected to Sephadex G 100 chromatography; the fractions were tested on mouse and human bone marrow (Fig. 3). Up to three human activities could be separated showing molecular weights of 70,000, 35,000, and 10,000 daltons. In addition, one CSAm (MW 70,000) was found in the cultures (see also Havemann et al. following contribution of this symposium). Spleen and AMoL cell supernatants revealed two activities, whereas mononuclear leukocytes produced up to three CSAh with changing combinations in different donors but with identical pattern in succeeding cultures of the same donor. Isoelectric focusing of the G 100 separated activities showed coincident isoelectric points of CSAh with corresponding molecular weight, suggesting identity between these activities from different leukocyte cultures (Fig. 4).

Furthermore, antisera were produced against the Sephadex G 100 fraction of CSAh 35,000 and 10,000 . Since CSAh 10,000

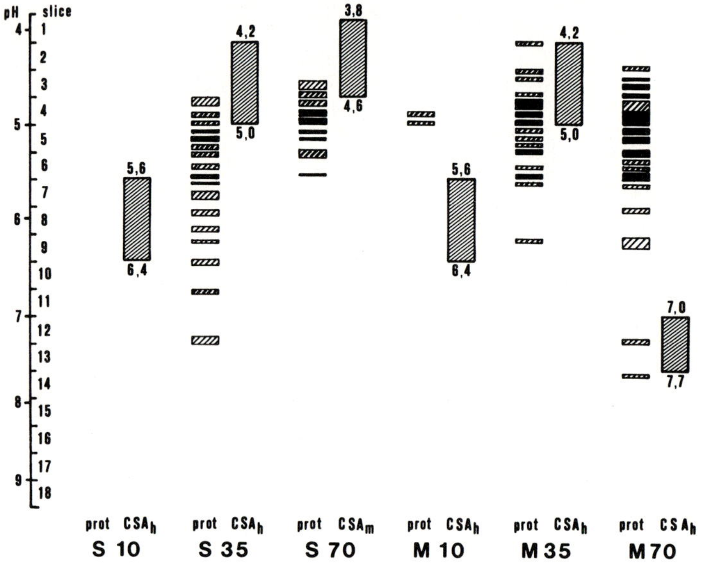

FIGURE 4. Scheme of isoelectric focusing of different CSA preseparated by Sephadex G 100 chromatography. S - spleen; M - peripheral mononuclear leukocytes; 10, 35, 70 - MW x 1000. The protein bands (prot) and the range of the eluted activity (CSA) are shown.

did not show detectable protein bands after IEF the AS exhibited no precipitation with serum proteins or the G 100 fractions. On the other hand, as expected from IEF AS-CSAh 35,000 still precipitated with a number of serum proteins. Experiments to inhibit colony formation by these antisera are in progress.

REFERENCES

Parker, J.W., Metcalf, D. (1974). J.Immunol. 112, 502.
Robinson, W.A., Kurnick, J.E., Pike, B.L. (1971). Blood 38, 500.
Bradley, T.R., Metcalf, D. (1966). Aust.J.exp.Biol.med.Sci. 44, 287.

DISCUSSION

LEON: I would like to offer for consideration a more general approach to the problem of studying factors such as CSF which apparently exist in a range of different molecular weights. *Partial* absorption with target cells might preferentially remove material of one molecular weight, in which case it would be assumed that this was the most active biological state of the factor. Alternatively, removal of equivalent amounts of each molecular weight form would be indicative of equivalent biological activity.

FARRAR: In our laboratory Harrar and Moore have induced macrophage-depleted T cells to make CSF following stimulation with Con A, under conditions in which the T cells do not make mitogenic factor. To me this suggests that murine T cells produce CSF.

INDICATION FOR IDENTITY OF MOUSE MYELOPOIETIC PROGENITOR CELL INDUCING ACTIVITIES (CSA) FROM HUMAN LEUKOCYTES AND HUMAN URINE

Klaus Havemann
Herbert Laukel
Wulf-Diether Gassel

Medizinische Klinik und Poliklinik
Universität Marburg
Marburg, W. Germany

Colony stimulating activity (CSAm) inducing mouse bone marrow cells (CFU-C) to form colonies of monocytes and/or granulocytes in semisolid medium (1) is produced by different human leukocyte culture systems (2,3). A factor identical in its biological behaviour called colony stimulating factor (CSF) is excreted in human urine. Because of this identical biological activity the question arises whether these factors are identical by biochemical and immunological means.

The technique employed to purify CSF is demonstrated in Tab. I. In the final step of isoelectric focusing (IEF) biological activity is distributed over a broad pH range. The bulk of activity with isoelectric point lower than pH 4.0 could be separated completely from remaining protein impurities (Fig. 1a). This material eluted from a preparative IEF run (slice 3) was used to raise an antiserum (AS) in rabbits. Immunoelectrophoretic analysis showed one distinct precipitation line with the eluted material from slice 4 of the same run whereas an AS against the Phenylsepharose step - inspite of its capacity to inhibit colony formation - showed no precipitation (Fig. 2). The AS against IEF slice 3 proved to be a potent inhibitor of colony formation in the culture system (Tab. II).

Different human unstimulated and stimulated leukocyte cultures from peripheral mononuclear cells (Ficoll mononuclear cells) and spleen cells are known to produce CSA active on mouse CFU-C. The yield of activity increases with the duration of culture (Fig. 3). To compare these CSA from the different leukocyte sources with urinary CSF (MW 70,000 D) concentrated culture supernatants were subjected to Sephadex G 100 chromatography. As shown in Fig. 4 CSAm always elutes at a MW of 70,000 D. Further chromatographic analysis employing anion-exchange and hydrophobic interaction chromatography showed an

ISBN 0-12-213950-X

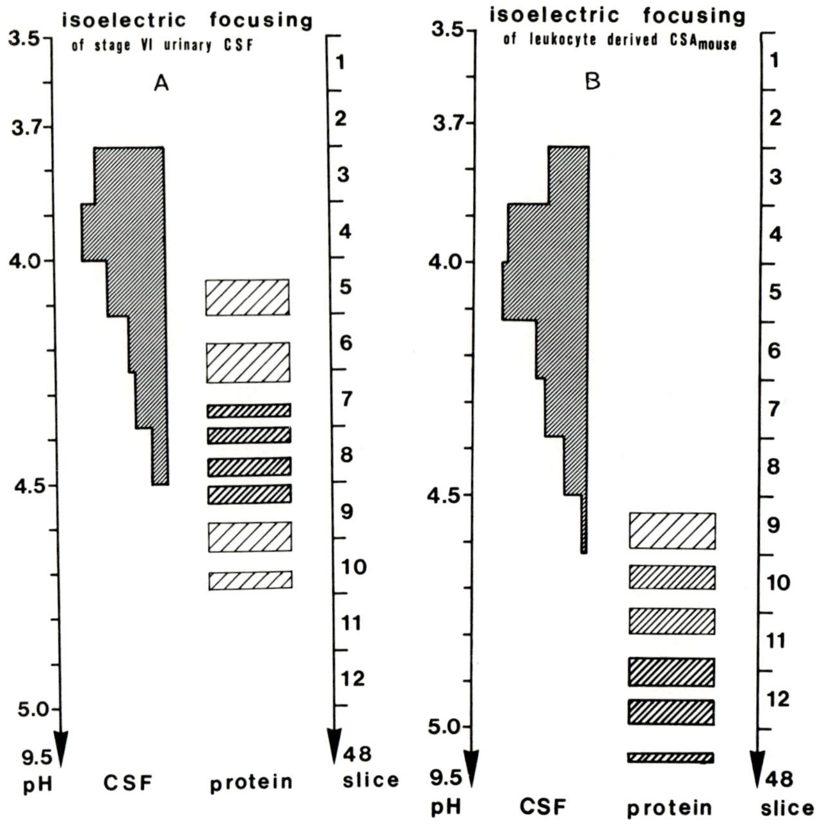

FIGURE 1. Isoelectric focusing pattern of human urinary CSF, immunoabsorption step (a) and human peripheral mononuclear cell derived CSA active on mouse bone marrow (b). The distribution of biological activity and the protein bands are shown schematically.

TABLE I **Purification procedure of human urinary CSF**

hemodialysis (artificial kidney)	NaCl $<$ 0.05 M
ionexchange (Whatman DE 32)	contin. 0.05-0.4 M NaCl gradient (0.13-0.18 M)
affinity chromatography (Con A-Sepharose)	0.15 M α methyl D mannoside
gelfiltration (Sephadex G 100)	MW: 70,000
hydrophobic interaction (Phenyl-Sepharose)	contin. 25 % sat. -0% $(NH_4)_2SO_4$ / 0 % - 50% ethyleneglycol gradient (13.5% sat. $(NH_4)_2SO_4$; 23% EG)
hydroxylapatit	contin. 0.005-0.1 M Na-phosphateb. pH 7.0 gradient (0.02-0.04 M)
immunadsorption IgG-antihumanserum-Seph.	elimination of serum proteins
isoelectric focusing (PAG plate pH 3.5-9.5)	IEP pH 3.8-4.6

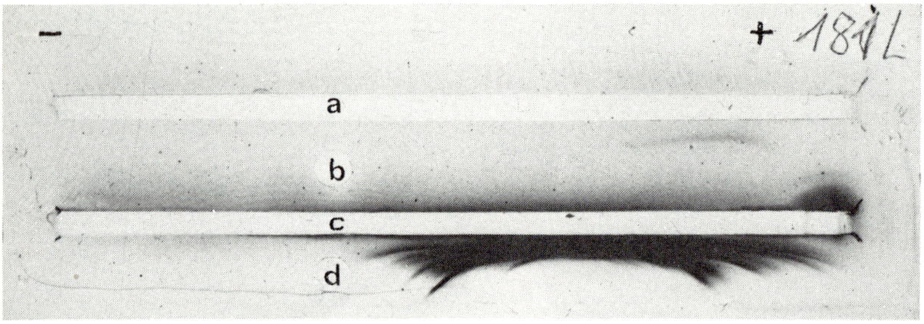

FIGURE 2. Immunoelectrophoretic analysis of antisera against different purification steps of human urinary CSF.
a rabbit antiserum against IEF slice 3 eluted material
b IEF slice 4 eluted material
c rabbit antiserum against the Phenylsepharose step material
d Phenylsepharose step material
Whereas b is precipitated by forming one single line with alpha1 mobility, there is no reaction with c because of its lower titer of anti-CSF. The much lower degree of purification of d is indicated by its reaction with c.

identical behaviour of leukocyte derived CSAm and urinary CSF. They elute from DEAE at 0.15M NaCl and from Phenylsepharose by a gradient concentration of 13.5% ammonium sulfate and 23% ethyleneglycol. In addition, the IEP of both the leukocyte and the urine derived factors are identical (Fig. 1).

TABLE II Antiserum inhibition of human urinary CSF and leukocyte derived CSA_{mouse}

500 (µl)	urinary CSF +		spleen + Con A +		blood MNC + Con A +		blood MNC - MLC +	
	NS	AS	NS	AS	NS	AS	NS	AS
100	82	-	73	-	78	-	80	-
50	87	-	78	-	81	-	88	-
10	99	-	87	-	89	-	93	-
7,5	101	-	96	-	94	-	97	-
5,0	98	5	100	3	102	-	95	3
2,5	105	41	102	46	106	39	101	54
1,0	107	80	98	74	103	71	97	78
0.5	103	93	106	87	99	86	108	89

Antiserum (AS):	rabbit antiserum against purified human urinary CSF (0.1 ml AS inhibits about 12.000 colonies of the urinary CSF)
Control:	normal rabbit serum (NS)
CSA preparations:	adapted to about 100 colonies /0.1 ml
Incubation:	1 h, 37°C
Colony counts:	colonies/0.1 ml

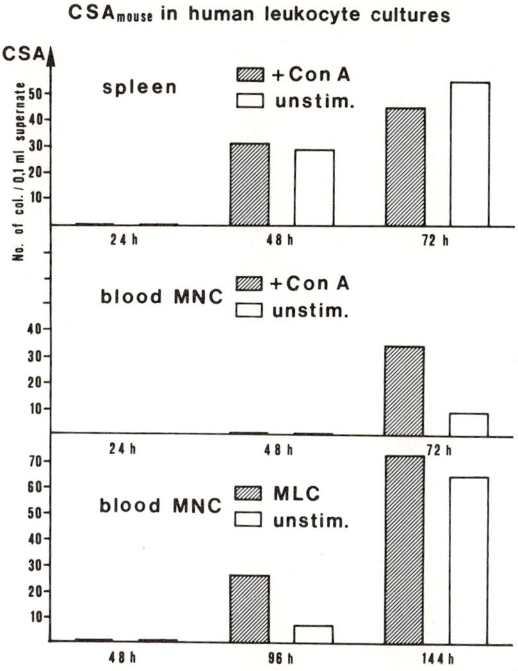

FIGURE 3. Kinetic of CSAm production of human stimulated and unstimulated cultures of spleen cells and peripheral mononuclear cells.

The IgG fraction of the described AS against purified urinary CSF (IEF slice 3) was tested in its capacity of inhibit CSAm from the different human leukocyte culture supernatants prepared by Sephadex G 100 chromatography. As shown in Tab.II complete inhibition of both mononuclear leukocyte and spleen cell CSAm was achieved by sufficient amounts of the antiserum. A 50% inhibition of the CSAm preparations inducing 1,000 colonies was obtained with about 50 μg protein of the IgG fraction. On the other hand the AS was completely inactive against CSA inducing human CFU-C (see Gassel, W.D. et al., preceeding contribution of this symposium).

The data indicate a complete identity of urinary CSF and human leukocyte derived CSAm. The cellular origin of this factor is uncertain. However, preliminary experiments employing the AS in immunofluorescence staining indicate that the monocytes present in the leukocyte preparation might be responsible for the factor production. The relation between CSAm and CSA inducing human CFU-C both generated in human leukocyte cultures is unknown. Since the described AS does not

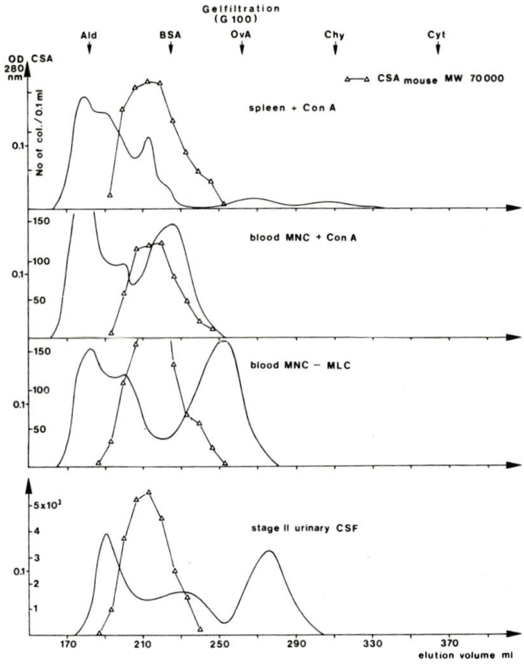

FIGURE 4. Sephadex G 100 elution profile of CSAm from different leukocyte sources.

inhibit human CSA common antigenic determinants between both groups of factors are unprobable. Furthermore the delayed production of CSAm in culture, its higher molecular weight and its higher degree of glycosilation (CSAm binds to Concanavalin A Sepharose) as compared to leukocyte derived CSA inducing human CFU-C suggest that both factors are not related to each other.

REFERENCES

Bradley, T.R., Metcalf, D. (1966(. Aust.J.exp.Biol.med.Sci. 44, 287.

Lind, E.D., Bradley, M.L., Gunz, F.W., Dickey, C.D. (1974). J.Cell.Physiol. 83, 35.

Parker, J.W., Metcalf, D. (1974). J.Immunol. 112, 502.

PRODUCTION OF COLONY-STIMULATING FACTOR AND ERYTHROID-POTENTIATING ACTIVITY BY A HUMAN T-LYMPHOCYTE CELL LINE

David W. Golde
Shirley G. Quan
Noelle Bersch
Aldons J. Lusis

Department of Medicine
UCLA School of Medicine
Los Angeles, California

Our laboratory has derived a human T-lymphocyte cell line that constitutively produces several T-lymphocyte products including colony-stimulating factor (CSF) and erythroid-potentiating activity (EPA). The cell line (Mo) was established from spleen cells from a patient with a T-cell variant of hairy-cell leukemia. The cells have been growing in culture for over two years and they maintain their T-lymphocyte properties. The CSF is continuously elaborated, and medium conditioned by the cells is 20% more potent than a human peripheral blood feeder layer in stimulating human granulocyte-monocyte colonies (CFU-C). The CSF has a molecular weight of about 35,000 daltons and stimulates monkey CFU-C but has no effect on rodent bone marrow. The Mo cell line also produces a material that potentiates human erythroid colony formation in vitro. The EPA is distinguishable from CSF on the basis of differential heat stability. The Mo EPA is a protein of approximately 50,000 daltons which is able to withstand at least 10 minutes of boiling without substantial loss of activity. The Mo EPA is ineffective against murine bone marrow. The Mo cell line should be an important source for the purification of human T cell-derived humoral factors involved in the regulation of hematopoiesis.

ISBN 0-12-213950-X

INTRODUCTION

T lymphocytes are known to have important functional interactions with stem cells in the regulation of hematopoiesis (1). A well-defined humoral interaction involves the T-cell production of CSF, a granulopoietic hormone necessary for the in vitro growth of precursors of monocytes and granulocytes (CFU-C) (2,3). Recently, evidence has accumulated to suggest that lymphocytes can release a factor which potentiates the growth of primitive erythroid precursors in vitro (4,5). Although erythropoietin is the primary humoral modulator of erythropoiesis, the lymphocyte-derived potentiator is thought to play an important role in the regulation of the early steps in erythroid development. We have derived a human T-lymphocyte cell line that produces both CSF and erythroid-potentiating activity (EPA).

METHODS AND RESULTS

A. Mo Cell Line

The Mo cell line was derived from the spleen of a patient with a T-cell variant of hairy-cell leukemia (6). The cells grow continuously in suspension culture, singly and in clumps, and exhibit the morphology of lymphoblasts. The cells are not infected with Epstein-Barr virus and they do not produce immunoglobulin (7). The Mo cells respond to phytohemagglutinin and are lysed by antithymocyte serum and complement. Over 60% of the Mo cells rosette with sheep erythrocytes and they contain the marker isozyme 5 of acid phosphatase characteristic of hairy-cell leukemia. The cell line can also grow in serum-free medium.

B. Production of Colony-stimulating Factor

The Mo cell line constitutively releases a protein (35,000 MW) capable of stimulating CFU-C (8). Activity is detectable in medium at concentrations below 5 μl/ml and maximum activity is usually seen at 25 μl/ml. At this latter concentration stimulation is 10 to 20% greater than that obtained using a feeder layer of peripheral blood leukocytes. In the presence of PHA there is augmented production of CSF (8). The Mo CSF is directly active in stimulating CFU-C from primate and human hematopoietic tissue but it does not directly stimulate rodent CFU-C.

C. Production of EPA

We used a standard methylcellulose technique for cloning small erythroid colonies (CFU-E) from normal human bone marrow and large erythroid clones (BFU-E) from peripheral blood (4,9,10). The culture system contained alpha medium with 30% fetal calf serum and 10^{-4} M α-thioglycerol. Mo EPA did not stimulate murine erythroid progenitors. As can be seen in Figure 1, Mo-conditioned medium caused a dose-dependent increase in CFU-E in cultures not containing added erythropoietin. Peak stimulation occurred at 50 μl/ml. At high concentrations of erythropoietin (> 1 U/ml) the Mo-conditioned medium had little stimulatory effect. If the Mo EPA was boiled for 5 minutes, the inhibition seen at high erythropoietin concentrations was removed and prominent potentiation of erythroid cloning could be observed at all erythropoietin concentrations up to 2 U/ml (Fig. 2). Mo EPA stimulated BFU-E from peripheral blood as well as bone marrow-derived CFU-E (Fig. 3).

The heat stability of EPA provided a simple means to separate the CSF and EPA molecules. After 5 minutes at 100°C

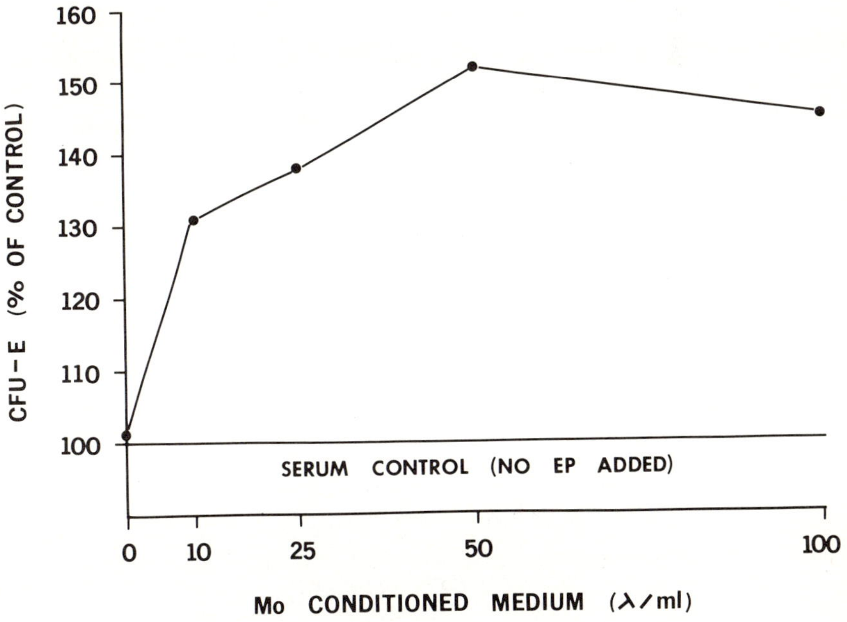

FIGURE 1. Effect of Mo-conditioned medium on human CFU-E without exogenous erythropoietin.

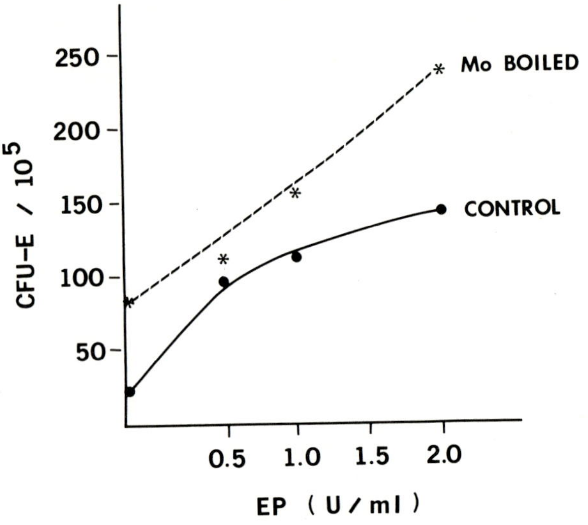

FIGURE 2. Effect of boiled Mo-conditioned medium on human CFU-E - erythropoietin dose-response relationship.

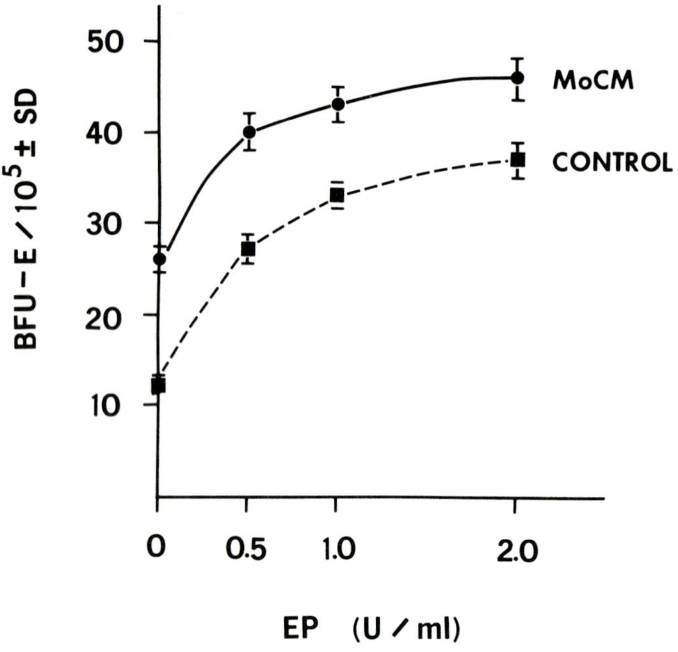

FIGURE 3. Effect of Mo-conditioned medium on growth of human peripheral blood bursts (BFU-E).

greater than 95% of the CSF activity was lost whereas EPA activity was fully retained. Mo EPA was sensitive to various proteases and had an apparent molecular weight of approximately 50,000 daltons as determined by gel filtration chromatography.

DISCUSSION

T-lymphocyte products have important effects on hematopoietic stem cells (1). The best characterized of the lymphocyte products affecting hematopoiesis are CSF and a factor which potentiates erythropoiesis in vitro. The Mo cell line is unique in that it is the only human T-cell line which constitutively produces both of these humoral mediators. The data reported here indicate that the Mo cell line produces high concentrations of both EPA and CSF and that these factors are separable by heat stability and size. The Mo cell line should provide the means to effectively purify and characterize these important hematopoietic hormones.

REFERENCES

1. Cline, M.J., and Golde, D.W. (1979). *Nature 277,* 177.
2. Cline, M.J., and Golde, D.W. (1974). *Nature 248,* 703.
3. Parker, J.W., and Metcalf, D. (1974). *J. Immunol. 112,* 502.
4. Iscove, N.N. (1978). *In* "Hematopoietic Cell Differentiation" (D.W. Golde, M.J. Cline, D. Metcalf, and C.F. Fox, eds.), p. 37. Academic Press, New York.
5. Metcalf, D., and Johnson, G.R. (1978). *J. Cell. Physiol. 96,* 31.
6. Saxon, A., Stevens, R.H., and Golde, D.W. (1978). *Ann. Intern. Med. 88,* 323.
7. Saxon, A., Stevens, R.H., Quan, S.G., and Golde, D.W. (1978). *J. Immunol. 120,* 777.
8. Golde, D.W., Quan, S.G., and Cline, M.J. (1978). *Blood 52,* 1068.
9. Golde, D.W., Bersch, N., and Li, C.H. (1977). *Science 196,* 1112.
10. Ogawa, M., Grush, O.C., O'Dell, R.F., Hara, H., and MacEachern, M.D. (1977). *Blood 50,* 1081.

INTERACTION BETWEEN MURINE LYMPHOID CELLS IN GENERATING A LPS-INDUCED LYMPHOKINE(CSF)

D.H. Pluznik, R.N. Apte, Ch.F. Hertogs & R. Lenz

Department of Life Sciences
Bar-Ilan University
Ramat-Gan, Israel

I. INTRODUCTION

Committed hemopoietic progenitor cells for granulocyte/macrophage differentiation, proliferate in soft agar cultures to form colonies of mature granulocytes and macrophages (1,2). Colony formation is dependent upon continuous presence of a regulatory glycoprotein designated colony stimulating factor (CSF) (3). Murine lymphoid cells incubated with a B-cell mitogen, bacterial lipopolysaccharide (LPS) elaborate CSF (4). The cellular interactions involved in generation of this LPS-induced CSF,as well as partial identification of the cellular receptors to this CSF will be described in the present study.

II. MATERIALS AND METHODS

Spleen cells or separated lymphoid cell populations were cultured in RPM1-1640 supplemented with 5% horse serum for different intervals of time. Splenic lymphocytes were obtained by passage of spleen cells through two successive pyrex wool columns. Macrophages were obtained from the peritoneal cavity of mice injected 3 days before with 10% proteose peptone. Soft agar cultures were performed according to Pluznik & Sachs (5). Supernatants of lymphoid cell cultures were incorporated into the base layer of the agar cultures as a source of CSF, at a final concentration of 15%. 10^5 bone marrow cells/plate were seeded onto the upper agar layer. Cultures were incubated for 7 days and thereafter colonies were counted microscopically. The number of colonies per plate reflects the colony stimulating activity in the tested

ISBN 0-12-213950-X

culture fluids. It was found that 15% CSF/plate gave maximal colony formation.

III. RESULTS AND DISCUSSION

Spleen cell cultures (2×10^6/ml), when incubated for four days in the presence of an optimal dose of LPS (50µg/ml), elaborated large amounts of CSF. When such cell suspensions were passaged through two successive pyrex wool adherence columns, in order to deplete adherent macrophages, the ability of the nonadherent effluent cells to secrete CSF in response to LPS decreased to 28 colonies/10^5 BM cells. Isolated splenic lymphocytes ($2\text{x}10^6$/ml), when mixed with $2\text{x}10^5$/ml of proteose peptone-induced peritoneal macrophages, and incubated for four days with LPS (50µg/ml), released optimal levels of CSF to culture fluids (181 colonies/10^5 BM cells). Macrophages themselves, when cultured at the same cell concentrations as those added to lymphocytes, secreted only small amounts of CSF (25 colonies/10^5 BM cells).

To elucidate the nature of the cellular interactions between macrophages and lymphocytes, in the process of generation of CSF, the following experiments were performed. Macrophage supernatants were prepared by incubating proteose peptone-induced peritoneal macrophages ($2\text{x}10^6$/ml for 24 h with or without LPS (50µg/ml), and the culture fluids were thereafter collected and diluted 1:2 in culture medium. Lymphocytes ($2\text{x}10^6$/ml) were suspended in such macrophage supernatants and were subsequently cultured for four days either with or without LPS (50µg/ml). The culture fluids of such lymphocyte suspensions were incorporated into the agar as a source of CSF at a final concentration of 15%. The results shown in Table I indicate that active macrophage supernatants were generated when LPS was added to cultures, and such supernatants could activate lymphocytes to secrete CSF even when

TABLE I. Effect of Supernatants from LPS-stimulated MØ or LY on Generation of CSF by MØ or LY

MØ-Sup	*Colonies/10^5 BM cells*		*LY-Sup*	*Colonies/10^5 BM cells*	
LY	*-LPS*	*+LPS*	*MØ*	*-LPS*	*+LPS*
-LPS	11	155	*-LPS*	11	34
+LPS	63	142	*+LPS*	18	23

the lymphocyte cultures were not stimulated by LPS. Supernatants prepared from macrophage cultures not stimulated by LPS manifested only a weak lymphostimulatory activity and addition of LPS to such lymphocyte cultures improved only partially the secretion of CSF.

In order to test whether the interactions between macrophages and lymphocytes are bidirectional, $2x10^5$ macrophages were suspended in lymphocyte supernatants and were cultured for four days with or without LPS (50μg/ml), and colony stimulating activity was tested in the culture fluids. Lymphocyte supernatants were prepared by culturing isolated splenic lymphocytes ($2x10^6$/ml) for 72 h in culture medium supplemented with LPS (50μg/ml). These cell concentrations of both macrophages and lymphocytes, used in the present experiments, were the optimal cell concentrations for LPS-induced CSF generation in the macrophage-lymphocyte mixed cultures. The results of such a representative experiment are shown in Table I. It is obvious, that macrophages were not activated to generate significant amounts of CSF by LPS-induced lymphocyte supernatants. Thus, generation of CSF in macrophage-lymphocyte mixed cultures seems to occur via unidirectional pathway whereby LPS-stimulated macrophages secrete soluble lymphostimulatory factor(s) which, in turn, activate lymphocytes to secrete CSF.

The availability of LPS-low and high-responder strains of mice provided us with a useful tool for further characterization of the mechanisms involved in generation of CSF in lymphoid cell cultures. C3H/HeJ mice are known to be low responders to the differential effects induced by LPS (6-8). LPS-induced macrophage supernatants were prepared from macrophage cultures of C3H/HeJ mice as well as from such cultures of LPS-high responder mice of the inbred strain C3H/eB. The activity

TABLE II. Lymphostimulatory Effect of LPS-stimulated Macrophage Supernatants from LPS Low (C3H/HeJ) and High (C3H/eB)-Responder Mice

Source of MØ-Sup	*Source of LY*	*Colonies/10^5 BM cells*
C3H/eB	*C3H/eB*	153
	C3H/HeJ	163
C3H/HeJ	*C3H/eB*	56
	C3H/HeJ	47

of each type of macrophage culture fluid was cross-tested on lymphocytes from both strains of mice. The results of these experiments are shown in Table II. Macrophages obtained from C3H/HeJ mice did not elaborate any significant lymphocyte helper activity. However, such macrophage supernatants generated by macrophages from LPS-high responder mice (C3H/eB) succeeded to activate lymphocytes from C3H/HeJ mice which, in turn, secreted large amounts of CSF. These data indicate that a soluble factor rather than residual LPS is the major stimulating moiety in the macrophage supernatants which activates B cells. In addition, these data strengthen the fact that the macrophages interact with LPS while the lymphocytes release the CSF.

Lymphocytes from congenitally athymic nude mice secrete normal levels of CSF when activated by LPS-stimulated macrophage supernatants from conventional mice. Thus, CSF can be regarded as a B-cell lymphokine.

Partial identification of the receptors of CSF, present on committed hemopoietic cells was elucidated by two types of experiments. In the first type of experiments cholera toxin was used. This toxin is known for its binding to membranal gangliosides (9). Bone marrow cells were preincubated at room temperature with increasing concentrations (10^{-7}M - 10^{-11}M) of this toxin for 20 min before cloning in soft agar supplemented with 15% CSF. Results of such experiments are shown in Table III. It can be seen that preincubation with cholera toxin reduced the precent of colonies growing in soft agar suggesting a competition with CSF on membranal gangliosides. The same results were obtained when a non-toxic preparation of cholera toxin was used. In the second type of experiments gangliosides were preincubated with CSF for 1 h

TABLE III. Competition Between Cholera Toxin and CSF on Receptors Present on Committed Hemopoietic Progenitor Cells

Cholera toxin (M)	*% Colonies/10^5 BM*
10^{-11}	100
10^{-10}	94
10^{-9}	53
10^{-8}	27
10^{-7}	0

TABLE IV. Inhibition of CSF Activity by Gangliosides

Gangliosides mg/culture	*% Colonies/10^5 BM cells*
0	*100*
0.25	*65*
0.50	*45*
0.75	*15*
1.00	*5*

at 37°C before incorporating it in the soft agar cultures. Data presented in Table IV show that such preincubation of gangliosides with CSF reduced the effectivity of CSF to stimulate clonal growth of BM cells.

REFERENCES

1. Pluznik, D.H., and Sachs, L., *J. Cell. Comp. Physiol. 66*, 319 (1965).
2. Bradley, T.R., and Metcalf, D., *Aust. J. Exp. Biol. Med. Sci. 44*, 287 (1966).
3. Stanley, E.R., Hansen, G., Woodcock, J., and Metcalf, D., *Fed. Proc. 34*, 2272 (1975).
4. Chervenick, P.A., *J. Lab. Clin. Med. 79*, 1014 (1972).
5. Pluznik, D.H., and Sachs, L., *Exp. Cell Res. 43*, 553 (1966).
6. Sultzer, B.M., *Infect. Immun. 5*, 107 (1972).
7. Watson, J., and Riblet, R., *J. Exp. Med. 140*, 1147 (1974).
8. Apte, R.N., Hertogs, Ch.F., and Pluznik, D.H., *J. Immunol. 118*, 1435 (1977).
9. Cuatrecasas, P., *Biochemistry 12*, 3547 (1973).

DISCUSSION

de WECK: Pluznik stated that CBA/N cells can produce CSF after LPS stimulation but that these cells do not produce mitogenic factors. I ask whether CBA/N cells are not merely insensitive to mitogenic factor(s)? Has he tested whether CBA/N cells are capable of producing mitogenic factors by testing the activity of CBA/N supernatants on third party cells?

PLUZNIK: What I said was that CBA/N mice do not respond to LPS by the regular mitogenic reaction; however, they are capable of responding to LPS as manifested by their generating CSF. I have no idea whether CBA/N mice produce LPS-induced mitogenic factors.

AX: Would Pluznik tell us more about the placenta as a source of CSF etc. What is known about the origin of this activity - is this produced upon cultivation, or merely released?

PLUZNIK: The CSF activity from mouse placenta is obtained by preparing an extract of the whole uterus of the pregnant mouse; this involves no need for cultivation of the tissues in vitro to release CSF into a culture supernatant.

MERGENHAGEN: CSF is regulated by prostaglandins. If one incorporates indomethacin in the culture medium of LPS-stimulated macrophages, CSF production increases up to 20-fold. The influence of indomethacin can be reversed by adding exogenous PGE_1 or E_2. The effect of prostaglandin on inhibiting CSF production is apparently mediated by its influence on c-AmP.

DAVID: Since macrophages and monocytes can make CSF, it is difficult to attribute mononuclear preparations of CSF to lymphocyte contamination. Can Pluznik give us the evidence that lymphocytes themselves make CSF? I was interested to learn of a ganglioside possibly acting as a receptor for CSF. We have been working on a putative receptor for MIF obtained from macrophages. This is a fucosyl ganglioside and requires both fucose and sialic acid for activity.

PLUZNIK: The evidence that lymphocytes actually release CSF is obtained from the experiments in which lymphocytes from C3H/HeJ mice (low responders to LPS) were incubated with supernatants from LPS-induced macrophages from C3H/eB (high responders to LPS). When the reverse experiment was done, namely lymphocytes from C3H/eB mice incubated with LPS-induced macrophages from C3H/HeJ mice, no CSF was generated. The macrophages used in these experiments were proteose peptone-stimulated peritoneal macrophages. Accordingly, the macrophage reacts with LPS, produces a lymphostimulatory factor, which activates the lymphocyte to release CSF.

LYMPHOKINE-INDUCED MACROPHAGE PROLIFERATION, ACTIVATION AND FUSION[1]

John W. Hadden
John R. Sadlik
Arthur Englard
Alwin H. Warfel
Elba M. Hadden

Laboratory of Immunopharmacology
Memorial Sloan-Kettering Cancer Center
New York, New York

The process by which macrophages of an immune animal become resistant to parasitization by facultative intracellular bacteria like *Listeria monocytogenes* is characterized by macrophage proliferation, macrophage activation with increased bactericidal capacity and granuloma formation with fusion of macrophages to form giant cells. The present studies were performed to elucidate the role of lymphokines in this process.

Our experiments in the guinea pig system (1,2) indicate that a lymphocyte-produced factor, macrophage mitogenic factor (MMF), acts to induce proliferation in monolayers of non-immune alveolar and oil-induced monocyte-derived peritoneal macrophages. The factor is elicited by antigen from lymph node lymphocytes sensitized with bovine gamma globulin (BGG) under conditions known to produce intense delayed hypersensitivity. It is not found in the supernatant of immune lymphocytes unstimulated by the antigen. While it is found in supernatants rich in migration inhibitory factor (MIF), treatment of the supernatants with vacuum dialysis and exclusion chromatography depletes much of the MIF or a co-factor required for MIF activity. MIF activity may be antagonistic to the initial expression of MMF activity, since its presence is correlated with less MMF activity. The factor induces tritiated thymidine incorporation, nuclear labeling and increases the number

[1] *Supported by grants CA-08748, CA-09149 & CA-20178.*

ISBN 0-12-213950-X

of peritoneal macrophages grown on monolayers. These three parameters correlate with each other, indicating a reliable detection system for macrophage proliferation. Visual determinations confirm that up to 60% of cells having a uniform macrophage morphology and exhibiting phagocytic vacuoles have nuclei labeled with ^{3}H-thymidine by radioautography. The proliferation of macrophages in this system is dependent on the concentration of MMF, low concentrations having earlier effects than higher concentrations. In general, peaks of thymidine incorporation occur between 3 and 5 days of culture. Factors which contribute to the magnitude and the kinetics of the response in this system include the animal, the serum source, the preparation of MMF, the amount of residual MIF in the MMF, the time of addition of MMF, and cell density.

Initial chemical characterization indicates that the mitogenic factor:

a) has a broad elution profile from sephadex G100 superfine between limits of 70,000 - 40,000 daltons
b) has an isoelectric focusing profile having a peak at pH 8.0 and several peaks between pH 3.0 - 5.5
c) is nondialysable and stable at pH 2 and in 0.8M NaCl
d) Precipitates between 50 and 80% saturated ammonium sulfate
e) is not adsorbed to Affi Gel 202

Of the other lymphokines examined by us and reported by others, only guinea pig fibroblast macrophage growth factor (MGF) shows close similarity. Lack of a reliable assay for colony formation by guinea pig bone marrow precursors has made it impossible for us to say at this time whether the mitogenic factor has macrophage colony stimulating factor activity. An identity of MMF and T cell MGF is a distinct possibility.

The production of prostaglandin by macrophages is regulatory in this system. Indomethacin, potent inhibitor of cyclooxygenase and of PG synthesis in macrophages, potentiates the effect of MMF in a manner which parallels the dose-response curve of the factor, and added PGE inhibits MMF action. If macrophages are cultured for 24 hours prior to MMF addition, MMF action is increased and indomethacin has less effect, suggesting that prostaglandin production by macrophages limits MMF-induced proliferation of peritoneal macrophages early in the culture period.

Assay of prostaglandin production by macrophages by radioimmunoassay at 1, 3, & 5 days of culture indicates a progressive increase in PGE_2 levels and relatively stable $PGF_{2}\alpha$ levels. Antigen-reconstituted control fractions increased PGE_2 levels to the same extent as MMF. Thus, while PGE production is limiting to MMF action, MMF does not induce significant PGE production under these circumstances. Since MMF increases cyclic GMP (3) and PGE_1 increases cyclic AMP in these macrophages, a dualistic regulation of macrophage proliferation by cyclic nucleotides similar to that observed in other immune and inflammatory cells is suggested (4).

Employing Sephadex G-100 and isoelectric focusing fractions containing MMF and depleted of MIF, we examined the effect of MMF on the activation of mineral oil-induced nonimmune guinea pig peritoneal macrophages. In the assay for activation, monolayers of macrophages are exposed to MMF for varying periods of time in LABTEK chambers, as described for the MMF assay. The monolayers are then subjected to a short exposure to virulent *Listeria monocytogenes* organisms at a low ratio of bacteria to macrophage. The monolayers are then washed and the number of phagocytized bacteria is confirmed visually by gram staining. At the onset of incubation following the pulsed exposure to the bacteria, approximately 30-40% of the macrophages have ingested an average of two organisms; over the ensuing 6 hrs of incubation, the ingested bacteria will replicate in the normal macrophage with a doubling time of < 2 hrs. When macrophages have been pre-treated with MMF for 4-6 days, they inhibit this replication of *Listeria* and proceed to digest them as judged by disintegration of the bacteria visualized by gram staining. Tumoricidal studies, in progress, indicate a relative lack of activity of MMF for cytocidal action in the guinea pig compared to interferon in the mouse. The evidence developed in this system suggests that MMF is the soluble mediator responsible for the activation of macrophages to kill pathogens and may perhaps play a role in killing tumor cells more effectively.

Scanning electron microscope studies on MMF treated and control macrophages after 4 days of culture revealed marked differences in surface morphologies between activated and control macrophages. MMF-treated macrophages were much larger overall than control cells. Activated macrophages exhibited marked spreading on the plastic cover slips, while control cells remained spherical in shape, although attached. MMF-treated macrophages presented a very complex and non-uniform surface morphology including micro blebs, membranous veil-like structures, pseudopodia, and extensive surface convolutions, resembling *roses*, not apparent in the control.

Studies (5) on the action of macrophage fusion factor (MFF) by BGG-sensitized lymph node lymphocytes have been performed in absence of serum on alveolar and peritoneal macrophages of both the guinea pig and the rabbit. In the guinea pig, MFF activity for alveolar macrophages was irregularly observed with supernatants tested at a 1:2 dilution. No activity was observed on peritoneal macrophages. MMF-rich, MIF-poor sephadex fractions showed no MFF activity. In contrast, in the rabbit, MFF-rich supernatant fused more than 80% of alveolar and peritoneal macrophages to form multinucleated giant cells. Sephadex fractionation of these supernatants yielded MFF activity eluting between 20,000-70,000 daltons. MFF activity correlated with an apparent migration inhibition resulting from fusion; however, preliminary experiments with fucose competition and cell adsorption of MFF indicate that MFF is distinct from MIF as well as MMF.

The biology of these soluble mediators would appear relevant in terms of the marked proliferation, activation and fusion of macrophages known to occur during states of intense T lymphocyte-mediated immunity, as occurs during infection with facultative intracellular bacterial pathogens. Precise molecular definitions are required in the future for studies of their mechanisms of action.

REFERENCES

1. Hadden, J., Sadlik, J., and Hadden, E. (1975) *Nature 257*, 483.
2. Hadden, J., Sadlik, J., and Hadden, E. (1978) *J. Immunol. 121*, 231.
3. Hadden, J., and Englard, A. (1978) In "*The Pharmacology of Immunoregulation*". (G. Werner and F. Floc'h, eds.), pp. 273, 369. Academic Press, London.
4. Hadden, Coffey, R., and Spreafico, F. (1978) "*Immunopharmacology*", Plenum Publ. Corp., New York.
5. Warfel, A. and Hadden, J. (1978) *Amer. J. Path. 93*, 753.

DISCUSSION

MIZEL: In suggesting an inverse relationship between MIF and MGF activities, has Hadden biochemically resolved MIF from MGF?

HADDEN: Biochemically we have depleted MIF activity by vacuum dialysis with collodion bags,with a molecular weight cut-off of 25,000,followed by Sephadex G 100 column chromatography or isoelectric focussing on a Sephadex bed (without added albumin to stabilize MIF). Under optimal circumstances we see 10% MIF activity at 9-fold concentrations relative to starting supernatants,meaning losses in excess of 95% for Sephadex chromatography and more than 99% with isoelectric focussing. Using these fractions, we can dilute the MGF activity out >1:500. Overall, we see greater MGF activity in the absence of MIF and a highly significant inverse correlation exists between the two activities suggesting antagonism. Biologically, we can distinguish the activities by showing that day 6 exudates and alveolar macrophages show little responsiveness to and binding of MIF but are very responsive to MGF.

WAKSMAN: What is the relationship of Hadden's factor to that described over a decade ago by Virolainen and Defendi? I thought CSF was defined in terms of its ability to make macrophages precursors *differentiate* to macrophages. MMF causes macrophages to *cycle*, i.e. to synthesize DNA and divide. These are quite different functions. I would hesitate to identify CSF and MMF on the basis of what has been said, since in general different signals induce these different effects. In a few well studied cases, differentiation is induced only by a signal given at the correct phase of the cell cycle, and in some instances the receptor for the mediator is only present in that particular phase of the cycle.

HADDEN: Mauel and Defendi described a fibroblast produced factor which Cohen has subsequently purified. This factor at 70,000 MW has both CSF and MGF activity not dissociable by biochemical or serological criteria. While we have been unable to date to show CSF activity of our MMF because of the lack of a workable assay for CSF on guinea pig marrow cells, we have compared MMF to guinea pig fibroblast MGF: they have similar dose response curves and are very similar on isoelectric focussing and with several other fractionation procedures. For the moment I think it is likely that MMF is a lymphocyte CSF/MGF and thus best called MGF. For both CSF assay on marrow cells and MGF assay on mature macrophages I think that both proliferation and differentiation are involved. Both factors must be constantly present. Little is known about their receptors let alone the timing of their presence.

DAVID: Since Hadden's MMF is found in the same Sephadex fractions as MIF but can also be found even when diluted 1:500 (while MIF activity was no longer discernible at 9-fold concentration) one could explain the data by assuming his MMF assay was much more sensitive than the MIF assay. This does not necessarily prove that they are different (they may of course *be* different). I want to emphasize that we do not lose guinea pig MIF by dialysis, neither do Stanley and Marion Cohen.

HADDEN: David's papers report concentration of MIF from Sephadex columns by 7-10 fold and the data show about 50% MIF activity. This constitutes an estimated loss of MIF activity by the two steps of over 90%; Remold (personal communication) lost MIF activity in isoelectric focussing when albumin was not added to stabilize the MIF. When albumin was added 10x concentration of the fractions relevant to starting volumes was necessary to detect MIF. I think the dissociation of the dose response curves makes it unlikely that MIF and MMF/MCF are identical. I do not exclude the possiblity that MIF activity results from a cofactor acting in conjunction with MMF/MGF.

DAVID: Hadden showed that MMF was one peak in isoelectric focussing at pH gradients 2-10. Remold also only gets one peak of MIF using broad gradients and can only differentiate two peaks on narrower gradients pH 2-6.

HADDEN: We observed two peaks on a pH gradient 2-10, one at pH 4.7 the other at pH 8 where no MIF activity has been described. Unlike MIF we see two peaks of MMF between pH 3 and 4 and none at pH 5.

OPPENHEIM: Moore (NIDR, NIH) has obtained a cytokine CSF from mouse L_{929} cells. This activity when eluted from Sephadex G 150 chromatography is in the 70,000-160,000 MW range. The same fractions also contain an activity which induces mouse peritoneal macrophages (PEC) to proliferate in suspension cultures (e.g. MGF). Furthermore, PEC are activated to produce LAF by the same eluted peak that contains the CSF and MGF activities as well as another 60,000 MW moiety. This data as well as published observations that CSF can increase the adherence, phagocytosis and plasminogen activator production by macrophages indicates that CSF coelutes with a factor that promotes differentiation of macrophages. Therefore CSF as well as SIRS, MAF and immune interferon all can activate macrophages in a variety of ways. Although CSF is classically defined as growth promoting, it also appears to have important regulatory effects on macrophages and must be differentiated from these other activating signals. These data also suggest that a given signal can promote both cell proliferation and differention and these two processes do not necessarily dissociate.

HAVEMANN: The question arises whether a similar elution from Sephadex G 150 is really sufficient to suggest identity between different factors. In a cooperative study of different German groups, we tested MIF, MCF, TRF and CSF active in the mouse system using mouse spleen cell supernatants, which were then separated by hydrophobic interaction chromatography. It was clearly shown that by their chromatographic behaviour there was no identity between these factors. In addition, our purified CSF (<50 pg protein necessary for induction of one colony; more than 100,000 fold purification) did not reveal MCF activity when tested by Lohmann-Matthes.

OPPENHEIM: I grant that with better purification CSF, MGF and LAF induction activities may be separated.

WAKSMAN: In responding to Oppenheim I want to emphasize that the temptation to confuse (or confound) the stimuli to cycling and to differentiation must be resisted. The well studied cases I referred to, were those of Hämmerling on differentiation in B cell precursors and T cell precursors of Schimpl and Wecker on TRF (to be discussed later), and of Varge on melanoma cells, all of which showed that differentiation only occurs in cells already cycling.

OPPENHEIM: My point was that a given signal such as CSF can probably drive cells both to cycle and to differentiate.

COHEN: There are several general issues that are important in studies on separation of mediator activity. First, in order to rule out differences in assay sensitivity as a cause of apparent dissociation of activities it is necessary to define experimental conditions under which an activity "A", but not activity "B" is present, and then define a second set of conditions in which B, but not A is present. This kind of "mirror" arrangement eliminates assay sensitivity as a problem. For example, Hadden could try limiting dilutions of his supernatant without dialysis to demonstrate that he can preserve detectable MIF activity to a greater (or at least the same) extent as MMF.

Another kind of problem is that different fragments of mediator may manifest different biologic properties. In our experience, the small piece of human MIF we described can not be separated from a molecule that specifically affects the migration properties of a variety of tumor cells. Hadden has provided evidence suggesting that the large segment of guinea pig MIF may be the same as MMF. In this regard, we are currently exploring the possibility that the small piece of human MIF exerts migration inhibitory activity following internalization. There is some evidence that in the case of epidermal growth factor (EGF), surface EGF-receptor interaction leads to the appearance of a new cytoplasmic factor or second signal that induces mitogenesis. Internalized EGF may not play a role. If similar mechanisms are involved in Hadden's system, then all these mechanisms begin to sort themselves out. It may well turn out to be that MMF, MIF, MAF and MCF activities represent neither distinct nor common molecular species, but instead represent different properties conferred by different pieces or subunits to a basic "mother factor".

As a final caveat, the same mediator acting on the same target cell may give different results in different assay systems. Thus the peptide 1-met-leu-phe is a well-defined, potent chemotactic factor for neutrophils. We have recently found that in comparable doses, this compound can be chemotactic for macrophages in the Boyden chamber, and cause migration inhibition from a capillary tube. The explanation of this phenomenon is beyond the scope of this discussion, but observations such as these attest to how assay-dependent our view of reality is.

SOME CHEMICAL PROPERTIES OF GUINEA PIG MITOGENIC FACTORS[1]

Carolyn L. Geczy

Kolling Institute of Medical Research
Royal North Shore Hospital
St Leonards, N.S.W. Australia

The possibility that mitogenic factors (MF) may be a heterogeneous group of molecules was raised after it was demonstrated that MF in supernatants from BCG-sensitized lymph node cells, stimulated with PPD, had a different M.Wt. and isoelectric point from MF from mixed leucocyte culture supernatants (MLC). The factors also differed in their ability to react with an anti-lymphokine serum and with L-fucose (1). These MF's are compared with those produced by lymph node cells stimulated with ovalbumin, IgG or Sepharose Concanavalin A (iCon A). Some proteases have been shown to be mitogenic (2) and we have found that a fraction containing an acid protease produced by lymph node cells stimulated with iCon A is mitogenic and has skin reactive factor (SRF) activity.

I. MOLECULAR CHARACTERISTICS OF THE FACTORS

Mitogenic factors were prepared by incubating guinea pig lymph node cells with either the sensitizing antigen (ovalbumin, OVA, human IgG or keyhole limpet haemocyanin, KLH), and serum as described previously (1) or with iCon A in the absence of serum (3). iCon A supernatants were filtered on a Sephadex G200 column (95x2.6 cm) to remove free Con A. Proteins in the M.Wt. range 15-70,000 were used for further separations. No MF activity was found in fractions of higher M.Wt. The pool of the G200 column was fractionated on a Biogel P100 column (95x1.6 cm), and the active peaks separated by flat-bed isoelectrofocusing using the LKB Multiphor apparatus. Table I

[1]*This work was supported by a grant from the National Health and Medical Research Council of Australia*

ISBN 0-12-213950-X

demonstrates that MF resulting from antigen stimulation of sensitized cells, regardless of the antigen used, had a M.Wt. of about 20-25,000. Small amounts of activity of M.Wt. 40-50,000 were observed in most cases. iCon A-MF, on the other hand, had an M.Wt. of 35-45,000 and sometimes minor activity at about 15,000. The major activities from iCon A fractions had isoelectric points at pH 4.4-4.6 and pH 5.4-5.6 with a minor peak at pH 6.5. Soluble Con A stimulated the formation of an even more heterogeneous MF profile, the major activities of which had similar properties to those of the iCon A factors. Activities with pI 4.4-4.6 and 5.4-5.6 were present in minor amounts in PPD, OVA and HGG-MF supernatants. The antigen-MF of M.Wt. 25,000, however, showed further heterogeneity in terms of pI, and differed with each of the antigens used for its preparation. All of these activities differed from MLC-MF which had a M.Wt. of 15-18,000 and pI of 6.5. The nature of this heterogeneity is still unknown. We have not investigated if the MF's bear Ia determinants because inbred guinea pigs were not available for this study. Preliminary attempts to demonstrate antigen-specificity of the antigen-induced factors have failed, in agreement with other authors (4). It is possible that molecules contain various amounts of sialic acid residues as described for interferon (5) and possibly migration inhibition factor (6) which may account for the differences in pI. However, it is unlikely that this is responsible for the marked difference in M.Wt. of iCon A-MF (35-45,000) to the major peak of antigen MF activity (20-25,000). The possibility that the latter may be active monomers which dimerize to produce characteristics of iCon A-MF has not been tested.

TABLE I. Chemical Properties of Guinea Pig Mitogenic Factors

Factor	*M.Wt*	*pI*	
iCon A-MF	*35-45,000*	*4.5*	
	25-45,000	*5.5*	
	nt	*6.5*	*minor activity*
PPD-MF	*20-25,000*	*7.5*	
	35-45,000	*4.5*	*minor activity*
Ovalbumin-MF	*20-25,000*	*9.3*	
	35-45,000	*4.5*	*minor activity*
HGG-MF	*20-25,000*	*9.0*	
	20-25,000	*8.6*	
	20-25,000	*7.2*	*minor activity*
	35-45,000	*5.4*	*minor activity*
	35-45,000	*4.4*	
MLC-MF	*15-18,000*	*6.5*	

2. STIMULATED LYMPH NODE CELLS PRODUCE AN ACID PROTEASE

It has been reported that human lymphocytes contain cell-bound proteases which are possibly involved in blast transformation (7), and that a number of protease inhibitors suppress lymphocyte responses to PHA (8). In addition, some polymorphonuclear leukocyte proteases (e.g., trypsin, cathepsin G) are mitogenic (2) and a variety of proteases are involved in tissue injury (9). These facts led to the investigations reported here.

iCon A-induced lymphokine fractions from supernatants (300 ml) filtered on Sepharose G200 (M.Wt. 25-60,000) were tested over a wide range of pH values for their ability to hydrolyse H^3-casein and H^3-haemoglobin to TCA-soluble peptides. Peak hydrolysis occurred at pH 3.5-4.0 and 5.6-6. Figure I shows examples of acid protease activity from two separate lymphokine preparations. Stimulated lymph node cells produced substantially more enzyme than the corresponding control culture supernatants.

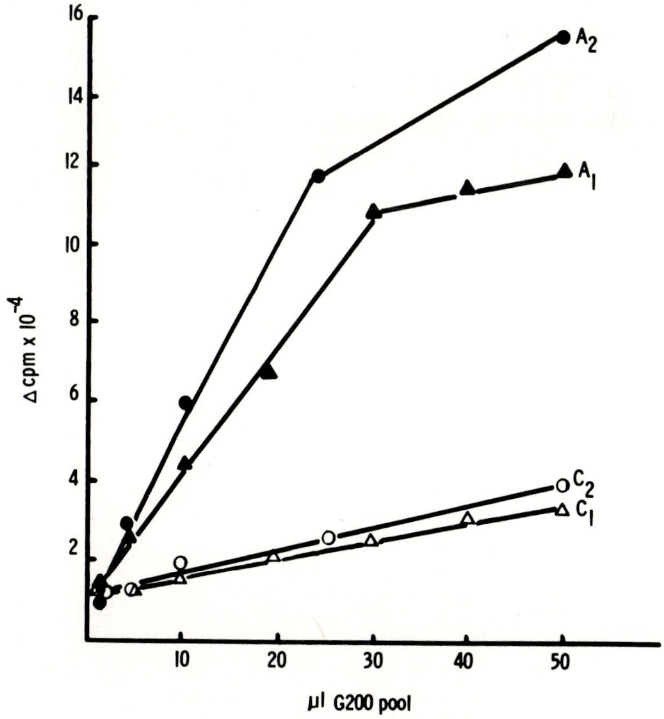

FIGURE 1. Acid protease activity from control (C_1,C_2) and Con A-induced lymphocyte supernatants.

3. PROPERTIES OF THE PROTEASE

The acid protease (pH 3.5-4.0) has been studied in more detail and it is still not clear whether the enzyme has two pH optima or whether another protease is present. The acid protease hydrolyses H^3-casein more readily than H^3-haemoglobin, H^3-guinea pig albumin only slowly and H^3-guinea pig IgG not at all. The enzyme obeys Michaelis Menten kinetics for the substrate H^3-casein. The enzyme is inhibited by 1 mM phenylmethylsulphonylfluoride (PMSF) and 1 mM EDTA; Ca^{++} and Mg^{++} only partially restore activity. Activity is not affected by soybean trypsin inhibitor, pepstatin, trasylol, N-ethylenediamine, 4-chloromercuribenzoate or dithiothreitol. The enzyme, therefore, does not appear to have cathepsin or collagenase-like properties and is probably a serine esterase with a requirement for a metal ion for activity.

The acid protease co-chromatographs with MF when the fraction from the G200 column is filtered on Biogel P100, indicating a M.Wt. of about 45,000; SRF activity is also detected in this fraction. Isoelectric focusing of the 45,000 M.Wt. fraction off Biogel P100 yielded a peak of SRF activity (assessed by measuring skin thickness; focussed fractions induced only slight erythema) with an isoelectric point of 4.4-4.6. A sharp peak of proteolytic activity is also observed in this region, which corresponds to the peak of pH 4.4-4.6 mitogenic activity. A broad proteolytic peak at pH 5.5-6.5 was also observed, but SRF could never be demonstrated in this pH range. Unfortunately, isoelectricfocusing leads to inactivation of the enzymes. Only about 10% of the activity applied to the focusing bed is recovered after the separation. The antigen-induced lymphokine preparations also contain small amounts of the pH 4.4-4.5 MF. It is not yet known whether the low M.Wt. peaks of antigen-MF are associated with protease activity.

The ability of the inhibited enzyme to elicit a skin reaction was tested. A Biogel P100 fraction with SRF and acid protease activity was incubated with 1 mM PMSF or 5 mM EDTA overnight at 20°, and excess inhibitor removed by dialysis. PMSF completely inhibited the induration caused by SRF although erythema was only partially inhibited. EDTA inhibited *in vivo* activity by about 50%, probably because dialysis of the fraction caused removal of some loosely chelated EDTA.

It is possible that SRF is a protease involved in the tissue injury observed at the site of a delayed hypersensitivity reaction. Release of chemotactic peptide fragments from protein substrates as yet unknown, may result in the mononuclear cell infiltrate observed in this reaction. A cathepsin B-like enzyme has been extracted from sites of Arthus reaction; this enzyme produces chemotactic fragments from IgM (10). SRF, itself a protease, may then be mitogenic for guinea pig lymphocytes thus causing localised lymphocyte proliferation and possibly increased lymphokine production (11) leading to an amplification of the response.

REFERENCES

1. Geczy, C., *J. Immunol. 119,* 2107 (1977).
2. Vischer, T., Bretz, U. and Baggiolini, M., *J. Exp. Med. 144,* 863 (1976).
3. Friedrich, W., Lazary, S., Geczy, C., and de Weck, A.L., *Int. Arch. Allergy Appl. Immun. 49,* 504 (1975).
4. Geha, R., Mudawwar, F., and Schneeberger, E., *J. Exp. Med. 145,* 1436 (1977)
5. Dorner, F., Scriba, M., and Weil, R., *Proc. Natl. Acad. Sci. 70,* 1981 (1973).
6. Sorg, C., and Geczy, C., *J. Immunol. 121,* 1199 (1978).
7. Grayzel, A., Hatcher, V., and Lazarus, G., *Cell Immunol. 18,* 210 (1975).
8. Hirschhorn, R., Grossman, J., Troll, W., and Weissmann, G. *J. Clin. Invest. 50,* 1206 (1971).
9. Hopsu-Havu, V., Fräki, J., and Järvinen, M., *in* "Proteinases in Mammalian Cells and Tissues" (A.J. Barrett ed.) pp. 545-581 North-Holland Publishing Co. (1977).
10. Higuchi, Y., Honda, M., and Hayashi, H., *Cell Immunol. 15,* 100 (1975).
11. Gately, C., Gately, M., and Mayer, M., *J. Immunol. 116,* 669 (1976).

DISCUSSION

MIZEL: Is Geczy suggesting that MF is a protease? Does MF function as a B cell mitogen, since a number of proteins are B cell mitogens?

GECZY: I am suggesting that the MF from insoluble con A-activated supernatants which has an isoelectric point of 4.5 could be a protease, but I do not yet know whether it is a B cell mitogen. This fraction also causes induration when injected into guinea pig skin.

BRETZ: We have shown that exogenous proteinases can stimulate lymphocytes in vitro and reported the data here in order to offer a possible mechanism of action of intercellular communication. It seems reasonable to look for proteolytic activity where mitogenic effects are concerned.

ALTMAN: I would like to mention that the production of allogeneic effect factor (AEF), originally described by Katz, is increased by pretreatment of the AEF-producing cells with PMSF (phenyl methylsulphonyl fluoride). In addition to the "classical" activity of AEF as a T cell-replacing factor, we found more recently that AEF is also a potent T cell mitogen and it appears that the mitogenic activity of AEF is also increased by PMSF pretreatment. Therefore, in this case, there appears to be a dissociation between proteolytic and mitogenic activities of a mitogenic factor.

WAKSMAN: Dessaint, in our laboratory, has shown that macrophage depleted T cells will not respond to PHA or Con A unless TAF (from macrophages) is added. This TAF appears to be carboxypeptidase B.

HAVEMANN: My comments refer to the same problem. The mitogenic factor with proteolytic activity Waksman describes may either induce direct mitogenicity or may just replace the macrophages which are necessary for the mitogenic response. Our experiments (Havemann & Janoff: Neutral proteases of human polymorphonuclear granulocytes, Urban & Schwarzenberg, Baltimore, 1978) with a number of proteolytic enzymes including granulocyte neutral proteases in human lymphocyte cultures stimulated with mitogen, antigen or allogeneic cells, show that the enzymes do not have direct mitogenicity but can replace the macrophages in the culture. If macrophages are present in the cultures, the enzymes markedly enhance the mitogenic response.

CHARACTERIZATION OF GUINEA PIG LYMPHOKINES BY ISOELECTRIC FOCUSING[1]

R. A. Wolstencroft, B. A. Ellis, S. Crome
Grace E. Restrick, Virginia Wolstencroft, D. C. Dumonde

Immunology Unit, The Rayne Institute,
St. Thomas' Hospital, London

I. INTRODUCTION

Guinea pig lymphokines (LK) that stimulate thymidine incorporation (STI) in cultured lymphocytes can be produced *in vitro* or *in vivo* under comparable immunological circumstances (1). In the present study LK, produced in guinea pigs with delayed hypersensitivity following parenteral challenge with specific antigen, were further characterized by preparative isoelectric focusing in granulated gel (PIGG).

II. MATERIALS AND METHODS

Guinea pigs were sensitised by footpad injection with bovine γ-globulin (100 μg) in Freunds complete adjuvant. Two weeks later LK were induced in the ascitic fluid of the animals by intraperitoneal injection of antigen (10 mg). The lymphokine-rich peritoneal exudate fluids (PEF) were recovered 6h after challenge, by irrigation of the peritoneal cavity with medium, and clarified by filtration. The PEF were pre-treated by stepwise precipitation with ammonium sulphate (AS) and the active material, between 50 and 90% saturation (AS 50-90), was solubilised in and dialysed against phosphate buffered saline (PBS).

Preparative flat-bed isoelectric focusing in granulated gel was performed using an LKB Multiphor system according to the manufacturers recommendations. The LK sample (AS 50-90) and carrier ampholytes (2%) were distributed throughout the gel bed. When focused the gel bed was divided using a

[1]*Supported by a grant from the Medical Research Council.*

ISBN 0-12-213950-X

30-position grid and individual fractions were recovered by elution from small columns; optical density and pH measurements were made on the eluted material. The fractions, either individually or as recombined pools, were dialysed and made to required volumes with PBS.

Lymphocyte STI activity was determined in cultures of guinea pig lymph node cells as described elsewhere (2). A minimum of three two-fold dilutions of the PIGG fractions, the corresponding 'starting material' (AS 50-90), and a laboratory LK standard (KILS 15) were tested in parallel in a single assay. Responses were computed in terms of quench-corrected disintegrations min^{-1} (dpm) per culture. Potency ratios of the starting material and the PIGG fractions were estimated in terms of KILS 15 using parallel line assay data in which log transformed values were used as the response and dose metameters.

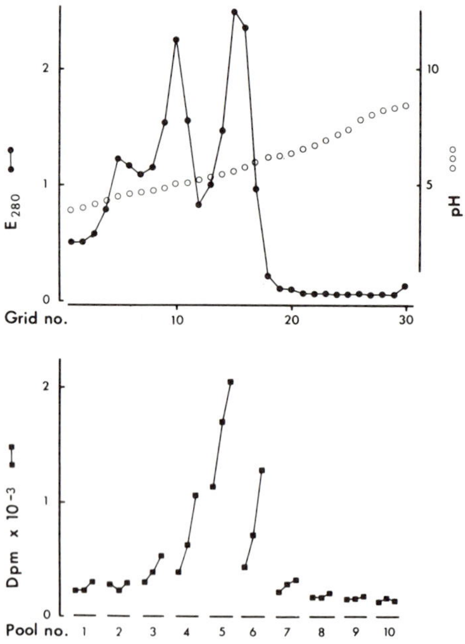

FIGURE 1. Fractionation of lymphocyte STI activity by PIGG. Upper graph: optical density and pH profiles. Lower graph: STI activity of fractions (pooled sequentially in groups of three) at doses (left to right) of 0.25, 0.5 and 1.0 fold with respect to the corresponding concentration in the PEF.

TABLE 1. Lymphocyte STI activity from sequential PIGG

pI	*5.00*	*5.26* ;	*5.35*	*5.60* ;	*5.62*	*5.88*
Grid no.	*(5)*	*(10)*	*(11)*	*(14)*	*(15)*	*(18)*
Potency[a]	*0.07*	*0.16*	*0.13*	*0.15*	*0.10*	*0.13*
Recovery[b]	*<5%*	*11.8%*	*8.7%*	*10.1%*	*6.7%*	*8.7%*

[a]*Potency ratio by reference to a LK standard (KILS 15)*
[b]*Recovery by reference to the starting material (AS 50-90)*

III. RESULTS AND CONCLUSIONS

Fractionation of active AS 50-90 by PIGG, using wide range ampholytes (pH 3.5-10.0), resulted in a relatively broad band of STI-active fractions between pH 5.0-6.0 with the maximum at about pH 5.5 (Fig. 1). In contrast, similar fractions obtained from control preparations, made by challenging sensitised guinea pigs with unrelated antigen, were virtually devoid of activity. Localisation of activity within pH limits of 5.0-6.0 was achieved using different active lymphokine preparations even though their optical density profiles were quantitatively disparate. Fractionation using narrower range ampholytes (pH 4.0-8.0 or 4.0-6.0) produced less symmetrical activity profiles indicating the presence of more than one peak of STI activity. Discrimination between separate peaks of activity was accentuated when 2-mercapto-ethanol was incorporated into the gel bed. A definitive separation of individual peaks of STI activity was undertaken by sequential PIGG. Table 1 summarises the results of an experiment, in which the active fractions - pools 3-7 inclusive as shown in Fig. 1 - obtained using wide range ampholytes were recombined and refractionated using narrow range ampholytes (pH 5.0-7.0). Assay of individual fractions showed four peaks of STI, each separated by at least one inactive fraction. The two major peaks of activity had mean pI values of 5.31 and 5.61; a third peak with lesser activity had a pI of 5.88; and a minor component had a pI of 5.00.

Preliminary evaluation of the fractions for additional lymphokine activities, viz. macrophage migration inhibitory and intradermal inflammatory, indicate that these separate activities are mediated by different molecular entities. This data provides further support for previous biochemical, biological and bioassay evidence of lymphokine heterogeneity (2).

REFERENCES

1. Wolstencroft, R.A., Wolstencroft, V. and Restrick, G.E. *Cell. Immunol. 27*, 356 (1976).
2. Bray, M.A., Dumonde, D.C., Hanson, J.M., Morley, J., Wolstencroft, R.A., and Smart, J.V. *Clin. exp. Immunol. 23*, 333 (1976).

DISCUSSION

PAPERMASTER: Some 15 years ago contention surrounded the biological activities of the immunoglobulin G class. Subsequent studies resulted in careful delineation of subclass structure and distinction of discrete immunologic activities among a group of molecules grossly similar in physicochemical properties. That we have lost sight of the confusing array of information which we had to contend with at that point is an indicator that immunologists exhibit immunologic amnesia, while the cells they study demonstrate a capacity for memory. Such procedures as isoelectric focusing, gel filtration on different chromatographic support materials and other separation procedures are subject to trailing and other artifacts. Guinea pigs are not likely ever to make enough material for molecular characterization and allow the fulfillment of structure-function criteria such as amino acid sequence correlation with proliferative capacity. Hopefully, in one or two years we will know with confidence whether type I and/or II interferon can function as MIF, and then apply the comparative structural information to other lymphokines in due time.

DVORAK: Are activities other than STI present in Wolstencroft's peritoneal exudates. For example, MIF, LIF, LAF and lymphotoxin etc.? If so, are they separable from STI?

WOLSTENCROFT: We have undertaken preliminary investigations of the PIGG fractions for macrophage migration inhibitory and intradermal inflammatory activities. The activity profiles for these activities are close to but distinct from the STI activity and from one another.

THE PRODUCTION AND ACTION OF T-CELL GROWTH FACTOR[1]

Kendall A. Smith
Steven Gillis[2]
Paul E. Baker[2]

Department of Medicine
Dartmouth Medical School
Hanover, New Hampshire

I. INTRODUCTION

T-cell growth factor (TCGF), derived from T-cell lectin- or antigen-stimulated mononuclear cells, selects for and supports the continuous exponential proliferative growth of T-cells (1,2). In addition to lectin-stimulated T-cells, antigen-specific, differentiated, murine and human cytolytic T-lymphocyte lines (CTLL) have been maintained for more than two years in TCGF-supplemented cultures (3,4). Furthermore, through cloning procedures, monospecific CTLL have been created (5).

II. THE PRODUCTION OF TCGF IS T-CELL SPECIFIC

The TCGF used for the initial reports on continuous T-cell growth was derived from phytohemagglutinin (PHA) or Concanavalin A (Con A)-stimulated human or murine mononuclear cells (1,2,3). Subsequent experimentation revealed that only T-cell lectins or antigens (alloantigens, tumor antigens) caused the

[1]*Supported in part by NCI grant #R01-CA-17643-04, NCI contract #N01-CB-74141, and a grant from the National Leukemia Association, Inc.*
[2]*Fellows of the Leukemia Society of America.*

ISBN 0-12-213950-X

release of TCGF activity (6). T-cells were shown to be required for TCGF production in that lysis of Thy-1-positive splenocytes markedly reduced TCGF production (6). Evidence that mature T-cells were required is shown in Figure 1. Splenocytes and cortisol-resistant thymocytes produced comparable quantities of TCGF whereas spleen cells from athymic nude mice produced no TCGF activity and normal thymocytes produced only 1% of that produced by spleen cells.

Adherent cells were also required in that removal of adherent cells by passage of splenocytes through a nylon wool column resulted in markedly diminished Con A-induced TCGF production (Fig. 1). Reconstitution of the nylon wool-passaged cells with 1% nonspecific esterase-positive adherent splenocytes completely restored the TCGF producing capabilities of the cells. The same number of adherent cells cultured without T-cells did not release measurable TCGF activity when cultured with Con A.

III. TCGF MEDIATES THE PROLIFERATION OF "ACTIVATED" T-CELLS

It was previously noted that both antigen-specific CTLL cells and lectin stimulated spleen cells depleted TCGF from culture media in a cell concentration- and time-dependent manner resulting in the cessation of proliferation and cell death (6,7). These observations suggested that TCGF was consumed by the proliferating cells and prompted a series of absorption experiments. Con A-stimulated splenocytes (10^8 cells/ml) absorbed TCGF within two hours at 37°C. The absorption of TCGF was cell concentration-dependent and only splenocytes or thymocytes which had prior exposure to a T-cell lectin or antigen absorbed TCGF activity (Fig. 2). Splenocytes exposed to lipopolysaccharide (LPS) or unstimulated splenocytes and thymocytes did not absorb TCGF.

Therefore, it appeared that upon ligand-cell membrane binding, both thymocytes and splenocytes acquired a specific reactivity for TCGF. These results implied that the proliferative effect of TCGF would only be manifested when T-cells had first been exposed to lectin or antigen. Indeed, in experimentation reported elsewhere (7), it was found that TCGF would only mediate the proliferation of T-cells which were "activated" by lectin or antigen. Once the primary activation signal had been received however, the ligand was no longer necessary, and continuous proliferative growth could be maintained solely in the presence of TCGF.

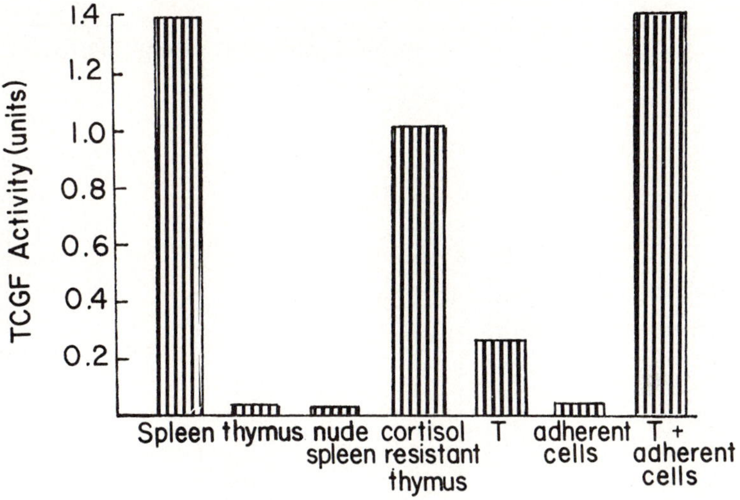

Fig. 1. The production of TCGF by different cell populations. Cells (1x10⁷/ml) were cultured with Con A (2.5 ug/ml) for 24 hrs. prior to TCGF assay.

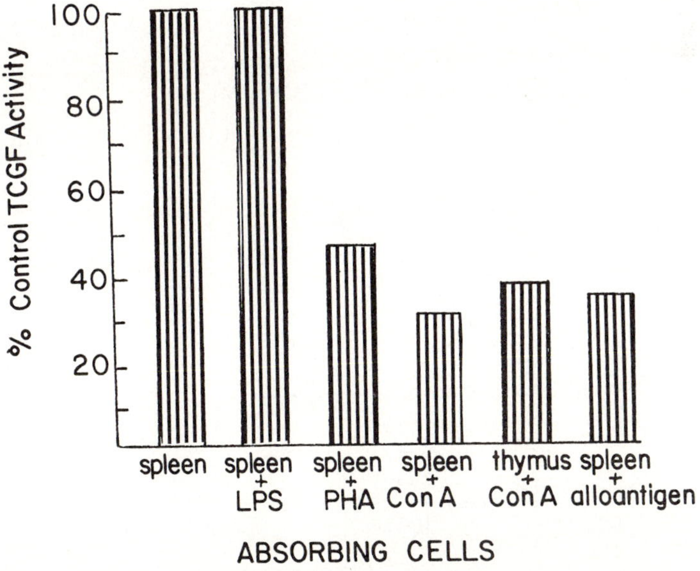

Fig. 2. The absorption of TCGF. Cells were incubated with TCGF ($1x10^8$ cells/ml) for 4 hrs. at 37°C.

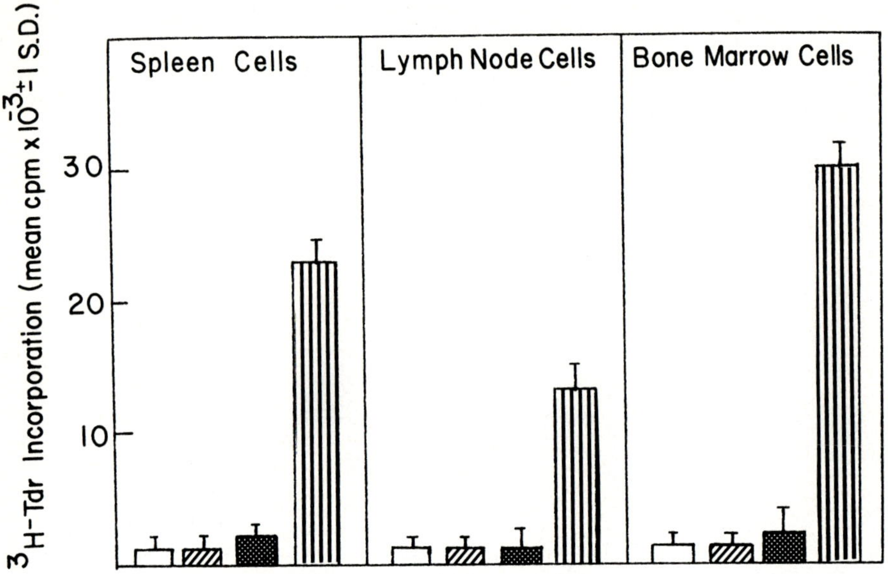

Fig. 3. The stimulation of BALB/c nu/nu cells. Medium = ☐ Con A = ▨ TCGF = ■ TCGF + Con A = ▥

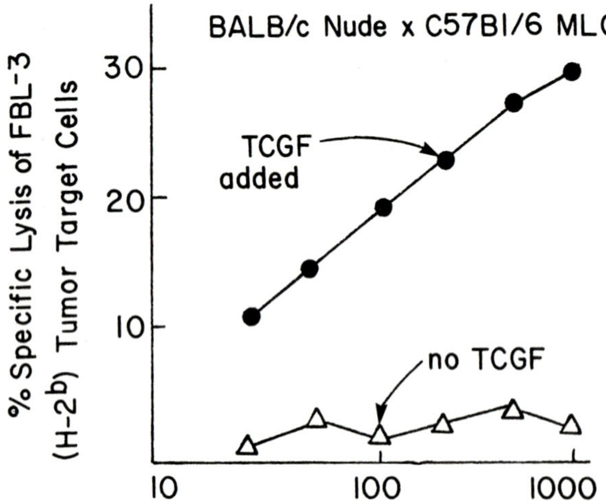

Fig. 4. Cytolysis mediated by BALB/c nu/nu splenocytes stimulated with C57Bl/6 splenocytes in the presence and absence of TCGF.

IV. TCGF RESTORES NUDE MOUSE T-CELL RESPONSES

The afore mentioned experimentation suggested that although thymocytes were incapable of producing TCGF, they were capable of a proliferative response to a T-cell lectin if TCGF was supplied exogenously. In addition, the marked difference between thymocytes and peripheral mature T-cells with respect to TCGF production, suggested that one function of the thymus was to effect the maturation of those T-cells which participated in TCGF production.

These observations suggested that prothymocytes might also be capable of a proliferative response if TCGF were supplied exogenously. Indeed, as shown in Figure 3, if nude mouse spleen, lymph node or bone marrow cells were exposed to both Con A and TCGF, a marked proliferative response was observed as quantified by tritiated thymidine incorporation. There was no response observed to Con A or TCGF alone.

Similar results were obtained when nude mouse splenocytes were stimulated by allogeneic spleen cells in the presence of TCGF. Furthermore, in addition to a proliferative response, the addition of TCGF to nude mouse mixed lymphocyte cultures (MLC) resulted in the generation of alloantigen-specific cytolytic effector cells as shown in Figure 4. Cells harvested from such TCGF-supplemented MLC have been maintained in TCGF-dependent proliferative culture for more than six months and continue to express Thy-1 antigen as determined by direct membrane immunofluorescence and the absorption of Thy-1 antiserum cytotoxic reactivity (8).

V. TCGF IS THE PROLIFERATIVE T-CELL SIGNAL

Based upon these observations, it appeared that as least two functional T-cell subsets existed. On one hand, prothymocytes, thymocytes, and mature peripheral T-cells were capable of responding to TCGF if activated to the responsive state by contact with a T-cell lectin or antigen. In addition, a separate functional T-cell subset which required thymic influence, appeared to be involved in TCGF production. The presence of both functional subsets was required for the generation of T-cell proliferative and effector responses unless TCGF was supplied exogenously.

It occurred to us that the assays for thymocyte mitogenic factor (TMF) (9), T-cell replacing factor (TRF) (10) and killer helper factor (KHF) (11), which made use of thymocytes or nude mouse splenocytes as the responding cell populations, were perhaps deficient in the appropriate T-cell subset required for TCGF production. Therefore, the addition of TCGF to such cultures would be expected to replace this deficiency and allow the clonal expansion of TCGF-responsive cells.

To explore this possibility, in collaboration with Dr. James Watson, we have examined these four assays (i.e. TCGF, TMF, KHF, and TRF) using conditioned media obtained from Con A-stimulated mouse and rat splenocytes, and PHA-stimulated human peripheral blood mononuclear cells. After each of three purification steps (Sephadex G-100 gel filtration, DEAE cellulose ion exchange chromatography, and preparative isoelectric focusing), the fractions obtained were assayed for activity in all of the assays. We found that the active material from all three sources co-purified when tested in all four assays (see Watson, J. et al., this volume). The biochemical characteristics of mouse, rat, and human TCGF are summarized in Table I.

TABLE I. BIOCHEMICAL CHARACTERISTICS OF TCGF

Procedures	Source of Conditioned Medium		
	Mouse	Rat	Human
Sephadex G-100[a]	30K	15K	15K
DEAE[b]	150 -200	15-35	15-35
pI	4.3,4.9	5.5	6.5

[a]Molecular size expressed in daltons
[b]mM concentration of sodium phosphate buffer (pH7.6) required for elution

Therefore, it appeared that each of these assays was capable of detecting the MF we have termed TCGF, most probably because the end-point of each assay depends upon the clonal expansion of functional T-cells.

VI. CONCLUSIONS

The implications of these studies may be summarized as follows: (1) The production and action of TCGF is obligatory for the generation of T-cell immune reactivity. (2) The production of TCGF requires the presence of a mature thymic dependent subset of T-cells and adherent mononuclear cells. (3) TCGF-responsive precursor T-cells are present in prothymocyte, thymocyte, and peripheral lymphoid cell populations.

REFERENCES

1. Morgan, D.A., Ruscetti, F.W., and Gallo, R. (1976) *Science 193*, 1007.
2. Ruscetti, F.W., Morgan, D.A., and Gallo, R.C. (1977) *J. Immunol. 119*, 131.
3. Gillis, S., and Smith, K.A. (1977) *Nature 268*, 154.
4. Gillis, S., Baker, P.E., Ruscetti, F.W., and Smith, K.A. (1978) *J. Exp. Med. 148*, 1093.
5. Baker, P.E., Gillis, S., and Smith, K.A. (1979) *J. Exp. Med. 149*, 273.
6. Gillis, S., Ferm, M.M., Ou, W., and Smith, K.A. (1978) *J. Immunol. 120*, 2027.
7. Smith, K.A., Gillis, S., Baker, P.E., MacKenzie, D., and Ruscetti, F.W. (1979) *Ann. N.Y. Acad. Sci.* in press.
8. Gillis, S., Union, N.A., Baker, P.E., and Smith, K.A. (1979) *J. Exp. Med.* in press.
9. Paetkau, V., Mills, G., Gerhart, S., and Monticone, V. (1976) *J. Immunol. 117*, 1320.
10. Watson, J.D., Aarden, L.A., Shaw, J., and Paetkau, V. (1979) *J. Immunol.* in press.
11. Farrar, J.J., Koopman, W.J., and Fuller-Bonar, J. (1978) *J. Immunol. 119*, 47.

CHARACTERIZATION OF MONOCYTE AND LYMPHOCYTE MEDIATORS MODULATING T LYMPHOCYTE COLONY FORMATION

L.A. Rozenszajn, A. Zeevi, I. Goldman, B. Sredni

Department of Life Sciences and Medical Laboratories,
Bar-Ilan University and Meir Hospital
Ramat-Gan and Kfar Saba, Israel

I. INTRODUCTION

The development of diverse culture systems for growing colonies of different classes of hemopoietic cells lead to the accumulation of much information and insight into the mechanisms and control of hemopoiesis and cellular kinetics. In order to have a better understanding of the mechanism that regulates the colony formation of the normal lymphoid cell system, we studied the interactions of hemopoietic cells and/ or products they secrete in culture fluid (CF) and examined their influence on colony growth.

II. METHODS

A. *Preparation of Conditioned Medium Containing Factors Affecting Lymphocyte Colony Growth*

1. *Lymphocyte Colony Enhancing Factor (LCEF).* Lymphocyte culture fluid (LCF) obtained from human PHA-stimulated lymphocytes or T-cells is a good source of T-lymphocyte colony stimulating activity (1).

2. *Lymphocyte Colony Inhibitory and Promoting Factors (LCIF, LCPF).* Culture fluids were prepared from murine, adherent peritoneal and spleen cells, and from human blood and spleen adherent cells (1,2).

ISBN 0-12-213950-X

B. *Isolation and Characterization of LCIF Secreted by Macrophages (MØ)*

Culture fluid prepared from human or murine spleen cells or from murine MØ were subjected to ultrafiltration through a UM-2 membrane, then dialyzed and subsequently extracted with a series of organic solvents. The active material was further purified by a silica gel column, and by TLC plates. Lymphocyte colony inhibitory activity was found in two fractions with 65% and 88% inhibition, respectively. The active materials were identified from their infrared, mass spectra, nuclear magnetic resonance and ultraviolet spectra. From these data the material was identified as PGE_1 and PGE_2.

C. *Isolation and Characterization of LCEF*

Lymphocyte culture fluid was precipitated at 40% $(NH_4)_2SO_4$ saturation and then centrifuged. The supernatant was dialyzed and applied to a DEAE-cellulose column. The fractions bearing LCEF activity were pooled, vacuum concentrated, dialyzed and subjected to a Bio-Gel P-150 column. Prior to use, the column was calibrated with molecular weight markers. Fractions containing LCEF activity were eluted at a Ve/Vo which corresponds to a M.W. of 90,000-100,000 daltons. The active fractions were pooled and electrophoresed on polyacrylamide gel. The LCEF migrated to the haptoglobin (2-2) post-transferrin region (3). The protein nature of the LCEF was established from its behavior with nucleases and proteases.

D. *Isolation of the LCPF*

Culture fluids from human mouse spleen cells were dialyzed through Diaflo ultrafiltration membranes PM-30, UM-10 and UM-2. The retentates were resuspended in Eagle's medium (EM). Two materials affecting lymphocyte colony growth were separated: 1) a dialyzable substance M.W.<1,000 daltons, exhibiting inhibitory activity and 2) M.W. 10,000-30,000 daltons which stimulated colony development. The LCPF was completely precipitated by 80% $(NH_4)_2SO_4$; it was sensitive to heat treatment and stable when stored at -20°C for a prolonged period.

E. *Colony Assays*

Lymphocyte colony stimulating activity was assayed in peripheral blood lymphocytes or mononuclear cells from healthy adult donors. Lymphocyte colony inhibiting activity was determined in human venous blood lymphocytes or mononuclear cells

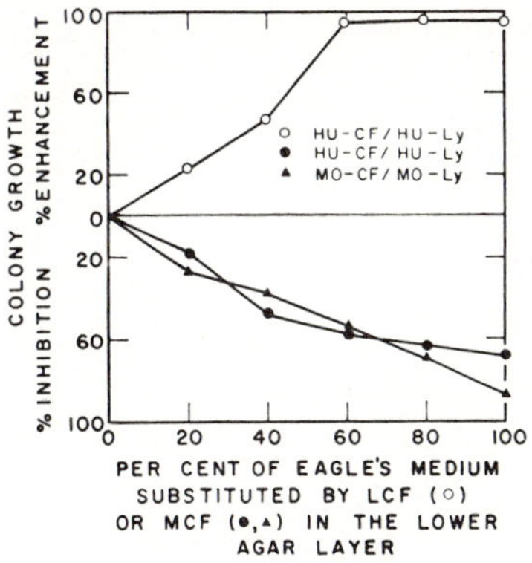

FIGURE 1. Effect of increasing concentrations of culture fluid (CF) prepared from human (Hu) lymphocytes —o (LCF), Hu blood adherent cells —● and mouse (Mo) adherent cells ▲ (MCF) on colony development of T cells (Ly).

and in murine lymph node cells. The lymphocytes were separated on glass columns and the mononuclear cells isolated by Lymphoprep and suspended as described earlier (4,5). The cells were sensitized with PHA 0.0125 ml/ml and seeded on the upper agar (0.3%) layer of a culture system whose lower agar (0.5%) layer contained LCF or monocyte-MØ CF or their isolated, active materials. The effects of the LCEF, LCPF and LCIF on lymphocyte colony growth were monitored from the number of colonies that developed and contained 50 or more cells 5-7 days after seeding.

III. RESULTS AND DISCUSSION

When the agar culture system was supplemented with LCF or with monocyte-MØ CF, enhancing and inhibiting effects, respectively, were observed. The effects were proportional to the number of cells used to prepare the CF and/or the amount of CF that was substituted for EM in the lower agar layer (Fig. 1), LCEF, M.W. 90,000-100,000 daltons, had a protein nature, and LCIF was identified as PGE_1 and PGE_2. This was substantiated by the facts that the inhibitory effect disappeared when indomethacin, a PG synthetase inhibitor, was added to MØ cultures and that synthetic PGE_1 and PGE_2 exhibit potent lymphocyte colony inhibitory activity. Ultrafiltration of material obtained from spleen CF contained LCIF, characterized as PG, and LCPF of M.W. 10,000-30,000 daltons. The addition of monocytes-MØ to purified MØ-depleted lymphocytes restored their colony formation capacity to that of undepleted lymphocytes. If

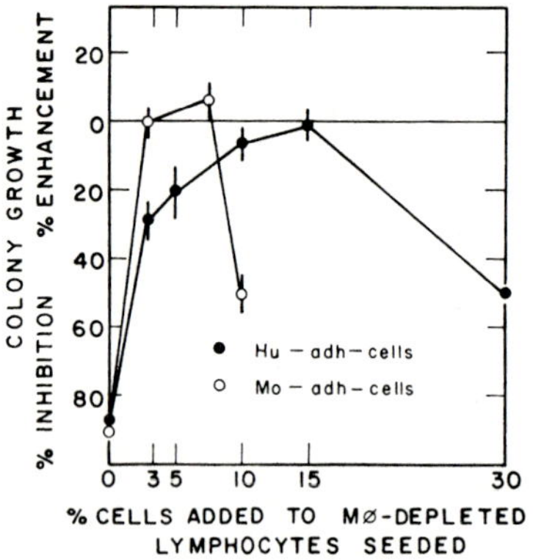

FIGURE 2. Effect on T-cell colony growth of human (Hu) blood adherent (adh) cells added to monocyte-depleted blood lymphocytes —• and mouse (Mo) spleen adherent cells added to MØ-depleted lymph node cells —o.

excessive numbers of MØ were introduced, colony development was markedly inhibited (Fig. 2). The colony growth of mitogen-sensitized mononuclear cells was 100% greater than that of isolated lymphocytes. Mitogen-stimulated T lymphocytes seem to secrete into the culture medium their own LCEF which, in the presence of monocytes-MØ, or their LCPF, augments lymphocyte proliferation and colony formation. The MØ, or their derivative, probably generate an additional signal that triggers the continued and/or accelerated production of LCEF. Our results on T cells point to the existence of a regulatory system in which stimulatory and inhibitory factors compete for T cells. Such a system might well also operate in controlling lymphocyte colony production under the influence of endogenous regulating substances. These include LCEF, LCPF and LCIF, the latter two released mainly by monocytes-MØ.

REFERENCES

1. Zeevi, A., Goldman, I., and Rozenszajn, L.A., *Cell Immunol. 28*, 235 (1977).
2. Sredni, B., Michlin, H., Kalechman, Y., and Rozenszajn, L.A., *Cell Immunol. 35*, 135 (1978).
3. Zeevi, A., Goldman, I., and Rozenszajn, L.A., *Immunology 34*, 523 (1978).
4. Rozenszajn, L.A., Shoham, D., and Kalechman, Y., *Immunology 29*, 1041 (1975).
5. Sredni, B., Kalechman, Y., Michlin, H., and Rozenszajn, L.A., *Nature (Lond.) 259*, 130 (1976).

DISCUSSION

WATSON: In collaboration with Gillis and Smith, we have been seeking to purify T cell growth factor from various sources. In short, murine T cell growth activity is associated with a protein 30,000 daltons in size and separable into two components by charge (pI 4.3 and 4.9). Rat and human T cell growth activity is contained in a smaller molecule (15,000 daltons), with an isoelectric point of 5.5 for rat and 6.5 for human.

FARRAR: We have shown that highly purified T cell mitogenic factor is also capable of enhancing the PFC response of nude mouse spleen cells, and augmenting the allo-antigen specific cytotoxic T cell response.

SCHIMPL: I would make a cautionary note about the "purity" of the factors mentioned by Watson and by Farrar, and indeed all the factors being discussed. Biosynthetically radioactively labelled TRF was subjected to PEG concentration, $(NH4)_2\ SO_4$ precipitation, phenyl-sepharose, and in some instances AH-sepharose and Gly-AH-sepharose purification. A single stainable spot is found in 2D-gel electrophoresis (IEF + SDS-PAGE) and this spot can be attributed to actin. Fluorography, however, reveals $\sim$50 spots, 8 of which are present in biologically active partial purified preparations only and are absent from identically treated biologically inactive control supernates. Obviously, we are too far away from pure preparations to make any statement whether different biological activities are associated with one and the same molecule or not.

MÜHLRADT: In reply to Watson's claim that TRF and costimulator activity reside in the same molecule, we have studied production of several lymphokines in mouse spleen cell cultures stimulated with Con A. We can find conditions which will allow high activity of costimulator and of practically no TRF and vice versa. This indicates that these two activities do not reside in the same molecule.

WEBB: First a comment on iodination of proteins. This procedure will only label proteins or peptides containing tyrosine. Therefore estimates of purity based on this procedure are of limited value. A second point is the issue of specific activity. Do either Watson or Farrar have any information on the specific activity of their preparations which would give us some idea of their level of purity?

WATSON: In murine, rat and human preparations of T cell growth factor, four lymphokine activities copurify: (1) T cell growth activity; (2) the stimulation of mitogenic responses to Con A in thymocyte cultures under conditions where the mitogen alone does not stimulate a response; (3) the stimulation of antibody responses to erythrocyte antigens in T cell-depleted cultures and (4) the generation of cytotoxic effector T cells in thymocyte or nude spleen cultures.

FARRAR: We have purified the mitogenic factor approximately 1000-fold and have found that this material is active in all three of the bioassays at approximately 10^{-10}M assuming a molecular weight of 30,000 daltons.

LYMPHOKINE AND MONOKINE REGULATION OF FIBROBLAST FUNCTION

Sharon M. Wahl
Larry M. Wahl
Stephan E. Mergenhagen

The National Institutes of Health
National Institute of Dental Research
Bethesda, Maryland

I. INTRODUCTION

Lymphocytes and monocytes are the primary cellular elements of chronic inflammatory lesions. Chronic inflammation is often accompanied by the formation of fibrotic tissue. The mechanism of induction of this fibrotic reaction is unknown, but current work suggests that the lymphocytes and monocytes may influence the enhanced fibroblast proliferation and collagen synthesis.

II. MATERIALS AND METHODS

The preparation of guinea pig macrophage and sensitized lymphocyte supernatants was carried out as described previously (1,2). Fibroblast culture methods, determination of their proliferation by tritiated thymidine uptake and increased cell numbers and the assay for protein synthesis have been reported elsewhere (1). Also described in detail elsewhere are the assays for cyclic AMP and prostaglandin E_2 (PGE_2) (2).

ISBN 0-12-213950-X

III. RESULTS AND DISCUSSION

Supernatants from DNP-OA sensitized T lymphocytes exposed to this antigen in vitro for 24-48 hr induced quiescent, serum-free fibroblast cultures to incorporate enhanced levels of tritiated thymidine (Fig. 1), while control lymphocyte supernatants were ineffective. The increased thymidine uptake correlated with increased numbers of fibroblasts in the cultures. Fibroblast proliferation was inversely proportional to the cell density in these cultures with maximal increases in subconfluent cultures (Fig. 1).

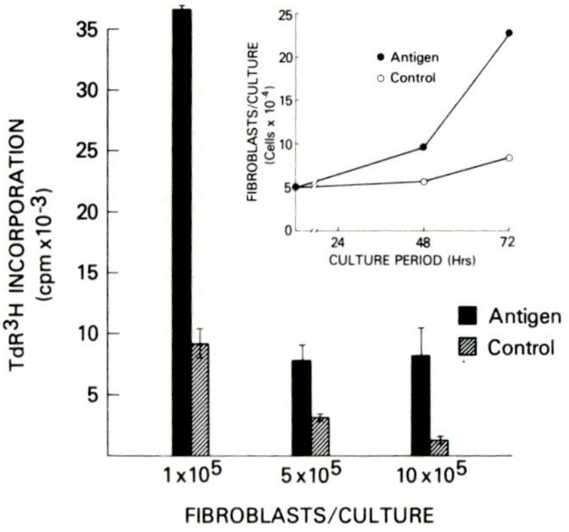

FIGURE 1. Antigen activated lymphocyte supernatants stimulated increased TdR^{3}H incorporation and cell numbers in fibroblast cultures.

In addition to stimulating the fibroblasts to proliferate, the T cell supernatants caused the fibroblasts to synthesize enhanced levels of PGE_2 ($\geq$ 20 fold increase). The elevated PGE_2 effected an increase in intracellular levels of cAMP which was blocked by indomethacin. Furthermore, these fibroblasts which were metabolically stimulated by the lymphocyte factor increased their output of collagen and noncollagenous protein (1). This soluble lymphocyte derived factor which activates fibroblasts was stable to dialysis, heating at 56°C for 30 min, lyophilization and freeze thawing. It was labile at 100°C for 15 min and precipitated by 40-60% ammonium sulfate. Thus, antigen activated lymphocytes may play a role in the control of fibroplasia associated with chronic inflammation through the release of this soluble mediator.

Macrophages which are abundant in chronic inflammation can also be activated to influence fibroblast function. Lipopolysaccharide stimulated macrophages to produce a soluble mediator of fibroblast proliferation. The activity was seen early after macrophage activation (1-2 hr) and continued to increase for 24-48 hr suggesting release of a preformed molecule followed by synthesis. Nonactivated macrophages did not produce this factor which stimulated both fibroblast protein synthesis (Table I) and proliferation (Table II).

TABLE I. Macrophage Stimulation of Collagen and Noncollagen Protein Synthesis by Fibroblasts

Macrophage Supernatant	^3H Proline (cpm) Incorporated into	
	Collagen	Noncollagen Protein
None	4,339	27,313
LPS	14,448	112,196
Control	5,502	27,804
Control + LPS	5,010	30,345

TABLE II. Effect of Dialysis of Macrophage Supernatants on Fibroblast TdR ^3H Incorporation and Proliferation

Macrophage Supernatant[a]	TdR ^3H Incorporation (cpm)	Cell Number (per culture)
Dialyzed		
1:2	21,610 ± 1,047	199,317
1:4	24,607 ± 1,318	171,683
Nondialyzed		
1:2	4,374 ± 230	218,850
1:4	9,328 ± 887	238,800

[a] *LPS activated macrophage supernatants were added to fibroblast cultures containing 5 x 10^4 cells.*

This macrophage derived fibroblast activating factor was inactivated at 100°C for 15 min and was precipitated at 40-60% ammonium sulfate. The approximate molecular weight as determined by gel chromatography was 40-60,000. In addition to this factor the macrophage supernatants contained a small, dialyzable molecule which inhibited the uptake of tritiated thymidine by the fibroblasts, but did not inhibit fibroblast division (Table II). Since it has been shown that macrophages release thymidine into their culture medium (3), we attempted to restore the inhibition of TdR^3H incorporation by adding cold thymidine to the dialyzed supernatants. Thymidine as low as 10^{-6} M caused an inhibition of TdR^3H uptake equivalent to that seen prior to dialysis without influencing actual cellular division.

Activated macrophages then can release a number of biologically active mediators including fibroblast activating factor which can trigger fibroblasts into active proliferation and protein synthesis. By this mechanism macrophages may play a functional role in the fibrosis seen in granulomatous and other chronic inflammatory diseases. Recent studies have shown that the granulomas in schistosomiasis produce a factor which causes enhanced fibroblast activity (4) and thus may influence the deposition of collagen associated with this liver disease.

REFERENCES

1. Wahl, S. M., Wahl, L. M. and McCarthy, J. B. (1978). *J. Immunol. 121*, 942.
2. Wahl, S. M., Wahl, L. M., McCarthy, J. B., Chedid, L. and Mergenhagen, S. E. (1979). *J. Immunol.* In press.
3. Stadecker, M. J., Calderon, J., Karnovsky, M. L. and Unanue, E. R. (1977). *J. Immunol. 119*, 1738.
4. Wyler, D., Wahl, S. M. and Wahl, L. M. (1978). *Science 202*, 438.

DISCUSSION

YOSHIDA: Does Mergenhagen have any data showing identity or differences of FAFs originating from in vivo granulomas with that produced in vitro?

MERGENHAGEN: None.

WAKSMAN: Proteases stimulate fibroblast proliferation. Is there proteolytic activity in Mergenhagen's active fractions? He might also look at the effect of protease inhibitors.

MERGENHAGEN: We know that collagenase is in the macrophage supernatants but have not looked for other activities that might be involved in fibroblast proliferation.

WAKSMAN: The schistosome granuloma contains large numbers of eosinophils, which are also known to release a variety of active mediators. One must be cautious about attributing the fibroblast stimulation to macrophage products, as Mergenhagen did.

MERGENHAGEN: We are certainly aware of the contributions of eosinophils to the granuloma. Waksman's point is certainly a valid one.

GRANGER: Does Mergenhagen's supernatant stimulate other cells to divide *in vitro*?

MERGENHAGEN: The only other activity we looked for is LAF. Mizel found no evidence of LAF activity in our Sephadex fractions containing fibroblast-activating factors.

BOROS: We have recently shown (Boros et al., Fed.Proc. 1979) that fibroblasts within artificial hypersensitivity lung granulomas generated by antigen-coupled Sepharose beads in a primed mouse, can be activated by systemic injection of the specific antigen. Stimulation has been proven by the removal of the lung granulomas, pulsing *in vitro* with ^{14}C-proline and proving incorporation of label and collagenase sensitivity of the labelled protein. Furthermore, dialyzed supernates of such hypersensitivity but not foreign-body (induced by bead alone in unprimed mice) granulomas injected into mice carrying foreign-body lung granulomas, induced enhanced fibroblast activity as outlined. These two pieces of evidence indicate that fibroblast activity within an imflammatory reaction *in vivo* can be manipulated by mediators probably produced by lymphocytes.

REGULATORY INFLUENCES OF THYMOSIN ON VARIOUS LYMPHOID POPULATIONS

Gailen D. Marshall, Jr.
Gary B. Thurman
Teresa L.K. Low
Allan L. Goldstein

Department of Biochemistry
The George Washington University
School of Medicine and Health Sciences
Washington, D.C.

I. INTRODUCTION

The role of the endocrine thymus in the initiation, maintenance, and regulation of the cellular immune system is being extensively investigated. Many investigators have described the existence of suppressor T cells which apparently function to regulate the appearance and/or magnitude of effector T and B cells (Gershon, 1974). The thymic dependence of suppressor T cells is suggested by the work of Reinisch (Reinisch and Andrew, 1978) and Simpson (Simpson and Cantor, 1975), who demonstrated that adult thymectomy abrogated thy 1.2 positive suppressor activity in spleens of mice.

Other studies (Dauphinee, 1974; Horowitz *et al.*, 1977) have shown that an extract from calf thymus, thymosin, can induce suppressor cell activity in murine and human situations where immune regulation appears to be lacking. These studies suggested an important regulatory role of the endocrine thymus in modulating immune functions.

Supported in part by grants CA-24974 and CA-25017 from The National Cancer Institute, Hoffman-La Roche, Inc., and The James W. McLaughlin Fellowship Fund.

ISBN 0-12-213950-X

II. REGULATORY EFFECTS OF THYMOSIN FRACTION 5

Recent studies have shown that the thymus is the major control organ for cell-mediated immunity (CMI). The T cell system, responsible for CMI, has the task of protecting self tissue by recognizing and destroying foreign or effete cells. The major T cell population responsible for this activity is the cytotoxic T lymphocytes (CTL). The study of CTL activity has been greatly aided by the technique of mixed lymphocyte tumor culture (MLTC) which allows *in vitro* generation of CTL. In addition, an accurate assessment of CTL activity is made possible by use of the *in vitro* ^{51}Cr release assay, which gives a sensitive measurement of target cell killing.

Investigation into the thymic control of CTL activity has yielded interesting information. Miller (Miller, 1961) paved the way for studies which demonstrated that neonatal thymectomy could prevent the appearance of CTL in mice. However, other investigators showed that adult thymectomy would result in enhanced CTL activity of murine splenic lymphocytes (Simpson, 1975). This implied that the thymus might have a regulatory function on CTL progenitors found in peripheral lymphoid tissue. Reinisch (Reinisch *et al.*, 1977) described a system, using complete Freund's adjuvant (CFA), whereby suppression of MLTC generation of CTL was possible. This effect was mediated by a cell population that was either thymus derived or thymus dependent, since adult thymectomy rapidly diminished the CFA effect. Other investigators showed similar regulatory defects in thymectomized animals (Asherson *et al.*, 1976). These studies and others led us to investigate the endocrine thymic dependence of suppressor T cells in two murine models.

A. *In Vitro Thymosin Induced Suppressor T Cells in Normal Murine Lymphocyte Populations*

The problem was approached based upon the understanding that normal animals have a certain number of suppressor cells that function on a routine basis. It was reasoned that *in vitro* MLTC might provide a means by which investigations into thymic hormonal dependence of suppressor cell function could be accomplished. Normal 6-8 week old BALB/c spleen or lymph node cells were cultured in a 5 day allogenic MLTC against RBL-5, a leukemia line of C57(B6) mice. Thymosin fraction 5 was added in various doses to appropriate cultures at the beginning of each experiment. Results showed that thymosin could suppress the generation of CTL by as much as 82 per cent (Table 1).

TABLE 1. Effect of Thymosin on In Vitro Generation Of CTL by BALB/c Lymphocytes

Cell source[a]	Thymosin[b]	Per cent cytotoxicity[c] (±SEM)[d]	Per cent suppression
Spleen	-	43.2 ± 0.9	-
	+	16.0 ± 0.7	63 ($p < .001$)[e]
Lymph Node	-	65.9 ± 1.4	-
	+	12.8 ± 1.5	82 ($p < .001$)

[a]Pool from 5 animals per group; [b]200 μg/ml thymosin fraction 5 (lot C100496); [c]effector:target ratio 25:1; [d]standard error of the mean; [e]Student's t test

Mixing of thymosin treated cells with fresh spleen cells in a second MLTC could suppress CTL generation again, indicating the presence of a thymosin-induced suppressor cell. Incubation of thymosin treated cells with anti-thy 1.2 and complement eliminated suppressor activity, confirming the thymosin-induced suppression was a T cell (Table 2).

TABLE 2. Effect of Anti-thy 1.2 Serum on Thymosin Induced Suppressor Activity

Cell treatment	Added to fresh spleen[a]	Per cent cytotoxicity (±SEM)
Media	-	52.0 ± 1.3
	+	54.3 ± 1.8
Thymosin	-	12.8 ± 1.5
	+	18.4 ± 1.0
Thymosin + Anti-thy 1.2[b]	-	4.3 ± 0.1
	+	54.6 ± 1.1

[a]Lymph node cells were obtained from 5 day primary MLTC incubated with media or media plus 200 μg/ml thymosin. Cells were harvested and added to fresh spleen cells in a 1:1 ratio and cultured in a second 5 day MLTC vs. RBL-5. [b]Anti-thy 1.2 treatment after 5 day MLTC with 200 μg/ml thymosin.

B. *In Vivo Thymosin Induced Suppressor T Cells in Nude Mouse Spleen*

It is well established that nude mice lack a thymic influence but do have normal T cell progenitors in bone marrow and peripheral lymphoid tissue (Kindred, 1978). Thus it was of interest to investigate the effects of *in vivo* thymosin treatment of CTL activity. Previous efforts had yielded seemingly negative results of thymosin-induced reconstitution of nudes (unpublished data). However, with the studies of Cantor and Boyse (Cantor *et al.*, 1975) showing stepwise maturation of T cells, our data was reviewed on the premise that partial restoration might have occurred in nudes treated with thymosin. Therefore, a series of experiments was initiated to determine whether or not thymosin had any effect on nude mouse lymphocytes. Groups of 10 nude mice were divided into two categories. Half received injections of saline and the other half received 400 µg of thymosin fraction 5. Thymosin treatment induced suppressor activity in nude spleens when mixed with normal spleens in a 5 day suppressor activity indicating that this suppressor cell was also a T cell (Table 3).

TABLE 3. Effect of Mixing Thymosin Treated Nude Mouse Spleen Cells With Fresh Normal Spleen Cells On In Vitro CTL Generation

Group	*Added to fresh normal spleen*	*Per cent cytotoxicity (±SEM)*	*Per cent suppression*
Norm	-	56.9 ± 1.5	
Nude	-	1.1 ± 0.1	
	+	56.2 ± 1.2	1 (NS)[b]
Nude-thymosin[a]	-	3.0 ± 0.6	
	+	27.2 ± 0.8	52 ($p<.01$)[c]
Nude-thymosin & Anti-thy 1.2	-	1.8 ± 0.4	
	+	52.7 ± 1.1	4 (NS)

[a]Nudes injected with 400 µg thymosin every other day for 14 days; [b]not significant; [c]student's T-test

III. DISCUSSION

The *in vivo* and *in vitro* regulatory effects of thymosin present a two-edged sword. The potentials for inducing regulatory cells in autoimmune diseases where regulation is absent is obvious. This information may someday be utilized clinically to regulate uncontrolled immunity. Another potential usefulness for thymosin-induced immunoregulation is iatrogenic induction of tolerance in transplant recipients. An *in vitro* induction of tolerance to a potential graft utilizing thymosin would allow the survival of allogeneic organ grafts without the immunosuppressive treatments that recipients must now receive.

However, a note of caution is also warranted in these findings. There are situations where suppression of the immune response is not desired. Most notable among these, cancer. Any agent, including thymosin, which has the capability of modulating the immune response must be utilized with proper caution. Our studies indicate that the effect of thymosin (augmentive or regulatory) is largely dependent upon the nature of the cell population on which it acts. The ultimate aim of the thymosin program is to define the peptide or peptides responsible for the various activities of the fraction 5 preparation. However, until this goal is accomplished, it is obligatory that the immune status of the individual or experimental system be determined prior to the use of thymosin to augment or regulate the immune response.

REFERENCES

Asherson, G.L., Zembala, M., Mayhew, B., and Goldstein, A.L. (1976). *Eur. J. Immunol. 6,* 699.

Cantor, H. and Boyse, E.A. (1975). *J. Exp. Med. 141,* 1376.

Dauphinee, M. (1974). *Proc. Natl. Acad. Sci. 71,* 2637.

Gershon, R.K. (1974). *In* "Contemporary Topics in Immunology" Vol. 3. (M.D. Cooper and N.L. Warner, eds.), p. 1. Plenum Press, New York.

Horowitz, S., Borcherding, W., Moorthy, A.V., Chesney, R., Schulte-Wissermann, H., Hong, R., and Goldstein, A.L. (1977). *Science, 197,* 999.

Kindred, B. (1978). *Immunol. Reviews 42,* 60.

Miller, J.F.A.P. (1961). *Lancet 2,*748.

Reinisch, C.L., Andrew, S.L., and Schlossman, S.F. (1977). *Proc. Natl. Acad. Sci. USA 74,*2989.

Reinisch, C.L., and Andrew, S.L. (1978). *J. Exp. Med. 148,*619.

Simpson, E. and Cantor, H. (1975). *Eur. J. Immunol. 5,* 337.

LT MOLECULES FORM A SUBUNIT SYSTEM OF CELL TOXINS[1]

G. A. Granger
J. C. Hiserodt
R. S. Yamamoto
M. W. Ross

Department of Molecular Biology and Biochemistry
University of California, Irvine
Irvine, California

Lymphotoxins (LT) are proteins of various molecular weight and charge released by activated lymphocytes in vitro from man and experimental animals. These substances cause growth inhibition and nonspecific protracted lysis of selected cell types in vitro (1). Lymphotoxins can be released by activated T and B cells or human B cell lines in vitro (1). The heterogeneity of lymphotoxins has been confusing; even different laboratories working with these materials from the same animal species have reported different sizes (2, 3). The inability to relate the various LT forms to one another within and between species has been difficult to understand. These molecules have been proposed as potential effectors of cell lysis in CMI reactions. Indeed, there is both positive and negative evidence concerning their role in these reactions (4, 5). There is clearly a need to resolve these components and define their role in CMI reactions.

Extensive biochemical and immunologic studies on human and murine LT forms reveal these molecules must be viewed in entirely new light, for while they are heterogeneous, they form an interrelated subunit system of molecules (6, 7). The total number of L cell lytic - human LT forms we have resolved by various biochemical techniques released by antigen or lectin activated human lymphocytes in vitro are shown in Figure 1. The situation appears very complex. The

[1]This research was supported by Grant No. AI-09460, from the Allergy and Infectious Diseases Institute, National Institutes of Health, Bethesda, Maryland.

ISBN 0-12-213950-X

particular forms detectable depend on a number of variables, such as culture conditions, the lymphoid cell type releasing, the time the supernatant is collected, etc. In addition, the forms marked with an asterisk are unstable and therefore only detectable when supernatants are handled rapidly. The

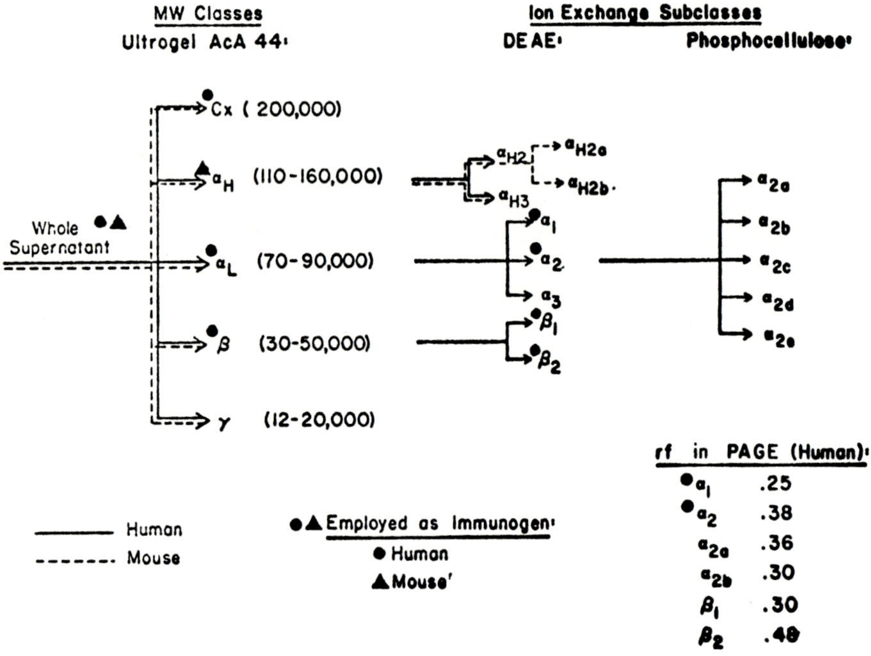

Fig. 1. Biochemical resolution of human and murine LT molecules.

major components in a given supernatant detectable on L cells are primarily the smaller molecular weight forms, α and β_2, because they are stable to storage and manipulation. It is not surprising, therefore, that these are the components that have been most studied by other investigators. The other forms detected by many investigators are either unstable or present as a small percentage of the total activity in a given supernatant. There are several types of heterogeneity: a) different molecular weight classes, each of which we have given a specific designation, Cx, α, β, and γ; b) α and β MW classes can be further separated into charge subclasses. Walker and Lucas, and our own studies revealed the α class can be separated into multiple charge subclasses. Our own studies indicate some of the charge heterogeneity of this class is due to sialic acid associated with these materials which can be removed with neuraminidase (8). The small dots and triangles indicate human and murine LT forms against which we have been able to induce antibodies. While the detailed proofs cannot be discussed thoroughly here, we have found the different MW classes are interrelated subunits. This relationship is shown in Fig. 2. It is clear the molecular heterogeneity can be resolved into a much simpler model. We have found the smaller molecular weight

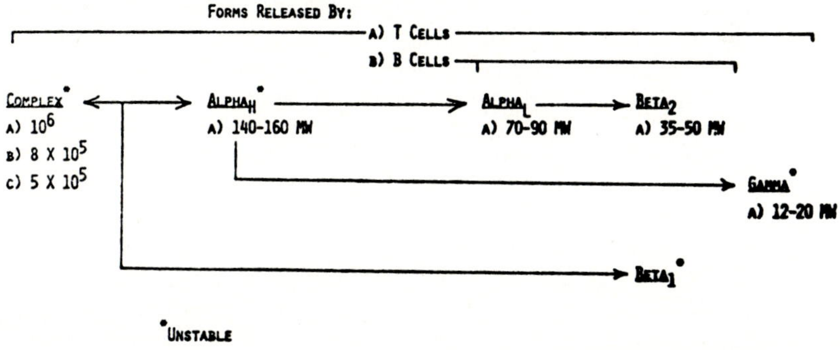

Fig. 2. Relationship of human LT MW classes lytic for L-929 cells released by lectin activated T and B cells in vitro.

forms can be dissociated from the larger MW forms by high ionic strength buffers, and each subunit has been identified by both physical and immunological methods. The association between the various subunits appears to be by noncovalent means of various degrees of strength. We also find that different lymphoid cells can release different LT forms. B cells or continuous B cell lines appear to release only the α_L form, whereas T cells are able to release all detectable forms. It should also be mentioned here that strikingly similar MW size and charge forms have recently been identified in the mouse.

The various human LT forms, not only can associate with themselves, but are capable of associating with antigen binding receptors, which appear to be of T cell origin. Antibodies reactive with human immunoglobulin molecules were first noted to interact with LT forms by Amino and colleagues (9). We found rabbit anti-F(ab')$_2$ prepared from human IgG Fab fragments is capable of inhibiting the LT activity in fresh human supernatants and certain MW LT classes obtained from lectin activated peripheral blood T cells or lectin activated 5-day MLC blasts. Antisera reactive with Fab fragments reacted strongly with the complex and alpha heavy forms. No reactivity was noted with anti-H chain sera. These results suggested the presence of an antigen binding receptor in the high MW forms. We collected supernatants and MW classes from alloimmune human (MLC sensitized) peripheral blood lymphocytes stimulated for 10 hr in vitro with PHA. We found supernatants and Cx MW LT forms from the alloimmune lymphocytes possessed the capacity to specifically bind to stimulator cells. Similar results were obtained with human lymphoid cells sensitive to soluble antigens bound to affinity beads. Our recent studies performed in the mouse revealed a similar situation, namely, identification of high MW LT receptor forms released in vitro by lectin activated alloimmune murine cells which can specifically bind to sensitizing allogeneic tumor cells in vitro (10). The receptor in these forms from human and mouse does not appear to be traditional immunoglobulin. The evidence to support this is: a) in human, it can be identified in supernatants from T "enriched" lymphocytes; b) in human, it is not reactive with antibodies reactive with H regions of serum antibodies; and c) in the mouse, the releasing cells are Ig negative and theta positive. The alpha heavy forms of 140-160,000 MW, derived from purified human T cells, appear to be the smallest LT form which contains R. The present evidence indicates about 100,000 MW of this form can be accounted for by α_L and γ LT forms. The remaining 40-60,000 MW may be assigned to the R, which is much smaller than a traditional Ab molecule. Our latest studies indicate that Cx forms are released by T cells in a precursor form which express Fab determinants and require further processing before the LT antigenic determinants are expressed. Fig. 3 contains a theoretical model which places the R and LT forms together.

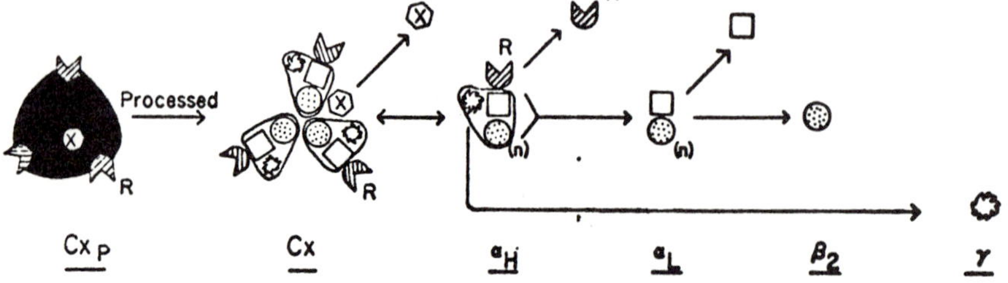

Fig. 3. Molecular model of LT subunits.

These molecules once released appear quite unstable and rapidly dissociate into the smaller MW classes.

The most recent studies indicate that various MW LT human and murine forms have different functional capacity (10, 11). In the human, the smaller forms, α, β, and γ are only weakly lytic and most effective on murine L-929 cells in protracted assays. The most recent studies indicate they are actually inactive and require an enzymatic activation step by target cell proteases. The larger forms, complex and α_H, are from 10 to 200 times more effective in a nonspecific fashion on other cell types than the smaller MW forms. In both the human, and the mouse system, we have identified that the high MW complex LT receptor forms from alloimmune cells are capable of causing rapid specific target cell destruction. This very brief summary indicates some important new concepts associated with the LT cell-lytic system of molecules, namely, that LT molecules are small, weakly lytic subunits, but can be assembled together, presumably by T cells to further associate with antigen binding receptors to form high MW complexes. These complexes are capable of rapid specific target cell lysis. They are very unstable and rapidly dissociate into the smaller less effective components.

REFERENCES

1. Granger, G. A., Daynes, R. A., Runge, P., Jeffes, E., and Prieur, A.-M. (1975). *Contemp. Top. Molec. Immunol.* *4*, 205.
2. Kolb, W. P., and Granger, G. A. (1968). *PNAS* *61*, 1250.
3. Trivers, G., Baumgart, D., and Leonard, E. J. (1976). *J. Immunol.* *117*, 130.
4. Hiserodt, J. C., and Granger, G. A. (1977). *J. Immunol.* *119*, 374.
5. Gately, M., Mayer, M., Henney, C. S. (1976). *Cell. Immunol.* *27*, 82.
6. Yamamoto, R., Hiserodt, J., Lewis, J., Carmack, C., and Granger, G. (1978). *Cell. Immunol.* *38*, 403.
7. Ross, M. W., Tiangco, G., Horn, P., Hiserodt, J. C. and Granger, G. A. (1979). *J. Immunol.* (*in press*).
8. Toth, M. K., and Granger, G. A. (1979). *Immunochem.* (*in press*).
9. Amino, N., Pipher, J., Mier, R., Moore, G., and DeGroot, L. (1974). *J. Immunol.* *113*, 1334.
10. Hiserodt, J., Tiangco, G., and Granger, G. A. (1979). *J. Immunol.* (*in press*).
11. Yamamoto, R., Hiserodt, J. C., and Granger, G. A. (1979). *Cell. Immunol.* (*in press*).

EFFECTOR MOLECULES IN DIRECT LYMPHOCYTE MEDIATED CYTOTOXICITY[1]

Carl F. Ware[2]
Gale A. Granger

Department of Molecular Biology and Biochemistry
University of California
Irvine, California

INTRODUCTION

Investigations into the role of lymphotoxins (LT) in direct lymphocyte mediated cytotoxic reactions by the use of LT-neutralizing antibodies have been complicated by the antigenic heterogeneity exhibited by the different components of the LT system (1). We have approached this problem by employing anti-human LT sera with different specificities and studying the properties of these antisera on the cytolytic capacity of alloimmune human lymphocytes *in vitro*.

METHODS

Lymphotoxin activity was measured on non-dividing mouse L929 cells (2). The production and characterization of xenogenic anti-LT sera have been described (1).[1] Briefly, anti-whole supernatant (anti-WS) was made against serum-free unfractionated supernatants from PHA-stimulated adenoid lymphocytes. Anti-LT class and subclass antisera were made against gel filtration and/or ion exchange resin purified LT. Membrane associated LT was detected by absorption of anti-LT activity (3). Direct lymphocyte cytotoxicity was assayed in a 4 hr ^{51}Chromium release micro-test employing 5 day one-way MLC-sensitized lymphocytes to human B-cell lines (4). Precursor-LT containing supernatants were obtained by co-culture of MLC-lymphoblasts with Conconavalin A (10 μg/ml) for 5 to 10 hrs.

[1] *This work was in part supported by grant AI-09460 from NIAID, NIH.*
[2] *Present address: Department of Biochemistry, The University of Texas Health Science Center, San Antonio, Texas, 78284*

ISBN 0-12-213950-X

RESULTS AND DISCUSSION

1. *Identification of an Antigenic Precursor Form of LT*

Investigations of the immunologic forms of cytotoxins released by MLC-sensitized ConA-activated T-lymphocytes revealed that the polyspecific anti-WS, but not anti-α or β LT sera, was capable of neutralizing the cytolytic activity. However, the gel filtration chromatographic pattern of the cytotoxic activity obtained from MLC-blasts indicated that these cytotoxins were biochemically and antigenically identical to LT obtained from lectin-stimulated (no prior MLC culture) lymphocytes (5). Treatment of the unfractionated supernatant with non-ionic detergents, urea, or freeze-thawing altered the antigenic nature of the cytotoxic activity such that anti α LT was now capable of neutralizing the cytotoxic activity. As shown in Figure 1, this antigenic form of LT was detectable on the membrane of both MLC-blasts and ConA-activated blasts, whereas the α LT antigenic determinant(s) was detectable only on activated cells (3). Collectively, these data suggest that the α and β antigenic determinants are derived from an antigenically distinct membrane-associated precursor form of LT (pre-LT).

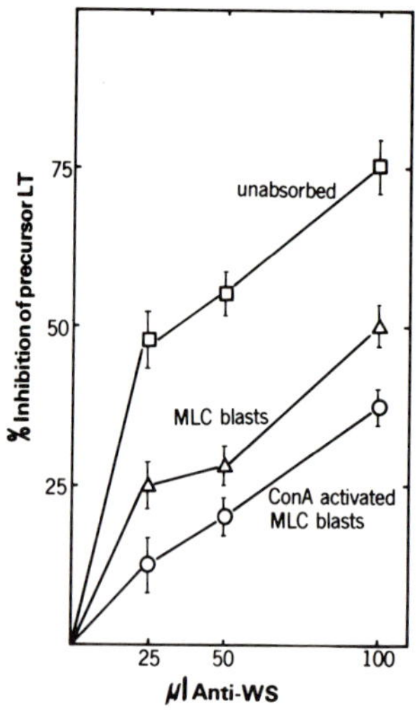

FIGURE 1. Detection of Membrane Associated Precursor LT (see reference 3 for details)

2. *The Effects of Anti-LT Sera on Direct Lymphocyte Mediated Cytotoxicity*

Presented in Table I is a summary of seventeen experiments in which the various anti-LT sera were added concurrently with cytotoxic lymphocytes and radiolabeled specific target cells. The results indicate the poly-

TABLE I. Summary of the Effects of Anti-LT Sera on Human T-Cell Mediated Cytotoxicity[a]

% Inhibition of Cytolysis by[b]			
Anti-WS	*Anti α class or α_1 and α_2 subcl.*	*Anti-β*	*Anti-LTcx*
60-100 (1:4-1:30)[c]	*0-3 (1:2)*	*−20-5 (1:2 to 1:10)*	*0-5 (1:2)*

[a]*20:1 effector:target cell ratio*

[b]*Heat inactivated, preabsorbed with target cells (WIL-2, RPMI-1788, 2 x 10^8/ml), serum proteins, PHA-P*

[c]*Effective dilution of antisera*

specific anti-WS was the only antisera capable of consistently inhibiting this cytotoxic reaction. Variable results were found with anti-class and subclass antisera of restricted specificity. Additional experiments revealed that absorption of the anti-WS with lectin-activated alloimmune lymphocytes preferentially removed the cytolytic-inhibitory antibodies when compared to non-activated lymphocytes and that the LT neutralizing capacity of both anti-WS and anti α for pre-LT and α LT activity was significantly reduced after incubation in the cytotoxic reaction. Previously published work has shown that the anti-LT sera do not inhibit the proliferation of lymphocytes to alloantigens or lectins (6). Collectively, these data support the concept that the anti-WS inhibits T-lymphocyte cytolytic activity by virtue of binding LT molecules, most likely associated with the pre-LT antigen(s).

3. *The Stage of the Alloimmune Cytotoxic Reaction Inhibited by Anti-WS*

By analogy to the murine alloimmune cytotoxic system we have attempted to define the site(s) of the inhibitory action of the anti-WS relative to the Ca^{2+} dependent phase of the cytotoxic reaction (7). Effector and target cells were centrifuged together to initiate contact and incubated at 37°C. At various intervals following centrifugation EGTA[3] (5 mM) or anti-WS (1:4 dilution) were added to the reaction mixtures. The reaction was then allowed to proceed for 3 hrs at which time the degree of inhibition

[3]*Ethyleneglycol-bis-(β-amino-ethylether)N,N′-tetraacetic acid, Ca^{2+} specific chelator*

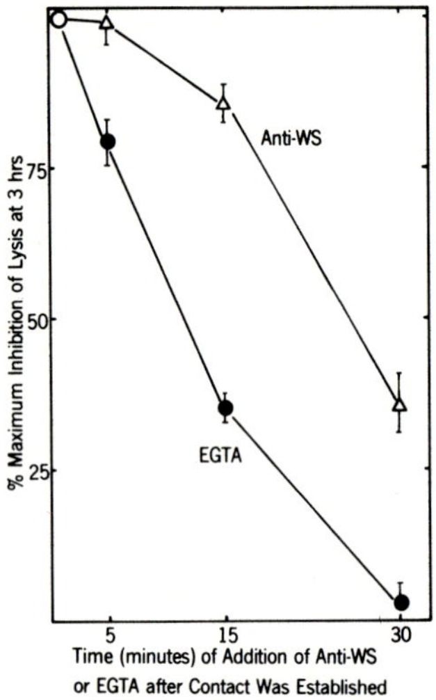

Figure 2. Kinetics of the Inhibitory Action of EGTA or Anti-WS on T-Cell Cytotoxicity. Human PBL:WIL-2 Target Cell Ratio of 20:1

of cytolysis was assessed. The data are presented in Figure 2 as the percent inhibition of the maximum inhibition obtained when these reagents are added to the reaction before the centrifugation step. The results indicate that the anti-WS inhibits lysis through a sequence of events into and following the Ca^{2+} dependent process, perhaps during the lethal hit.

4. *Biochemical Characterization of the Antigen(s) Recognized by Anti-WS*

Abrogation of the cytolytic-inhibitory activity of the anti-WS by absorption of the antisera with selected fractions of LT containing supernatants provides a method to physically characterize the antigen(s) recognized by this complex antiserum. An example of this method is shown in Figure 3. Anti-WS was absorbed with gel filtration fractions obtained from lectin-stimulated adenoid lymphocytes (5). The absorbed antisera were then tested for their capacity to inhibit human T cell cytotoxicity. This method is limited to fractionation techniques that preserve antigenic structure. The results indicate the antigenic determinant(s) recognized by the anti-WS are heterogenous, but predominantly associated with a high MW component, present in the LTcx fraction. This evidence supports our concept that the LT form most probably employed by an effector T-lymphocyte is a high MW LT complex.

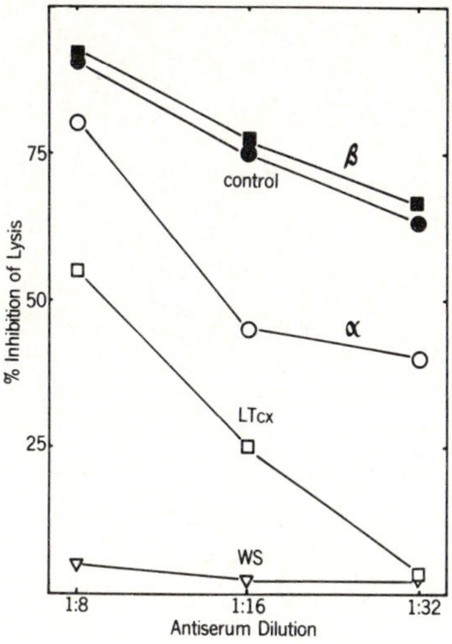

Figure 3. Abrogation of the Cytolytic-Inhibitory Action of Anti-WS by Gel Filtration Purified LT Molecules. Adenoid Lymphocytes:WIL-2 ratio of 20:1

ACKNOWLEDGEMENTS

The authors wish to thank Mr. Bob Yamamoto and Mr. Paul Harris for their contributions. The excellent assistance of Linda Winchester in preparing this manuscript is appreciated.

REFERENCES

1. Yamamoto, R. S., J. C. Hiserodt, J. E. Lewis, C. E. Carmack, and G. A. Granger, Cell. Immunol. 38, 403 (1978).
2. Spofford, B. T., R. A. Daynes, and G. A. Granger, J. Immunol. 12, 2111 (1974).
3. Hiserodt, J. C., C. F. Ware, P. C. Harris, and G. A. Granger, Cell. Immunol. 34, 326 (1977).
4. Svedmyr, E., H. Wigzell, and M. Jondal, Scand. J. Immunol. 3, 499 (1974).
5. Granger, G. A., R. S. Yamamoto, D. S. Fair, and J. C. Hiserodt, Cell. Immunol. 38, 388 (1978).
6. Hiserodt, J. C. and G. A. Granger, J. Immunol. 119, 374 (1977).
7. Martz, E., Contemporary Topics in Immunobiology 7, 273 (1977).

AN IMMUNOLOGIC COMPARISON OF HUMAN INTERFERONS AND LYMPHOTOXINS

Carl F. Ware
Thomas H. Reidarson
Gale A. Granger

University of California, Irvine
Irvine, California

INTRODUCTION

The physiochemical resolution of lymphotoxins (LT) and interferons (IF) obtained from antigen or lectin stimulated lymphoid cells has been complicated by the molecular heterogeneity exhibited by these lymphokines (1,2). We have recently reported that continuous lymphoblastoid cell lines can be employed as a source of IF or LT that are restricted in physiochemical heterogeneity (2,3). Thus, employing the PGLC-33h B-lymphocyte line, α-LT activity could be resolved from immune IF-like activity by physiochemical and immunologic techniques. These same techniques were not successful in resolving LT and IF activities obtained from lectin-stimulated peripheral blood lymphocytes (PBL).

The IF activity obtained from the PGLC-33h cell line shares physiochemical properties with both viral induced leukocyte IF (IFle), (MW 25,000) and immune IF (type II) (acid and heat lability) (2). This evidence has led us to further investigate the immunologic relationships between the different types of lymphoid cell produced interferons and the relationships of these different types of IF to lymphotoxins.

RESULTS AND DISCUSSION

The different IF preparations were then tested for their capacity to be neutralized by an anti-IF_I or anti-LT antibodies. Two types of anti-LT IgG preparations were employed in this study (4). 1) Anti-WS, a polyspecific LT neutralizing antiserum directed against whole unfractionated

ISBN 0-12-213950-X

TABLE 1. Neutralization of Human Immune or Viral-Induced Interferons by Anti-LT or Anti-IF Antibodies[a]

Source of IF	% Neutralization of IF Activity by[b] (μl of Antisera)						
	Anti-α_2LT	Anti-WS			Anti-IF_I		
	100	100	50	25	100	50	25
A. PGLC-33H	1. ----	72±5	50±3	30±6	50±2	68±7	70±3
	2. 5±2						
	3.[d] 3±4						
	Anti-α_2LT	Anti-WS			Anti-IF_I		
	100	100	50	25	100	50	25
B. ConA Induced	1. ----	41±3	43±1	23±5	3±5	−1±3	−5±4
	2. −15±8						
	3.[d] 3±4						
	Anti-α_2LT	Anti-WS			Anti-IF_I		
	100	100	25	5	35	10	5
C. Leukocyte Viral Induced	1±4	55±10	91±4	15±2	98±2	62±4	16±2

[a]*Rabbit anti-leukocyte IF globulin fraction (anti-IF_I) is the NIAID reference standard (No.24) produced against Sendai virus induced leukocyte IF. Rabbit anti-human LT IgG preparations are characterized in reference (4).*

[b]*Neutralization of IF activity was conducted by incubating 1-2 units of the IF preparation with various amounts of the indicated antibody preparation (500 μg/100 μl anti-LT sera) for 1 hr at 37°C. Residual IF activity was then measured on HeLa cells (D98) by the VSV plaque reduction assay (2). The percent neutralization was calculated relative to the effect of normal rabbit IgG ± one standard deviation.*

[c]*PGLC-33H, a human B-lymphoblastoid cell-line that spontaneously releases IF activity (2). ConA induced, human peripheral blood lymphocytes were stimulated with Conconavalin A for 72 hrs (immune IF). Leukocyte IF, the NIAID reference standard (No.G-023-901-527) was Sendai virus induced.*

[d]*A sheep anti-rabbit IgG was employed as a second antibody.*

serum free supernatants from PHA stimulated human adenoid lymphocytes. 2) Anti-α_2LT antiserum prepared against gel filtration and DEAE ion exchange resin purified α-LT. The results of these experiments are presented in Table I and they indicate: 1) Anti-WS and Anti-IF_I recognize similar (both neutralize IF_I) and distinct (only anti-WS neutralizes IF_{II} activity) IF-associated antigenic determinants. 2) PGLC-33h IF activity contains immunologic similarity with both IF_I and IF_{II}. 3) Both type 1 and 2 IF are immunologically distinct from α-LT. The partial reactivity of anti-WS or anti-IF_I for PGLC-33h or IF_{II} activities indicates that an additional specie(s) of IF may be present in these preparations. Whether this additional species is fibroblast like-IF is unclear (5). It would seem unlikely since the anti-IF_I has both anti-leukocyte and anti-fibroblast IF activity (6). These data indicate an immunologic heterogeneity among IF_{II} species.

REFERENCES

1. Granger, G. A., R. S. Yamamoto, D. S. Fair, and J. C. Hiserodt, Cell. Immunol. 38, 388 (1978).
2. Ware, C. F. and G. A. Granger, J. Immunol. 122, 1763 (1979).
3. Fair, D. S., E. W. B. Jeffes, and G. A. Granger, Immunochemistry (in press) 1979.
4. Yamamoto, R. S., J. C. Hiserodt, J. E. Lewis, C. E. Carmack, and G. A. Granger, Cell. Immunol. 38, 403 (1978).
5. Parker, K., In: The Interferon System, S. Baron and F. Dianzani, eds. Texas Reports on Biology and Medicine 35, 23 (1977).
6. Berg, K., C. A. Ogburn, K. Parker, K. E. Morgensen, and K. Cantell, J. Immunol. 114, 640 (1975).

DISCUSSION

HENNEY: Does the antiserum which inhibits T cell-mediated lysis react with lymphocytes? Is it simply an antilymphocyte serum? If that were the case it should not surprise us if it were to inhibit cell-mediated cytotoxicity. However, in that event, it would certainly not necessarily implicate LT in the process.

WARE: To answer this question in the proper perspective requires that I point out the data that indicate lymphotoxins are lymphocyte membrane components. First, absorption of anti-LT antibodies with alloimmune or lectin-activated lymphocytes will remove LT neutralizing antibodies. Second, the LTCX and α_H components in solution possess alloantigenic determinants present on the normal lymphocyte cell surface. Our data indicate that activated cells are quantitatively more efficient in absorbing the cytolytic inhibitory action of anti-LT for T-cell cytolysis. However, we do not feel this inhibitory activity of the anti-LT is a non-specific effect since this antiserum does not block MLC or lectin induced proliferation and inhibits cytolysis at a stage beyond recognition (post Ca^{++} dependent). Furthermore, antisera reactive with B2, HLA, H-2, or anti-T cell sera etc., do not inhibit T-cell cytolysis.

DVORAK: What is the spectrum of target cells on which the various lymphotoxins act? Is killing limited only to L-cells or is there a broader variety of target cells? If only L-cells are affected, the role of lymphotoxins in vivo might well be questioned.

GRANGER: This is indeed an important question and one of our areas of active research. The results are very exciting and can be summarized for human and murine LT forms as follows: (A) The smaller MW forms ($\leq$ 70 - 90,000) are only weakly lytic and cause protracted (12 - 20 hr) lysis of selected cells *in vitro*, i. e. the L 929 cell. In fact recent data reveal that these subunits are not inherently lytically active but require an enzymatic activation step via a target cell protease. (B) The α_H and Cx forms are potent cell toxins and can cause protracted nonspecific lysis (16 - 20 hr) of many cell types *in vitro*. (C) Unstable Cx forms associated with receptors from alloimmune human or murine T-cells can cause rapid specific *in vitro* lysis of various target cell types in 6 - 9 h. This evidence supports the view that the complex LT forms are more likely candidates as cell lytic effector molecules in CMI reactions. Moreover the reason for the instability of Cx forms is probably that in solution they rapidly dissociate into weakly lytic subunits and therefore do not distroy host tissues.

GOODMAN: Granger indicated that normal B cells produce lymphotoxin. Since this has been a controversial issue, would he describe how he established that B cells produce LT?

GRANGER: This concept is supported by two types of data. The first is the demonstration of α_L LT activity in supernatants from established continuous human B cell lines, PGLC-334 and RPMI-1788 (this has been published). The second type of study is the demonstration of LT activity in supernatants derived from lectin-stimulated human adenoid B cells, purified by anti-Ig affinity columns. These cells are 98 - 100 % Ig positive and SRBC-rosette negative. However, LT activity was not evident until late in the culture period, i. e. 5 - 7 days.

LEON: Could a small contaminating T cell population have grown during the 6 day culture period and be responsible for the LT activity? Has Granger done marker studies on the culture to exclude this possibility?

GRANGER: We have not checked the phenotype of the cells responding in these cultures at 6 - 7 days. It is possible that this represents the proliferation of a small percent of contaminating cells.

LOHMANN-MATTHES: Sundsmo and Goetze have recently shown that in a MLR, lymphocytes synthesize the lytic complex of complement components comprising C5b, C6, C7, C8, C9. Has Ware looked for correlation between his lymphotoxin preparations and this lytic complement complex?

WARE: To my knowledge, the terminal complement components are present on B lymphocytes or macrophages. In collaboration with Kolb we have studied the relationship between lymphotoxins and C by studying the effects of several monospecific anti-C antisera on LT activity. Anti-C3 or -C5, -C6 or -C5-9 did not block LT-cytolysis. However, we did see some inhibition of LTcx cytolysis with an anti-Cl_q. We do not know whether this represents a physiologic interaction in view of the propensity of Cl_q to bind to many substances. It is interesting to speculate that a Cl_q "like" molecule may serve to link the cytotoxin moieties of LT to the antigen specific receptor in the LTcx, just as the function of humoral Clq is to link C and immunoglobulin.

LITTMAN: If I understood Granger correctly, anti-Fab (of immunoglobulin) binds to some forms of lymphotoxin (LT). If this binding is due to idiotypic determinants on LT and if, as reported, idiotypic determinants are related to the T-lymphocyte antigen receptor, then lymphotoxin may play a role in modulating the T-lymphocyte response to antigen as well as its classic cytotoxic activity. LT may also contain the T-lymphocyte antigen receptor. Would Granger care to comment on this possibility?

GRANGER: Littman has raised two interesting questions. It is now clear that both human and murine Cx and α_H LT forms can associate with Ag-binding receptor(s). This is demonstrated by anti-Fab reactivity or by specific binding to the relevant antigen. It is most likely that these receptor forms are of T-cell origin because: (A) These forms are released by highly purified T cell preparations and not preparations in which T cells have been removed. (B) They have no reactivity with antisera reactive with traditional immunoglobulins. Physicochemical studies indicate the α_H form is the smallest which contains receptor (R) activity and will readily dissociate into an α_L (70 - 90,000 MW) and γ (12 - 20,000 MW). If we assume that one α_L and one γ LT subunit are associated together with the receptor in the α_H form, the receptor, if separate, must be about 40 - 60,000 MW and smaller than a regular Ig molecule. Collectively these data strongly support the association of LT with the T cell-receptor itself. Since the α_H will associate together to form complexes, we feel these forms may represent multimeric structures of R-LT (α_H) subunits. While we are very excited about the role of these components in cell killing we have not tested their role as regulating molecules in the immune system. That they could have a role in the latter situation is an interesting speculation.

ON THE CHANNEL HYPOTHESIS OF ANTIBODY-DEPENDENT CELL-MEDIATED CYTOTOXICITY (ADCC): Evaluation of a Liposome Model System

Manfred M. Mayer
Judith B. Willoughby

Department of Microbiology, Johns Hopkins University School of Medicine, Baltimore, Maryland

Moon L. Shin

Department of Pathology, University of Maryland School of Medicine, Baltimore, Maryland

Henkart and Blumenthal showed that the electrical conductivity across planar bilayers of "oxidized cholesterol", containing dinitrophenylphosphatidyl ethanolamine complexed with IgG antibody, was increased many hundred-fold on interaction with human peripheral blood lymphocytes (1). Among three alternative mechanisms, they favored the hypothesis that this is due to release of a channel-forming substance from the lymphocytes. As pointed out by us, this hypothesis is supported by similarities between the cytotoxic action of lymphocytes and the lysis of target cells by complement (2,3).

In order to explore this hypothesis, we have conducted a model study in which multilamellar liposomes containing dimyristoyl phosphatidyl choline, cholesterol, dicetylphosphate (molar ratios 2:1.5:0.3) and Forssman hapten in the lipid phase, as well as $^{86}Rb^{+}$ marker in the aqueous phase, were treated with anti-Forssman IgG and non-adherent cells from mouse spleen (4). Unlike other recent experiments on ADCC with liposomes as targets (5-7), our studies were designed to detect synergistic marker release as an indication of joint membrane attack by antibody and cells. As shown in the following table, synergistic marker release was observed under certain experimental conditions. Furthermore, as shown in (3), the synergistic release proceeded directly from the liposomes into the medium, as would be expected if the lipid bilayer is damaged.

ISBN 0-12-213950-X

1	2	3	4	5	6	7	8	9	10
			MARKER RELEASE (%)						
Experiment Number	Volume Antibody (µl)	Incubation Time (Hours)	Liposomes Alone	Liposomes + Antibody	Liposomes + Cells	Liposomes + Antibody + Cells	Antibody Contribution (5 - 4)	Cell Contribution (6 - 4)	Synergistic Effect (7 - 8 - 9 - 4)
1	50[a]	4	8.6	13.6	9.1	25.9	5.0	0.5	11.8
2	50[a]	4	8.7	13.7	8.3	25.3	5.0	-0.4	12.0
3	75[a]	4	8.7	25.1	8.3	39.6	16.4	-0.4	14.9
4	75[a]	1.5	7.4	18.6	7.4	21.7	11.2	0	3.1
5	75[a]	3	7.5	26.3	10.2	36.5	18.8	2.7	7.5
6	75[a]	4	7.7	29.4	11.2	41.4	21.7	3.5	8.5
7	75[a]	24	11.2	31.3	33.4	48.1	20.1	22.2	-5.4
8	50[a]	4	4.4	10.7	9.9	26.4	6.3	5.5	10.2
9	50[a]	1.5	3.1	9.6	2.5	18.6	6.5	-0.6	9.6
10	50[a]	4	2.6	13.1	4.4	24.3	10.5	1.8	9.4
11	50[a]	24	4.2	16.9	9.1	41.6	12.7	4.9	19.8
12	50[a]	4	6.7	15.9	7.5	17.2	9.2	0.8	0.5
13	50[a]	4	10.6	10.0	23.1	16.4	-0.6	12.5	-6.1
14	50[a]	4	5.0	10.8	4.8	13.8	5.8	-0.2	3.2
15	50[b]	4	5.0	5.7	4.8	6.7	0.7	-0.2	1.2
16	10[b]	4	6.2	6.1	6.4	6.8	-0.1	0.2	0.5
17	25[b]	4	6.2	5.8	6.4	6.6	-0.4	0.2	0.6
18	50[b]	4	6.2	5.3	6.4	7.0	-0.9	0.2	1.5
19	100[b]	4	6.2	5.5	6.4	7.0	-0.7	0.2	1.3
20	300[b]	4	6.2	5.6	6.4	6.7	-0.6	0.2	0.9
21	700[b]	4	6.2	5.1	6.4	6.8	-1.1	0.2	1.5
22	100[b]	20	8.2	6.8	13.2	14.5	-1.4	5.0	2.7
23	50[b]	4	8.0	6.3	9.7	9.7	-1.7	1.7	1.7
24	50[b]	4	8.0	6.3	9.8*	10.8	-1.7	1.8	2.7
25	100[c]	4	8.0	7.2	9.7	11.1	-0.8	1.7	2.2
26	100[c]	4	8.0	7.2	9.8*	11.7	-0.8	1.8	2.7
27	50[b]	4	7.1	6.4	7.2	10.0	-0.7	0.1	3.5
28	50[b]	4	7.1	6.4	8.0*	9.0	-0.7	0.9	1.7
29	100[c]	4	7.1	6.2	7.2	9.4	-0.9	0.1	3.1
30	100[c]	4	7.1	6.2	8.0*	9.7	-0.9	0.9	2.6

Spleen cells from C3HeB/FeJ mice were depleted of adherent cells with glass beads or carbonyl iron. Human peripheral blood lymphocytes (in Table) were purified with Ficoll-Hypaque and carbonyl iron. Antibody lot "a" contained 15-20% sucrose. Lot b was prepared without sucrose gradient frac-*

tionation. Lot c was the same as a, but dialyzed. Hemolytic titers of a and b were 1460 and 3700 per ml, respectively. Protein concentration was ca. 3 mg/ml in all three lots. Reaction set-up: 20 μl liposomes + IgG + RPMI; total volume 700 μl. After 30 min at 27°, 2 x 10^7 cells were added in 100 μl and the mixture was incubated at 37°. Released marker was separated on a 50 m agarose column. Lines in the table indicate experimental groups.

It is evident that only nine experiments showed a significant synergistic effect. In all of these, marker release by antibody (column 8) was high, probably due to the presence of sucrose in IgG lot *a*. The final sucrose concentration, 0.04-0.15 *M*, would disturb the osmotic balance and perturb the membrane bilayer, thus rendering it leaky. This perturbation would also be expected to increase the efficiency of insertion of hydrophobic peptides (8). We suspect that the synergistic release and the high antibody blanks in the work of Juy *et al.* (5) were also due to some kind of membrane perturbation. Since a significant synergistic effect was demonstrable only with perturbed membranes, we conclude that a liposome system of this type is an inefficient model for ADCC, probably due to the large size disparity between liposomes and lymphocytes (9). Therefore, it appears better to use targets of similar size, like resealed erythrocyte ghosts (10). The demonstration of 120-165 Å diameter lesions in their membranes (10), in conjunction with the synergistic marker release from liposomes that can be seen in the work of Juy *et al.* (5), and that was observed by us, lends strong support to the hypothesis that trans-membrane channels are formed in the target bilayer by insertion of hydrophobic peptides from activated lymphocytes. (Supported in part by a contract with ONR N00014-75-C-0142 and a grant from NCI 9 RO1 CA24441-04 ALY.)

REFERENCES

(1) Henkart, P., and Blumenthal, R. (1975). *Proc. Natl. Acad. Sci. USA. 72, 171.*

(2) Mayer, M. M. (1977). *J. Immunol. 119, 1195.*

(3) Mayer, M. M., Hammer, C. H., Michaels, D. W., and Shin, M. L. (1978). *Immunochemistry 15, 813.*

(4) Shin, M. L., Willoughby, J. B., Shin, H. S., Whitlow, M. B., and Mayer, M. M. (1978). *Fed. Proc. 37, 1272.*

(5) Juy, D., Billecocq, A., Faure, M., and Bona, C. (1977). *Scand. J. Immunol. 6, 607.*

(6) Ozata, K., Ziegler, H. K., and Henney, C. S. (1978). *J. Immunol. 121, 1383.*

(7) Geiger, B., and Schreiber, A. D. (1979). *Clin. Exp. Immunol. 30, 149.*

(8) Miller, C., Arvan, P., Telford, J. N. and Racker, E. (1976). *J. Membrane Biol. 30, 271.*

(9) Henkart, P. Personal Communication.

(10) Simone, C. B., and Henkart, P. (1979). *Fed. Proc.38,926.*

DISCUSSION

MIZEL: I am somewhat confused. What is the relationship of these observations to LT killing? Is the effect of LT only in long-term killing? In which instance is pore formation important?

MAYER: Cytotoxicity by guinea pig LT begins only after a lag of about 4 hr. Therefore, cell mediated cytotoxicity is thought to proceed by a different, more rapid, mechanism. It is this rapid mechanism that is thought to involve channel formation.

HENNEY: One comment on the adequacy of the liposome model for cell mediated cytotoxicity. The data Mayer presented are reminiscent of those of Ozata and myself (J. Immunol., 1978) but we carried out two further controls that caused us to become disenchanted with the model: (1) Depletion of Fc receptor-bearing cells totally abrogated the ability of the resulting cells to lyse antibody-coated target cells but had no effect on their ability to cause 88Rb release from antibody-coated liposomes; (2) Liposome destruction took place, in an unimpeded manner, in the presence of EDTA and cytochalasin B, both of which totally inhibit antibody-dependent cell mediated cytotoxicity.

MAYER: Juy et al. already demonstrated the Fc receptor requirement in a liposome system similar to ours. The results of the Ozato/Henney experiments cannot be interpreted because controls without antibody are lacking. We too, are disenchanted with liposomes as a model target, but for different reasons, namely their inefficiency. Accordingly we have switched to resealed erythrocyte ghost targets for which Henkart has demonstrated an Fc receptor requirement.

SHIN: In support of the general concept proposed by Mayer, I would add that we have recently isolated a cytotoxic factor from macrophage membranes. The molecular weight of this factor is about 30,000 daltons. It causes a rapid release of radiolabelled Rb from the cell target. This event is followed by cytolysis. During this period there is no cytolysis as measured by the release of ^{51}Cr. The factor also causes release of Rb from liposomes suggesting that the site of action may be the lipid bilayer.

MAYER: Shin's observation would be in accord, by analogy, with my proposal that on activation lymphocyte membranes release a channel-forming agent.

WARE: Results in the guinea pig and human cytotoxic systems are difficult to compare directly. However, there are two points I would make with respect to the failure of anti-guinea pig LT to inhibit alloimmune cytotoxicity. First, as will be shown in an upcoming report (M. Ross, J. Immunol.) guinea pig LT is not a single substance as reported by Gately et al.; rather it exists as a multicomponent system with biochemical characteristics similar to the human system. Thus, the anti-guinea pig LT serum is reactive with only a subunit component (β). This result agrees with ours in that anti-subunit antibodies (anti α or β) failed to inhibit human alloimmune cytotoxicity. Secondly, and most importantly, the LT forms released by T cells do not express subunit determinants (i. e. α and β antigens are hidden) and are thus not accessible to neutralizing antisera. Our results indicate that for an antiserum to inhibit T-cell killing it most likely has to react with the precursor LT antigens.

BIOLOGICAL AND BIOCHEMICAL CHARACTERIZATION OF A CYTOTOXIC FACTOR FROM MURINE MACROPHAGES

Daniela N. Männel
John J. Farrar
Stephan E. Mergenhagen

National Institutes of Health
Bethesda, Maryland

The serum of BCG infected mice (C3H/HeN) treated with LPS (7 to 14 days later) contains a factor that is cytotoxic for tumor cells (1). CF activity was measured by the release of ^{3}H-thymidine into the culture supernatant from prelabeled tumor target cells (mouse L 929 cells). Peak serum CF activity was detected 1 to 2 hours after LPS injection; no activity was found after 6 hours. CF was stable for 30 minutes at 56° C. Gel filtration of CF-containing serum on Sephacryl S-200 indicated that the factor had an apparent MW of 125,000. The CF coeluted with a helper factor which restored the anti SRC PFC response of Balb-C nude mice (2). CF was bound by DEAE Sephacel (pH 7.1) and was eluted with 0.2 M sodium chloride. After DEAE chromatography or ammonium sulfate precipitation the MW of CF was changed to 60,000 and was clearly separated from the helper factor (MW 12,000 to 15,000) when chromatographed under high ionic strength (1.6 M sodium chloride) conditions (Figure 1). Fractions containing the helper activity also had mitogenic activity for mouse thymocytes. These findings suggest that the helper factor was presumably identical to lymphocyte activating factor (LAF) (3).

CF with similar biochemical properties was also obtained in the supernatant from adherent peritoneal cells of BCG infected mice (2 hours after in vitro stimulation with ng amounts of LPS). Adherent peritoneal cells from healthy mice also released CF into the supernatant when pulsed with a lym-

ISBN 0-12-213950-X

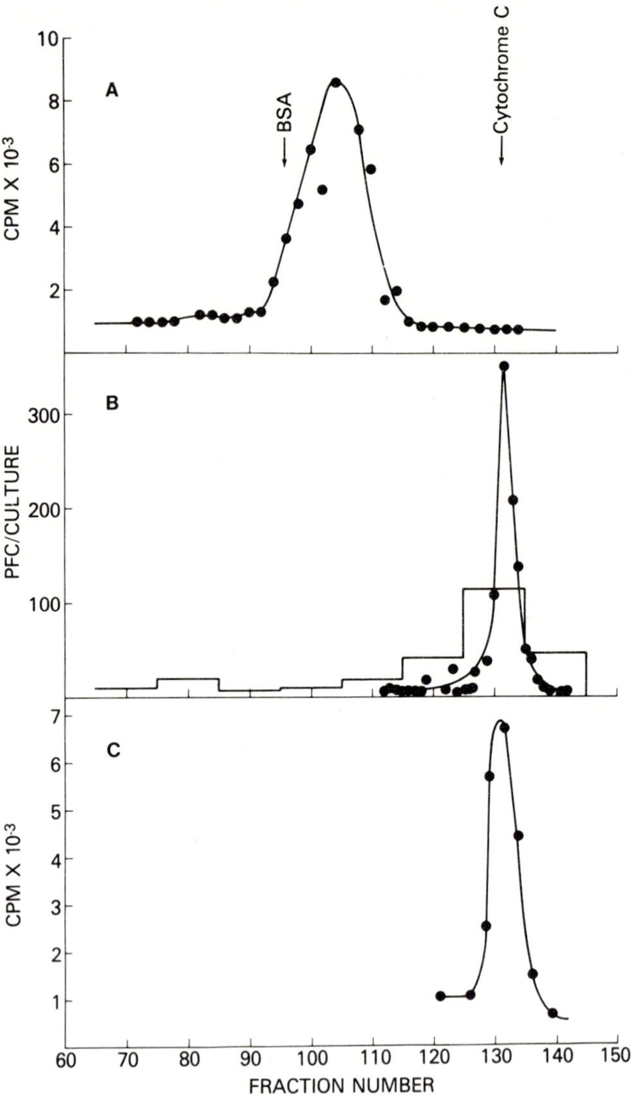

Fig. 1. Sephacryl S-200 chromatography of ammonium sulfate precipitated serum from BCG infected mice after LPS injection. CF activity (panel A) is expressed as cpm label release; helper activity in the anti SRC PFC response (added hour 0) as PFC per culture, and mitogenic activity (panel C) as cpm ^{3}H-thymidine uptake by mouse thymocytes.

phokine containing supernatant[1] for 3 to 6 hours followed by incubation with ng amounts of LPS for 2 to 3 hours. Furthermore the cells of the macrophage like cell line PU 5-1.8 released CF into the supernatant after 2 to 3 hours of stimulation with LPS.

These results indicate that CF is a macrophage product, its production may be regulated by other lymphokines, and finally that it is biochemically distinct from the helper factor.

REFERENCES

1. Carswell, E.A., Old, L.J., Kassel, R.L., Green, S., Fiore, N., and Williamson, B. (1975). *Proc. Nat. Acad. Sci. U.S.A. 72*, 3666.
2. Hoffmann, M.K., Green, S., Old, L.J., and Oettgen, H.F. (1976). *Nature 263*, 416.
3. Männel, D.N., Farrar, J.J., and Mergenhagen, S.E. (Submitted for publication).

[1]*Lymphokine containing supernatant was obtained by stimulation of spleen cell cultures of BCG infected mice with PPD.*

EFFECTS OF RABBIT TUMOR NECROSIS FACTOR (TNF) ON CELLS

George E. Gifford
Jeffrey Ostrove
Michael R. Ruff

Department of Immunology and Medical Microbiology
University of Florida College of Medicine
Gainesville, Florida

TNF is found in the serum of animals infected with *Mycobacterium bovis*, strain BCG, when challenged 2 weeks later with endotoxin (1). *Corynebacterium parvum* and zymosan also prime animals for TNF production. TNF causes a hemorrhagic necrosis of tumors *in vivo* and cytotoxic effects on transformed and/or tumor cells *in vitro* but does not have any effect on normal cells. TNF lacks species specificity (2,3). Evidence has implicated the mononuclear phagocyte as the source of TNF (1,4) and TNF may thus be a monokine.

Interferon, B cell differentiating factor, bone marrow colony stimulating factor, and lysosomal enzymes are released under conditions used to induce TNF (5-7). We realized the necessity to purify TNF from other effector molecules. Our initial goal was to purify TNF and to accumulate information on the properties of the molecule as well as the kinetics of the cellular effects (8). The necessity of developing sensitive assays for TNF action was apparent so that we could monitor purification procedures. Our initial observations studying RNA synthesis showed a 6-fold stimulation in L-929 cells after TNF addition (9). TNF had no effect on RNA synthesis in normal mouse embryo cultures. When RNA synthesis was inhibited by treatment with Actinomycin D, an enhancement of cell killing was obtained. Fig. 1 shows the enhanced killing effect of simultaneous treatment with TNF and Actinomycin D. The dose response curve is shifted 3 logs. Furthermore, cell killing in the presence of Actinomycin D was measured at 18 hours; in its absence killing was measured at 48 h.

ISBN 0-12-213950-X

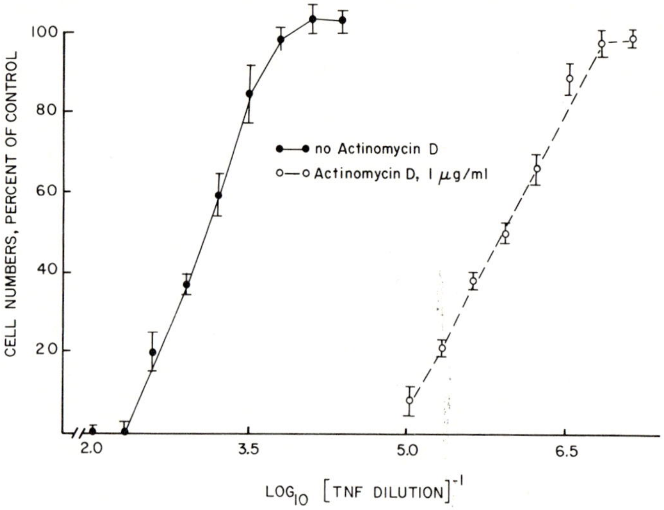

FIGURE 1. The effect of various dilutions of TNF on the growth of L-929 cells in the presence and absence of Actinomycin D, 1μg/ml.

We have also measured the effect of TNF on DNA synthesis (Fig. 2). TNF has a greater effect on DNA synthesis than on cell killing indicating that at high dilutions of TNF a cytostatic rather than a cytocidal activity may result. Cells also appear to become leaky as shown by the release of ^{32}P. This effect seems to be manifested at still higher dilutions and may indicate damage to the cell membrane.

Our purification procedure consisted of a gel filtration step followed by two ion exchange fractionations (DEAE and carboxymethyl cellulose). These procedures resulted in a final 650-fold purification with 40% recovery of activity and 700 μg of protein. The homogeneity and activity of the sample was verified by several gel electrophoretic steps. The protein migrated as a single homogeneous band on a native acrylamide gel just to the anodic side of the BSA marker. This material was eluted from the native gel and run on an SDS-polyacrylamide gel with various protein markers. TNF ran as a single homogeneous band with molecular weight of 62,000 daltons. Other properties are shown in Table 1.

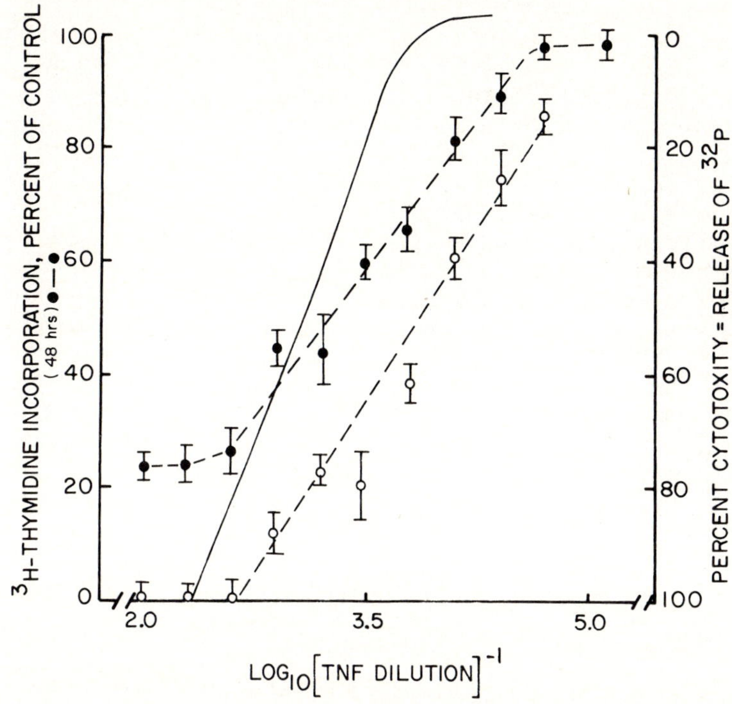

FIGURE 2. Effect of various doses of TNF on DNA synthesis and on isotope release from cells (^{32}P. carrier free, 1 μC/ml). The solid line is taken from Fig. 1 for cell killing.

TABLE I. Properties of Rabbit Tumor Necrosis Factor (8)

Hemorrhagic necrosis of some tumors in vivo
Selective cytotoxicity for transformed cells in vitro
Activity not due to nutritional depletion
Activity is temperature and serum dependent
Does not lyse erythrocytes
Not species specific
Stimulation of host RNA synthesis: Transformed cells only
Activity enhanced by Actinomycin D
Mass: 62,000 daltons; no reductive subunits; Trypsin sensitive
Isoelectric point: ca. 5.5 pI
Thermostable: 70°, 1 hr.; loss of activity at 80°, 15 min.
Requirement for metal ions: Co, Cu, Mo

REFERENCES

(1) Carswell, E.A., Old, L.J., Kassel, R.L., Green, S., Fiore, N., and Williamson, B. (1975). *Proc. Nat. Acad. Sci. (U.S.A.) 72*, 3665.

(2) Helson, L., Green, S., Carswell, E., and Old, L.J. (1975). *Nature (Lond.) 258*, 731.

(3) Matthews, N., and Watkins, J.F. (1978). *Br. J. Cancer 38*, 302.

(4) Matthews, N. (1978). *Br. J. Cancer 38*, 310.

(5) Sauter, C., and Gifford, G.E. (1966). *Nature (Lond.) 212*, 623.

(6) Hoffman, M., Oettgen, H.F., Old, L.J., Chin, A.F., and Hammerling, U. (1977). *Proc. Nat. Acad. Sci. (U.S.A.) 74*, 1200.

(7) Hoffman, M.K., Green, S., Old, L.J., and Oettgen, H.F. (1976). *Nature (Lond.) 263*, 416.

(8) Ruff, M.R., and Gifford, G.E. (1979). Manuscripts in preparation.

(9) Ostrove, J., and Gifford, G.E. (1979). *Proc. Soc. Exp. Biol. and Med. 160*, 354.

DISCUSSION

KIRCHNER: One of the most interesting features of TNF is its apparent "selectivity" for "malignant" cells. This mimics somehow the situation which has been reported when macrophages manifest a certain preference for "malignant" target cells. Obviously there must be some kind of recognition for the malignant phenotype. Three more experiments would be worth while:

1. Comparison of SV 40 (or any other virus) - transformed cells with its untransformed counterpart.

2. Comparison of mouse embryo fibroblasts at various passage numbers.

3. Testing the effect of TNF on mitogen-induced lymphoblasts.

GIFFORD: I, too, am impressed with the selectivity of activated macrophages for killing of malignant and transformed cells, particularly that this effect seems to lack immunological specificity and is not species specific. These effects are similar to TNF except that for killing, macrophages require close proximity to their target cells. We have considered a comparison of a SV40-transformed cell and its normal counterpart to study the phase during transformation when the cell becomes sensitive to TNF action. Unfortunately the SV40 transformed cells that we have so far tested have *not* been sensitive to TNF but we plan on using other viral and chemical transforming agents for this purpose. We also plan on studying the effect of TNF on normal cells just prior to, during and after the "crisis" period in which they spontaneously transform. Lastly, TNF does not have any effect on DNA synthesis of mitogen-stimulated lymphocytes using both a B cell (endotoxin) and T cell (PHA) mitogen.

PICK: I would like to ask Gifford three questions:

1. Does he know the cellular origin of TNF and whether it can be produced in vitro by stimulating macrophages derived from BCG-injected rabbits?

2. Is his factor present in both plasma and serum or does he need the clotting sequence activated in order to have detectable TNF?

3. Does his factor have any protease-like activity? Since his TNF will only kill tumor cells in the presence of Cu^{++}, I would like to suggest that TNF might activate the endogenous tumor cell superoxide dismutase and by producing H_2O_2 cause cell death.

GIFFORD:

1. We have not been able to induce TNF production in spleen cell cultures, peritoneal exudate cells or liver slices from BCG-infected rabbits or *Corynebacterium parvum* primed mice when these suspensions were treated with endotoxin. However, alveolar macrophages from such animals, when placed in culture and exposed to endotoxin, release a factor which kills L-929 cells. We assume that this is TNF and we are in the process of further characterizing it.

2. We have only looked for TNF activity in serum. I think Pick has a good point and we shall certainly ascertain whether the clotting sequence is involved in TNF generation.

3. We do have evidence suggesting an enzymatic action for TNF activity. We have considered the possibility of it being a protease and have used several inhibitors of protease activity to see if they would block TNF activity. O-phenanthroline was employed for this purpose since it chelates heavy metal ions and thereby inhibits metallo-proteins. We were able to show a

TNF requirement for Cu^{++}, Co^{++} or Mo^{++} to manifest activity. I like Pick's idea about the activation of the endogenous tumor cell enzyme and we will explore that possibility.

MIZEL: Since interferon has a MW of 67,000 (one species), has anti-tumor activity and binds Cu^{++} and Zn^{++}, is it conceivable that what Gifford calls TNF is really interferon?

GIFFORD: Interferon is indeed present in serum containing TNF and it will also inhibit cell proliferation. We were initially concerned with this finding and elected to use rabbit TNF for our studies on human and mouse cells. Interferon is relatively species specific in its action; accordingly rabbit interferon has no effect on human and mouse cells. Furthermore, rabbit interferon activity is destroyed by heating at 70°C for 30 minutes whereas TNF is stable. Another point is that interferon does *not* discriminate between normal and transformed and /or tumor cells in its cytostatic activity as does TNF. Purification also separates the two activities. Thus, we can say with confidence that TNF is not interferon.

STEWART: In collaboration with Old (Sloan-Kettering Institute) we, too, have looked at the question of whether Tumor Necrosis Factor (TNF) might be an interferon. Mouse cells sensitive or resistant to TNF were both equally sensitive to either type I or type II mouse interferons. Similarly, several mouse cells with markedly different sensitivity to mouse interferons were equally sensitive to TNF.

INTRODUCTORY STATEMENTS ON INTERFERON

DE MAEYER, J.: Interferons are a group of vertebrate glycoproteins with broad antiviral activity synthesized either (a) in any cell of the organism (immune system included) when induced by a virus or double-stranded RNA (type I interferon) or (b) in lymphoid cells of the immune system by antigen or mitogen (type II interferon). Interferons are heterogeneous, not only in terms of their origin and mode of induction, but also in terms of species specificity. In contrast to many lymphokines, interferons appear to be *strictly* species specific. Within the same species, interferons also appear to be heterogeneous in terms of molecular species.

DE MAEYER, E.: Type I mouse interferon has recently been purified to homogeneity in three different laboratories. Pure type I mouse interferon consists of two molecular forms; one of 35,000 and another of 22,000 daltons. Both have the biological activities of mouse interferons. An interesting calculation which can be made from knowing the specific activity of pure interferon (2.4 x 10^9 units/mg), and its molecular size, is that interferon is active at 10^{-15} molar concentration. Interferon is therefore an active substance of extreme potency since one antiviral unit corresponds to 0.19 fentomole or roughly 10^6 molecules. Considering that in the interferon assay, one uses about 10^5 - 10^6 cells, one can estimate that for expression of its antiviral activity, interferon is active at a level of one to a few molecules per cell. This should not be so surprising, since it is not interferon itself which is responsible directly for the antiviral activity but rather the cascade of events it induces in the cell. It also induces many biochemical changes, i. e. activates protein kinase, interferes with initiation factors, induces endonucleases and a number of other events not all of which may be known. For comparative purposes it is also possible to block antigen sensitization in the mouse by interferon; here as little as 8.4 x 10^5 units suffice, which corresponds to 13 ng/g mouse.

Another consideration should be encouraging to those working with still impure lymphokines and monokines. Why did it take 20 years to purify interferon? In 1958, our production systems yielded about 10 units/ml and most people were working with 1 : 2 to 1 : 5 dilutions of active supernatants. At that time, to isolate 1 mg of interferon from crude supernatant would have required 250,000 liters! By selecting high producer cells, probably more through luck than wisdom, and also by

ISBN 0-12-213950-X

studying the fundamental aspects of interferon induction, the field has arrived at the point where the production has reached 10^5 - 10^6 units/ml and 1 mg interferon requires but 25 liters of culture medium. Thus one of the major factors in achieving purification has been the great increase in efficiency of production.

With electrophoretically pure mouse interferon (in collaboration with Gresser and Fridman) various in vitro effects such as priming of interferon synthesis, inhibition of cell multiplication, enhanced cytotoxicity of double-stranded RNA, enhancement of natural killer cell activity and enhanced expression of H-2 antigens as well as inhibition of antibody formation in the Mishell-Dutton system have been confirmed as being due to one and the same interferon molecule. In vivo, not so many experiments have been performed because of the scarcity of purified material, but the antitumor activity also appears to be due to pure interferon, as measured by inhibition of early ascites. Inhibition or enhancement of delayed-type hypersensitivity depending on the time at which interferon is given, has also been obtained with pure interferon.

In contrast to the situation up to now in lymphokine investigation where there is a multitude of factors, each seemingly with its own effects, we have in interferon one substance with a spectrum of different effects in vivo and in vitro on the immune and other systems.

HUMAN INTERFERON: THE MESSENGER RNA AND THE PROTEINS

Sidney Pestka
Marian Evinger
Philip Familletti
Mitchell Gross
Shuichiro Maeda
Russell McCandliss
Menachem Rubinstein
Sara Rubinstein
Alan Sloma
John Tabor
Hideo Takeshima

Roche Institute of Molecular Biology
Nutley, New Jersey 07110

Several programs involving interferon are underway. We have been interested in the synthesis of interferon, its regulation, and in the interferon proteins themselves.

To study interferon biosynthesis, we have isolated mRNAs from various cells synthesizing interferon and have translated them in cell-free extracts as well as in frog oocytes to synthesize biologically-active interferon. The availability of an assay for interferon mRNA permits its purification. Accordingly, these mRNAs have been characterized and partially purified.

In addition, we have prepared and purified human leukocyte interferon to homogeneity. The overall degree of purification was 80,000 fold and the specific activity, 2-4 x 10^8 units/mg. A single protein band of molecular weight 17,500 $\pm$ 1,000 coinciding with a single peak of antiviral activity on sodium dodecyl sulfate polyacrylamide gel electrophoresis was observed. The homogeneous interferon exhibited antigrowth activity as well as antiviral activity.

ISBN 0-12-213950-X

STUDIES WITH INTERFERON mRNA

Our studies on interferon first centered on isolation and translation of mRNA. Interferon mRNA from human cells was translated in cell-free extracts (1,2) as well as in frog oocytes (3-6). Biologically-active interferon was synthesized in these extracts and in oocytes. That the activity was indeed human interferon was demonstrated by its species and antigenic specificity as well as additional characteristics of the interferons. These studies with interferon mRNA provided a number of useful insights. Since our cell-free extracts were not capable of synthesizing carbohydrates *de novo* (7), we speculated that the carbohydrate moiety was not essential for activity of the interferons.

Interferons made in cultures of human buffy coat cells (leukocyte interferon) or in human fibroblasts (fibroblast interferon) have a number of distinct properties. Differences between human leukocyte and fibroblast interferons could originate in at least two ways. There may be two distinct structural genes for interferon, each coding for a protein with unique primary sequence. Alternatively, if there were a single structural gene for interferon, differences might result from distinct post-translational modifications carried out by lymphoid and non-lymphoid cells (e.g., glycosylation, proteolytic cleavages, etc.). In this case, the same polypeptide sequence would be synthesized, but processed differently into the final active product in the different types of cells. To distinguish between these alternatives, we isolated mRNA from human lymphoblasts and fibroblasts induced to produce their characteristic interferons and injected the mRNA into *Xenopus laevis* oocytes. *Xenopus* oocytes have been shown to translate a variety of injected mRNAs and to carry out a number of post-translational modifications. Because the secondary modifications produced by the oocytes would be expected to be the same for a single translational product, any differences observed in the interferon produced by the oocytes should represent differences in their mRNA sequences.

Interferon synthesized when fibroblast mRNA was injected into oocytes was neutralized by antiserum to fibroblast interferon, but not by antiserum to leukocyte interferon. Interferons synthesized when lymphoblastoid mRNA was injected were either not neutralized or were only partially neutralized by either antiserum alone. A mixture of both antisera was required for complete neutralization. Interferons produced in intact fibroblasts or Namalva cell cultures showed the same neutralization patterns as the corresponding oocyte products. Thus, the oocyte products resemble the products of the cells from which the mRNA was derived. The fact that complete neutralization of lymphoblastoid cellular interferon required a mixture of anti-leukocyte and anti-fibroblast interferon sera suggested that lymphoblastoid interferon as well as the oocyte product synthesized after injection with mRNA from lymphoblastoid cells contained a mixture of leukocyte and fibroblast interferons.

In addition, the cellular specificity of interferon produced by oocytes injected with the various messages resembled the cellular specificity of the interferon preparations produced by those same cells (3).

We thus concluded that lymphoblastoid interferon is a mixture of two types of interferon, leukocyte and fibroblast interferon and that the preparations of lymphoblastoid mRNA injected into oocytes contained mRNA for both types of interferon since the oocytes synthesized both interferons. These results indicate that human interferons produced in oocytes with mRNA preparations extracted from fibroblast or lymphoblastoid cells showed the same characteristic molecular weights, antigenic properties, and cellular specificities as the products of the intact cells from which the mRNA was derived. These findings support the conclusions that the mRNAs are different, and, therefore, the amino acid sequences of the interferons synthesized on these mRNA templates must be different. We speculate that these mRNAs are products of separate human interferon genes, *ifn*Le and *ifn*F. Both of these genes are expressed in induced lymphoblastoid cells, but only one of these genes appears to function in the fibroblast. However, it also is conceivable that the genes may be overlapping and that the individual mRNAs for leukocyte and fibroblast interferons are the result of distinct splicing mechanisms characteristic of the cells from which the mRNAs are derived.

PURIFICATION OF HUMAN LEUKOCYTE INTERFERON

Recently, interferon research has generated great interest because of promising clinical studies in which they have exhibited antiviral and antitumor activities. Because no pure preparations of interferon were available for these studies, it is not yet clear that both these activities reside in the same molecular species. Furthermore, human interferon was not available in homogeneous form in sufficient amounts for chemical characterization. Complete physical, chemical, and biological characterization of the molecules depends on obtaining homogeneous interferon in sufficient amounts. We have purified one species of human leukocyte interferon to homogeneity in amounts sufficient for physical and chemical characterization. Details of the purification and initial characterization, including amino acid analysis, of the homogeneous species have been described (8,9). As can be seen in Fig. 1, a single protein band of molecular weight 17,500 was obtained upon staining with Coomassie blue on sodium dodecyl sulfate-polyacrylamide slab gel electrophoresis. After being stained, the gel was cut into 1-mm slices and each fraction was assayed for interferon activity. A single peak of activity coinciding with the protein band was obtained.

So far, most of the interferon used for clinical studies was produced by induction of leukocytes obtained from blood donors. Other sources of interferon include lymphoblastoid cell cultures and fibroblast cells. Leukemic patients with high leukocyte counts could serve as a rich source of white blood cells. Leukocytes can be selectively removed from such patients by leukopheresis. By this method, an amount of leukocytes equivalent to that obtained from 100 to 300 units of blood can be obtained from a single patient with a count of 10^5 leukocytes/μl.

Initially, leukocytes from various sources were tested for their ability to produce interferon upon induction with viruses. We found that leukocytes obtained from patients with chronic myelogenous leukemia (CML) produced higher levels of interferon than leukocytes from patients with chronic lymphocytic leukemia or the acute leukemias as previously reported by Lee *et al.* (10) and Hadházy *et al.* (11).

Interferon produced by leukocytes from CML patients was compared with interferon produced by leukocytes from normal donors (12). The elution patterns from the various high performance liquid chromatographic (HPLC) columns were highly reproducible and therefore could serve as an analytical tool for comparing interferon preparations (9,12). It was found that interferon obtained from leukemic leukocytes exhibits the same elution characteristics on various HPLC columns and the same amino acid composition as that from normal leukocytes. We, therefore, conclude that these two interferons are essentially identical.

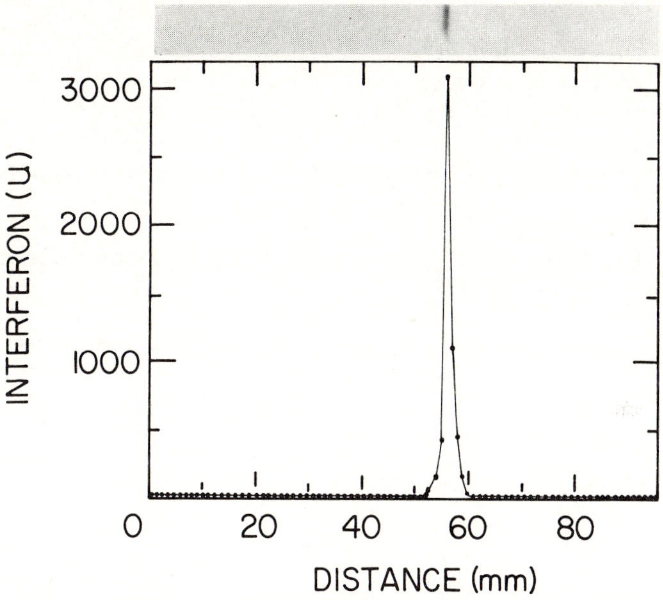

FIGURE 1. Sodium dodecyl sulfate polyacrylamide slab gel electrophoresis of human leukocyte interferon. A photograph of the polyacrylamide slab gel after staining with Coomassie blue is shown above the figure. A duplicate gel was cut into 1-mm slices and assayed for interferon activity. Interferon activity is expressed as units (u) on the ordinate. Details are described elsewhere (8).

COMPARISON OF ANTIVIRAL AND ANTIGROWTH ACTIVITY

Interferons have been reported to have a large number of effects. For example, antiviral, antitumor, growth inhibitory and immunosuppressive activities have been described. Because most of these assays were performed with relatively crude preparations, less than 1% of which was human interferon, the results could have been due to components other than interferon. The availability of homogeneous interferon makes it possible to resolve these uncertainties.

To determine whether the homogeneous leukocyte interferon exhibited antigrowth activity as well as antiviral activity, the effect of the pure material on growth of lymphoblastoid (Daudi) cells was examined (13). It was shown that the homogeneous human leukocyte interferon exhibited antigrowth activity as well as antiviral activity (Table I). Thus, we conclude that the antigrowth activity is an inherent property of the interferon molecule.

With the availability of homogeneous interferon, we shall soon be able to determine if the additional activities ascribed to interferon are exhibited by the pure material.

TABLE I. Growth-inhibitory Activity of Human Leukocyte Interferon[a]

Addition to Culture Medium	*Growth (% of Control)*
Unfractionated Interferon	*15%*
Homogeneous Leukocyte Interferon	*12%*
No Additions	*100%*

[a]*Unfractionated human leukocyte interferon was added to Daudi cell cultures to a final concentration of 25 and 50 units/ml. Homogeneous human leukocyte interferon was added to cultures to a final concentration of 36 units/ml. Growth of cells are expressed as a percentage of the growth of control cells after three days. Details of the procedures are described elsewhere.*

ACKNOWLEDGMENTS

The early studies of interferon mRNA were performed in collaboration with Jan Vilček, Ralph Cavalieri, Edward Havell, and James McInnes (1-6). We thank Dr. Julius Horoszewicz for providing a flask of the lymphoblastoid Daudi cells to perform the growth-inhibition studies.

REFERENCES

1. Pestka, S., McInnes, J., Havell, E., and Vilček, J., *Proc. Natl. Acad. Sci. U.S.A. 72,* 3898 (1975).
2. Pestka, S., McInnes, J., Weiss, D., Havell, E.A., and Vilček, J., *Ann. N.Y. Acad. Sci. 284,* 697 (1977).
3. Cavalieri, R.L., Havell, E.A., Vilček, J., and Pestka, S., *Proc. Natl. Acad. Sci. U.S.A. 74,* 3287 (1977).
4. Cavalieri, R.L., Havell, E.A., Vilček, J., and Pestka, S., *Proc. Natl. Acad. Sci. U.S.A. 74,* 4415 (1977).
5. Cavalieri, R.L., and Pestka, S., *Tex. Rep. Biol. Med. 35,* 117 (1977).
6. Pestka, S., *in* "Symposium: Dimensions in Health Research - Search for the Medicines of Tomorrow" (H. Weissbach, ed.), p. 29. Academic Press, New York, (1978).
7. Tucker, P., and Pestka, S., *J. Biol. Chem. 252,* 4474 (1977).
8. Rubinstein, M., Rubinstein, S., Familletti, P.C., Gross, M.S., Miller, R.S., Waldman, A.A., and Pestka, S., *Science 202,* 1289 (1978).
9. Rubinstein, M., Rubinstein, S., Familletti, P.C., Miller, R.S., Waldman, A.A., and Pestka, S., *Proc. Natl. Acad. Sci. U.S.A. 76,* 640 (1979).
10. Lee, S.H.S., van Rooyen, C.E., and Ozere, R.L., *Cancer Res. 29,* 645 (1969).
11. Hadházy, Gy., Gergely, L., Tóth, F.E., and Szegedi, Gy., *Acta Microbiol. Acad. Sci. Hung. 14,* 391 (1967).
12. Rubinstein, M., Rubinstein, S., Familletti, P.C., Hershberg, R.D., Brink, L.D., Gutterman, J., Hester, J., and Pestka, S., *Proc. Sixth Amer. Peptide Symp.,* in press.
13. Evinger, M., Rubinstein, M., and Pestka, S., in preparation.

CHARACTERISTICS OF INTERFERONS PRODUCED IN CULTURES OF HUMAN LYMPHOCYTES BY STIMULATION WITH *CORYNEBACTERIUM PARVUM* AND PHYTOHEMAGGLUTININ

Jan Vilcek
Ioan T. Sulea
Franklin Volvovitz
Y.K. Yip

Department of Microbiology
New York University School of Medicine
New York, New York

Interferons produced by lymphocytes in response to mitogens, or by sensitized T lymphocytes in response to antigens, are often referred to as "immune" or "type II" interferons. The term "T-type" interferon has been proposed recently (1). We prefer the designation *T* interferon over the other two terms because (i) the induction of this interferon is obviously not always based on immune recognition and (ii) two other species of interferon, designated *Le* and *F*, are already known in the human system (2).

Apart from the somewhat confusing terminology, there is no generally accepted definition of *T* interferon. Any meaningful definition must include some properties of the molecule that allow its differentiation from other interferons. Lack of stability at pH 2 and lack of affinity for antisera to *Le* or *F* interferons serve as the major distinguishing properties of human *T* interferon.

Inactivated *C. parvum* organisms were shown to induce a lymphoproliferative response as well as interferon production in human lymphocyte cultures (3, 4). According to one report the interferon produced appeared to represent type II interferon (3). Another group concluded that the sensitivity to heat and low pH exhibited by the *C. parvum*-induced interferon was similar to that of human immune interferon (5). In the present study we compared the properties of interferons produced in cultures of human lymphocytes stimulated with *C. parvum* or phytohemagglutinin (PHA).

Two methods were employed for the purification of lymphocytes from freshly collected heparinized venous blood. Unless indicated otherwise in the text, leukocyte-rich plasma was passed through a column of sterile adsorbent cotton (6; F. Va-

ISBN 0-12-213950-X

TABLE I. Antigenic differences between interferons induced with C. parvum or PHA

Interferon preparation			Per cent neutralized by[a]	
Inducer	Cell source	Units/ml	Anti-Le	Anti-F
C. parvum	Lymphocytes	128	96.8	0
PHA	Lymphocytes	64	0	0
Sendai virus	Buffy coat cells	512	≥99.6	25
Poly(I)·poly(C)	FS-4 fibroblasts	1,536	0	≥99.8

[a]Each of the interferon preparations was mixed with an excess of antibody against human Le or F interferon, incubated for 1 hr at 37°C and titrated to determine residual interferon activity.

lentine, personal communication) and the eluted nonadherent cells were employed for the seeding of cultures. Sedimentation through ficoll-hypaque was used as the alternative method of lymphocyte purification. Optimal culture conditions for interferon production with *C. parvum* and PHA were worked out in preliminary experiments. In short, 96-well plastic tissue culture plates were seeded with 600,000 mononuclear cells/well in 0.2 ml of RPMI 1640 medium. The medium was supplemented with 1% heat-inactivated fetal bovine serum (FBS) for stimulation with PHA (6.2 μg/ml unless otherwise indicated, Wellcome

TABLE II. pH 2 stability of interferons induced with C. parvum or PHA

Interferon preparation			Per cent inactivated at pH 2[c]
Inducer	Cell source	Units/ml	
C. parvum	Lymphocytes[a]	128	50
	Lymphocytes[b]	128	0
PHA	Lymphocytes[a]	128	97
	Lymphocytes[b]	64	94
Sendai virus	Buffy coat cells	768	0
Poly(I)·poly(C)	FS-4 fibroblasts	768	0

[a]Purified on cotton column.

[b]Purified by ficoll-hypaque sedimentation.

[c]Dialyzed for 24 hr against HCl-KCl buffer, pH 2, then re-adjusted to pH 7.4.

TABLE III. Antiviral activity of C. parvum and PHA-induced interferons in bovine EBTr cells

Interferon preparation		*Interferon titer in*		*Ratio*
Inducer	*Cell source*	*GM-258*	*EBTr*	*GM-258/EBTr*
C. parvum	*Lymphocytes*[a]	*2,048*	*512*	*4*
	Lymphocytes[b]	*256*	*16*	*16*
PHA	*Lymphocytes*[a]	*384*	*<4*	*>96*
Sendai virus	*Buffy coat cells*	*2,560*	*384*	*6.6*

[a, b] *See Table II.*

Reagents Ltd., Beckenham, England) or with 1% human AB serum when the cells were stimulated with 140 μg/ml of heat-killed *C. parvum* (strain CN 6134, received from Dr. R.L. Tuttle, Burroughs Wellcome Co., Research Triangle Park, NC). Culture fluids were collected after 24 hr of incubation with the inducer at 37°C in 5% CO_2. Interferon titrations were done by a microassay based on inhibition of vesicular stomatitis virus in human GM-258 cells with trisomy 21 (7). In this highly sensitive assay 1 unit corresponds to approximately 0.1 reference units of human leukocyte interferon.

Over 95% of the antiviral activity of interferon produced with *C. parvum* was neutralized by antiserum against human *Le* interferon. Only a small fraction of the *C. parvum*-induced interferon remained active after mixing it with an excess of serum against *Le* interferon (Table I), suggesting the possible presence of a minor component antigenically heterogeneous from *Le* interferon. In contrast, no detectable neutralization of PHA-induced interferon activity was seen with either of the two antisera employed.

C. parvum-induced interferon was essentially stable at pH 2, while PHA-stimulated interferon was not (Table II). However, in contrast to the control preparations of "leukocyte" and "fibroblast" interferon included in the experiment, a 50% drop in activity was seen with one of the two *C. parvum*-induced preparations. This difference may not be significant; nevertheless, in view of the results of other investigators (3, 5) it remains to be determined whether *C. parvum*-induced interferon, while antigenically homologous with *Le* interferon, is perhaps more labile at pH 2 than virus-induced *Le* interferon.

Human *Le* interferon is known to exert a high degree of antiviral activity in bovine cells (8). In this respect too

TABLE IV. Effects of TPA on interferon production stimulated with C. parvum or PHA

Exp. No.	*Inducer*	*Interferon yield (units/ml)*	
		Control	*TPA*[a]
	None	*<4*	*12*
1	*C. parvum*	*3,840*	*64*
	PHA (6.2 μg/ml)	*40*	*3,840*
2	*PHA (6.2 μg/ml)*	*128*	*1,280*
	PHA (31 μg/ml)	*128*	*960*

[a]*TPA (final conc. 5 ng/ml) was added to the lymphocyte culture medium along with the inducers.*

C. parvum-induced interferon resembled the control preparation of "leukocyte" interferon. PHA-induced interferon showed no detectable activity in bovine cells (Table III).

Biological activity of human *Le* interferon can be fully recovered after treatment with sodium dodecyl sulfate (SDS). This property is very convenient for the analysis of *Le* interferon (and some other interferons as well) by SDS-polyacrylamide gel electrophoresis (9). When analyzed by SDS-PAGE, virus-induced *Le* interferon and *C. parvum*-induced interferon preparations (produced both from cotton or ficoll-hypaque gradient purified lymphocytes) showed virtually identical patterns. In all of these preparations interferon activity was recovered in two bands corresponding to apparent molecular weights of approximately 20,000 and 27,000 (results are not shown).

The tumor promoting agent phorbol-12-myristate-13-acetate (PMA) or 12-0-tetradecanoylphorbol-13-acetate (TPA) was recently shown to stimulate interferon production in some lines of human lymphoblastoid cells (10). TPA also induces a lymphoproliferative response (11). These findings prompted us to examine the effects of TPA (a kind gift of Dr. Toby Rossman) on interferon production stimulated with PHA or *C. parvum*. PHA-induced interferon production was enhanced in the presence of a wide range of TPA concentrations; maximum enhancement occurred with a concentration of 5 ng/ml. At this dose of TPA, interferon production with PHA was enhanced from about 5- to 100-fold. In contrast, *C. parvum*-induced interferon production was greatly inhibited by TPA (Table IV). Other experiments showed that NDV-induced interferon production in lymphocyte cultures was also inhibited and interferon production stimulated with tuberculin-PPD in sensitized lymphocytes was essentially unaffected. Other mitogens have not yet been examined. Interferon stimulated by PHA in the presence of TPA was not neutralized by anti-*Le* and anti-*F* interferon sera. Thus, the use of TPA appears to be a helpful tool for the augmentation of *T* interferon production with PHA in human lymphocytes.

In sum, PHA-induced interferon shows properties characteristically associated with *T* interferon. However, the bulk of interferon activity produced after stimulation with *C. parvum* appears to be very similar or identical to *Le* interferon. Although induction with *C. parvum* probably involves immune recognition, the product is not "immune" interferon.

ACKNOWLEDGEMENTS

We thank Lyn Gradoville and Dorothy Henriksen for technical assistance, and Michele Cassano for typing. Antiserum to *Le* interferon was prepared by Dr. L. Borecký and provided to us by Dr. E.A. Havell. This study was supported by Grants AI-07057, AI-12948, and Contract NO1 AI-02169 from the U.S. Public Health Service.

REFERENCES

1. Wietzerbin, J., Stefanos, S., Falcoff, R., Lucero, M., Catinot, L., and Falcoff, E., *Infect. Immun. 21,* 966 (1978).
2. Havell, E.A., Berman, B., Ogburn, C.A., Berg, K. Paucker, K., and Vilček, J., *Proc. Nat. Acad. Sci. USA 72,* 2185, (1975).
3. Hirt, H.M., Schwentek, M., Becker, H., and Kirchner, H., *Clin. Exp. Immunol. 32,* 471 (1978).
4. Epstein, L.B., and Sugiyama, M., *Clin. Res. 25,* 501A (1977).
5. Sugiyama, M., and Epstein, L.B., *Cancer Res. 38,* 4467 (1978).
6. Lamvik, J., *Acta Haemat. 35,* 294 (1966).
7. Havell, E.A., Yip, Y.K., and Vilček, J., *J. Gen. Virol. 38,* 51 (1978).
8. Gresser, I., Bandu, M.-T., Brouty-Boyé, D., and Tovey, M. *Nature 251,* 543 (1974).
9. Stewart, W.E. II, and Desmyter, J., *Virology 67,* 68 (1975).
10. Klein, G., and Vilček, J., *J. Gen. Virol.* (in press).
11. Touraine, J.L., Hadden, J.W., Touraine, F., Hadden, E.M., Epstein, R.D., and Good, R.A., *J. Exp. Med. 145,* 460 (1977).

DISCUSSION

COHEN, S.: Pick pointed out that PMA mimics MIF. This means that it probably activates macrophages as well. Thus it may induce endogenous mitogenic or other kinds of stimulatory factors (LAF, etc.) which could provide a synergistic effect with PHA. Does Vilcek think this is a plausible mechanism for the enhancing effect of PMA on interferon production?

VILCEK: I do not know whether there are other mediators involved in the stimulation of interferon production by PMA. On the other hand, interferon *might* be involved in the activation of macrophages by PMA reported by Pick. Interferon is known to cause macrophage activation and we do find that PMA induces some interferon production in lymphocyte cultures.

FRIDMAN: We have shown that TPA, provided by Castagna, "mimics" interferon effects such as inhibition of the antibody response to SRBC or enhancement of NK cell activity. Accordingly the mechanism of these effects could well be by induction of interferon by TPA.

VILCEK: Absolutely. One of my tables showed that TPA alone, without another mitogen, induced some interferon in lymphocyte cultures. Thus the effects observed by Fridman could well be mediated by interferon.

EPSTEIN: What kind of interferon results from the stimulation of T lymphocytes by PHA and PMA? We also were able to more than additively enhance the amount of interferon produced by PHA when we also used C. parvum (Sugiyama and Epstein, Cancer Research 38: 4467, 1978).

VILCEK: The interferon produced in lymphocytes exposed to PHA and PMA is not neutralized by antisera to *Le* or *F* interferons; accordingly its properties conform to those associated with *T* (type II) interferon.

MIZEL: Mizel, Oppenheim and Rosenstreich published a paper (Cell Immunol., 1978) demonstrating that PMA is a potent inducer of macrophage LAF production. LAF and PHA could activate T cells to make IF.

EPSTEIN: If I understood Mizel properly, he is suggesting that LAF could induce interferon. Oppenheim was kind enough, with Mizel's help, to provide us with some LAF, which, in two experiments, failed to induce interferon in human T lymphocytes.

DE WECK: Could Vilcek tell us what increase in yield of IF is brought about by superinduction and has it been applied to increase the production of lymphokines?

VILCEK: Superinduction does not work with every interferon inducer and with every cell type. In those instances where superinduction does cause an enhancement of the interferon yield, the increase can be up to 1,000-fold. I am not aware of the successful application of the superinduction technique to lymphokine production. However, interferons are not at all the only proteins whose synthesis can be augmented by superinduction. In fact superinduction as a result of actinomycin D treatment was first observed by Gordon Tomkins for synthesis of the enzyme tyrosine aminotransferase in rat hepatoma cells induced by dexamethasone. I do not know whether anyone has yet developed similar information on a combination of procedures that would enhance LK production.

BELLER: Unanue has studied the effect of superinduction by cycloheximide on the production of LAF (J. Immunology, 1978).

NETA: We have shown that subcutaneous treatment of mice with complete Freund's adjuvant prior to intravenous sensitization with BCG enhances the titers of interferon released on OT challenge 100 - 1,000-fold.

GRANGER: We have found that by using combinations of non-specific (lectin) and specific triggering of antigen-primed cells we obtain rapid (4 - 5 h instead of 4 - 5 days) high level release of LT forms from murine or human cells. Thus there are a number of mehtods that conceivably could be employed to induce high levels of LK.

COMPARISONS OF THE PHYSICOCHEMICAL AND BIOLOGICAL PROPERTIES OF HUMAN, MURINE AND BOVINE INTERFERONS, TYPES I AND II[1]

Marzenna Wiranowska-Stewart
Leo S. Lin
Irwin A. Braude
William E. Stewart II[2]

Interferon Laboratories
Memorial Sloan-Kettering Cancer Center
New York, New York

I. PRODUCTION OF INTERFERONS TYPES I AND II

A. *Human Interferons*

Human fibroblast interferon (HuFiIF-I) prepared from diploid skin fibroblasts induced with poly rI•poly rC and superinduced (Havell and Vilcek, 1972) was provided from the NIH at a specific activity of about 10^6 units/mg protein. Human leukocyte interferon (HuLeIF-I) prepared from Sendai virus induced buffy coat leukocytes was also obtained from the NIH at a specific activity of about 10^6 units/mg protein (Cantell and Hirvonen, 1978). Human leukocyte suspensions were also induced with phytohemagglutinin (PHA) as indicated in TABLE I, and the antiviral activity obtained was designated as a presumptive human type II interferon (HuLeIF-II). The routine induction scheme developed was addition of partially purified PHA (Burroughs-Wellcome) at 3 μg/ml to human leuko-

[1] *Supported in part by NIH grant # CA-20863 from the National Cancer Institute*

[2] *Supported by USPHS Research Career Development Award AI-00219 from the National Institute of Allergy and Infectious Diseases*

ISBN 0-12-213950-X

TABLE I. Production of Human Type II Interferon[a]

Induction Scheme	*Interferon (Units/ml)*			
	Day: 1	*2*	*3*	*4*
PHA	*<10*	*60*	*300*	*2500*
Priming + PHA	*20*	*50*	*1000*	*4200*
2-ME + PHA	*<10*	*125*	*300*	*1400*
2-ME + Priming + PHA	*<10*	*100*	*400*	*800*

[a]*Human leukocyte suspensions were incubated at* 10^6 *cells/ml in RPMI 1640+10% fetal calf serum with 3 μg/ml of PHA.*

cyte suspensions at 10^6 cells/ml. Interferon reached maximum levels by 4 days. When cultures were primed by exposure to 100 units/ml of HuLeIF-I for 2 hrs before induction, interferon yields were slightly - but consistently - increased. Addition of 2-mercaptoethanol (5×10^{-5}M) to culture medium did not enhance interferon production, and inhibited the priming effect. Thus, HuLeIF-II preparations used for the purification and characterization studies were routinely produced in primed leukocyte suspensions induced with PHA and harvested after 4 days incubation.

B. *Murine Interferons*

Mouse type I interferon was induced in primed L_{929} cell cultures by Newcastle disease virus and was purified to approximately 10^6 units/mg protein as previously described (Stewart II et al., 1978). Mouse spleen cell suspensions were prepared from C57Bl mice and were incubated with PHA (at 3 μg/ml) as indicated in TABLE II. The suspensions produced maximal interferon yields by 48 hrs. In contrast to HuLeIF-II, production of mouse type II interferon was not increased by priming with mouse type I interferon; but again in contrast to the HuLeIF-II production scheme, mouse type II interferon was significantly enhanced by inclusion of 5×10^{-5}M 2-mercaptoethanol in the medium. Thus, mouse type II interferon for the purification and characterization studies was produced in unprimed spleen cell suspensions in cultures stimulated with PHA and 2-mercaptoethanol, harvesting after 2-day incubation.

TABLE II. Production of Mouse Type II Interferon[a]

Induction Scheme	*Interferon (Units/ml)*	
	Day: 1	*2*
PHA	*80*	*160*
Priming + PHA	*80*	*100*
2-ME + PHA	*300*	*800*
2-ME + Priming + PHA	*300*	*800*

[a]Mouse spleen cell suspensions were incubated at 3 x 10^6 cells/ml in RPMI 1640+10% fetal calf serum with 3 μg/ml of PHA.

C. *Bovine Interferons*

Bovine interferon was induced in primary bovine kidney fibroblasts with Newcastle disease virus. This interferon was presumptively designated as bovine interferon type I. Bovine interferon, designated type II, was induced in bovine leukocyte suspensions by PHA.

II. DESIGNATION OF INTERFERONS AS TYPE I AND TYPE II

All these inhibitors were classified as interferons on the basis of their abilities to induce a virus non-specific resistance in cells, through cellular metabolic processes (Stewart II, 1979). HuLeIF-I and HuFiIF-I were designated as type I interferons on the basis of their complete stabilities to pH2 treatment. HuLeIF-II was designated as a type II interferon on the basis of its complete inactivation at pH2 (>99% loss), by either direct addition of acid or by dialysis against pH2 buffer.

Mouse interferon from L cells was completely stable at pH2, thus a type I interferon; mouse spleen cell interferon induced by PHA was completely destroyed by this acidification, therefore it is a type II interferon.

The bovine interferons, however, were less easily classified as type I or type II. Both the virus-induced bovine fibroblast interferons and the mitogen-induced bovine leukocyte interferons lost at least 90% of their antiviral activities at pH2. Thus, even bovine fibroblasts can produce an "immune" interferon, "T" interferon or "mitogen-type" interferon in response to a viral stimulation. These data suggest that the best criterion for interferon designations is not inducer type or cell type but rather the properties of the interferon produced, being type I if stable - or type II if unstable - at pH2.

III. PURIFICATION OF TYPE II INTERFERONS

The human type II interferon was clarified by low-speed centrifugation and was dialyzed against 0.01M tris buffer, pH7.5 and was applied to a column of poly U-Sepharose, as described for type I mouse interferon (DeMaeyer-Guignard et al., 1977). The bulk of protein passed unretarded through column, while the interferon was retained. The applied interferon was then quantitatively recovered by elution with 0.07M tris + 1M NaCl giving a purification of approximately 300-fold purification to a specific activity of about $10^{4.5}$ units/mg protein. This method has the disadvantage of requiring dialysis of large volumes of culture fluid prior to chromatography; therefore, we undertook to find a purification method allowing direct application of culture fluids to chromatographic columns. Such a method has been described for type I human and mouse interferons by Edy et al. (1978) using controlled-pore glass beads (CPG). However, the adsorbed type I interferons were eluted with pH2 buffer, which would destroy type II interferons. Alternatively, we attempted release of type II interferon by stepwise elution with ethylene glycol. Human type II interferon applied directly to a CPG column (350Å) harvested in culture medium, was completely retained while most of the loaded protein passed through the bead column. Elution with 20% ethylene glycol in 1M NaCl at pH7.0 released a sharp peak of protein with almost complete recovery of interferon. Further elution with 60% ethylene glycol released another large peak of protein with little or no interferon activity. Thus, CPG-chromatography provides a simple and efficient method for both concentration and purification of crude human type II interferon giving about 100-fold purification to a specific activity of about 10^4 units/mg protein.

When the human type II interferon activity peak from the CPG column was dialyzed against 0.01M tris, pH7.5, and applied to a poly U-Sepharose column, the sequential chromatographic purification combined to give virtually complete activity recovery with a total purification to approximately 10^6 units/mg. Mouse type II interferon can be similarly purified by this chromatographic scheme.

TABLE III. Comparative Properties of Type I and II Interferons

Property	*Human LeIF-I*	*Human FiIF-I*	*Human LeIF-II*	*Mouse IF-I*	*Mouse IF-II*
Stability at pH2:	+	+	-	+	-
Neutralized by:					
Anti-HuLeIF-I	+	-	-		
Anti-HuFiIF-I	-	+	-		
Anti-Mouse-IF-I				+	-
Cross-Species Activity:					
-on bovine cells	+	-	-		
-on Guinea Pig cells				+	-

IV. PROPERTIES OF PARTIALLY PURIFIED TYPE II INTERFERONS

The type II mouse and human interferons so purified were compared to type I mouse and human interferons of similar specific activities (TABLE III). Thus, type II interferons are distinguishable from type I interferon by pH2 lability, antigenicities, and activities on heterologous cells. Further characterizations will require improvements in both production and purification of these interferons.

REFERENCES

Cantell, K., and Hirvonen, S. (1978). *J. Gen. Virol. 39*, 541.

DeMaeyer-Guignard, J., Thang, M.N., and DeMaeyer, E. (1977). *Proc. Natl. Acad. Sci. U.S.A. 74*, 3787.

Edy, V.G., Braude, I.A., DeClercq, E., Billiau, A., and DeSomer, P. (1976). *J. Gen. Virol. 33*, 517.

Stewart II, W.E. (1979). "The Interferon System". Springer-Verlag, Vienna-New York.

Stewart II, W.E., Chudzio, T., Lin, L.S., and Wiranowska-Stewart, M. (1978). *Proc. Natl. Acad. Sci. U.S.A. 75*, 4814.

DISCUSSION

DE MAEYER, J.: Does Stewart feel that in human leukocyte interferon preparations as presently used for clinical trials, the antitumor activity can be ascribed to interferon itself?

STEWART: This question should be adressed to Edy, who is preparing human leucocyte interferon for clinical use.

EDY: According to recent results obtained in collaboration with Schook in de Weck's group, crude and partially purified leukocyte interferon does not contain lymphokine activities such as MIF or LAF.

SCHOOK: Both crude and purified IF (type I) preparations were tested for MIF, LIF, MF (mouse thymocytes) and LAF activity. Both stimulated and mock preparations were devoid of these activities.

PAPERMASTER: In the matter of a relationship between lymphokine activities and interferon I can add that Baron at University of Texas, Galveston , has tested our concentrated supernatant preparations from the human lymphoblastoid cell line RPMI 1788 and found no evidence of type I interferon anti-viral activity.

What increase in specific activity did Stewart obtain in the two dimensional electrophoresis over the previous SDS gel strip? What was the final specific activity of his most purified preparation?

STEWART: Approximately 10-fold, to about 10^8 units/mg.

McDANIEL: I use the Namalwa cell line for production of MAF (evokes tumoricidal macrophages). It produces both MAF and MIF. However, it does not produce interferon at concentrations less than 10^7 cells/ml. Anfinsen is currently using this cell line to produce leukocyte interferon for sequencing.

OGBURN: In this matter of the relationship between antiviral activity and other biologic activities we associate with interferons, I would like to mention that even though the purification of mouse and human interferons may have been achieved, the question of the relation to other activities still needs further consideration. Reports concerning the relationship of antiviral and growth inhibitory activity fall into three categories:

(1) reports stating no separation

(2) reports showing inconstancy in the antiviral and growth inhibitory effects

(3) reports that antiviral and growth inhibition activities are completely separable.

STEWART: Studies with deglycosylated human leukocyte interferons have shown that species of interferons can be separated by isoelectric focussing but not by SDS-PAGE. This is not seen in control interferon preparations. This seems to indicate that separation is based on *charge* not molecular weight. It is interesting to speculate that interferon molecules may exist that vary in antiviral/growth inhibitory ratios. These may result from cell of origin, induction etc.

HALLER: Does the efficiency of priming depend on the type of interferon used for priming, e. g. is type I interferon more effective in priming cells for type I interferon than for type II interferon?

STEWART: We have been able to prime production of type I mouse interferon by pretreatment of cells with *either* type I or type II mouse interferon.

KIRCHNER: Would Wietzerbin comment on his recent findings that spleen cell cultures of nude mice produce interferon in response to PHA?

WIETZERBIN: PHA is able to trigger interferon synthesis in spleen cell cultures from nude mice just as effectively as in splenic cell cultures from heterozygous nude mice or from normal mice. A minor theta-bearing cell population present in the spleen of nude mice appears to be essential for PHA interferon production although cooperating cells are also required. The properties of PHA interferon induced in nude mice are indistinguishable from those displayed by PHA interferons induced in normal mice. Both interferons are acid-unstable and cannot be neutralized by an antiviral interferon serum (so it behaves as T-type interferon). I should point out that spleen cells from nude mice did not show enhancement in ^{3}H thymidine incorporation into DNA when exposed to PHA. So, ^{3}H thymidine incorporation can also be dissociated from interferon production.

WAKSMAN: My comment relates to Wietzerbin's findings. So called T-cell mitogens (PHA, Con A) are defined by the fact that they induce *mitogenesis* in T cells and not in other lymphocytes. However, the fact is they bind strongly to *all* lymphocytes, as well as many other cells. They may well induce types of activation not associated with cycling.

HUMAN LEUKOCYTE INTERFERON: SEPARATION OF BIOLOGICALLY DIFFERENT SPECIES BY MODIFICATION OF THE CARBOHYDRATE MOIETY.

Clifton A. Ogburn
Marc G. Salit
Kurt Paucker

Department of Microbiology
The Medical College of Pennsylvania
Philadelphia, Pennsylvania

These data examine antiviral and growth inhibitory activities in partially purified human leukocyte interferon in which the carbohydrate has been modified by enzymatic or chemical cleavage. The preparations were then fractionated by methods that separate sub-populations of interferons based on molecular weight or electrostatic charge. More exact quantitation of growth inhibition by 50% endpoint determinations and comparisons with antiviral titers allowed better examination of the relationship between growth inhibition and antiviral effects than has been reported previously (1-5).

I. EXPERIMENTAL PLAN

Human leukocyte interferon (5-10X10^5 units/mg protein) was supplied by the National Cancer Institute and as a generous gift of Dr. H.L. Kauppinen, Finnish Red Cross Blood Transfusion Service, Helsinki, Finland. Antiviral activity was determined by a microplate assay (6) using FS-4 cells and encephalomyocarditis virus. Growth inhibition activity was measured in serial two-fold dilutions of the test sample using a ^{14}C-thymidine incorporation assay (7) and Daudi cells. Fifty percent endpoint titers were computed by the method of

This work was initiated by Grant C598-01F awarded by the Biomedical Research Support Grant Program, National Institutes of Health, and supported by Grant PC17 76-20133 awarded by the National Science Foundation.

ISBN 0-12-213950-X

Reed and Muench (8). Untreated interferon, and interferon deglycosylated by glycosidases (9) or metaperiodate (10) were subjected to polyacrylamide gel electrophoresis in sodium dodecyl sulfate (SDS-PAGE)and to isoelectric focusing in a pH 5-7 gradient. All gels were cut into 2mm slices and extracted for several days into buffer containing antibiotics. The relative proportions of antiviral and cell growth inhibitory activity (AV:GI ratio) were determined for each gel fraction. The use of AV:GI ratios is an operational way of describing the number of antiviral units of a sample needed to inhibit the growth of Daudi cells by 50%.

II. RESULTS

Complete recovery of antiviral and growth inhibitory activity was found after treating interferon for 3 hours with glycosidases, whereas 4 hours with metaperiodate caused a 60% loss of both activities. The AV:GI ratios in untreated preparations were in the 3:1 range. Crude, partially purified and more highly purified samples gave similar results which indicated that these ratios were not influenced markedly by impurities in the preparations.

The three preparations after exposure to SDS and urea were subjected to SDS-PAGE to determine if deglycosylation procedures had altered the distribution and molecular weights of the constituent molecules. The untreated preparation gave two peaks of antiviral-growth inhibition activity at about the 21000 and 15000 dalton positions relative to standard protein markers. Glycosidase treatment resulted in a modest decrease to 18,000 and 14,000 daltons in the respective peaks. Metaperiodate treatment resulted in one band at the 15,000 dalton position. Comparison of results showed that AV:GI ratios were not significantly different between untreated and treated samples which agreed with previous reports that these biologic activities are not dissociated on the basis of molecular weight (3, 4).

Isoelectric focusing of untreated interferon yielded four peaks (pI 5.34, 5.52, 5.67, 5.97) in which the AV:GI ratios were similar to those of native interferons (4:1). The heterogeneity of the enzyme-treated sample was only modestly reduced (3 peaks). However, the AV:GI ratios in these peaks were 16.4:1, 5.6:1 and 0.7:1 with pI values of 5.02, 5.32 and 5.6 respectively. Thus, the alteration in charge properties in some molecules, presumably caused by cleavage of carbohydrate moieties, was accompanied by separation of molecular species with different AV:GI ratios. Both biologic activities placed on the gels were recovered quantitatively. The four hour periodate-treated samples of the same interferon preparation were subjected also to isoelectric focusing. More than 80% of the antiviral activity was found in one sharp peak (pI 5.2) whereas more than 70% of the growth inhibitory activity was in multiple peaks associated with smaller amounts of antiviral activity (pI 5.3, 5.5, 5.6, 5.85). The AV:GI ratio in the pH 5.2 peak was 9.4:1 and that of the remaining peaks 0.5:1.

III. SUMMARY

Previous studies have noted the heterogeneity of antiviral activity of leukocyte interferons after isoelectric focusing (11), but none has explored systematically the growth inhibitory activity or the relationship of these two activities after deglycosylation procedures. Modification of carbohydrate by enzymatic or chemical means followed by fractionation through isoelectric focusing yielded 2 species of molecules, one enriched, the other depleted in terms of antiviral activity. These results indicate that under the conditions used, molecules can be obtained that differ significantly in antiviral and growth inhibitory properties. These molecular populations were also observed in untreated interferon fractions obtained by hydroxylapatite chromatography and SDS-PAGE (12), thus indicating that they may exist prior to deglycosylation.

REFERENCES

1. Borecký, L., Fuchsberger, N., Hajnicka, V., Stanček, D. and Žemla, J. (1972). Acta Virol. 16, 356.
2. Ohwaki, M., and Kawade, Y. (1972). Acta Virol. 16, 477.
3. Stewart II, W.E., Gresser, I., Tovey, M.G., Bandu, H.T. and LeGoff, S. (1976). Nature, 262, 300.
4. Knight, E. (1976). Nature, 262, 302.
5. Dahl, H. and Degre, M. (1975). Nature, 257, 279.
6. Havell, E.A. and Vilček, J. (1972). Antimicrob. Agents Chemo., 2, 476.
7. Hilfenhaus, J., Damm, H., Karges, H.E. and Manthey, K.F. (1976).
8. Reed, L.J. and Muench, H. (1938). Amer. J. Hyg., 17, 493.
9. Bose, S., Gurari-Rotman, D., Ruegg, L., Corley, L., and Anfinsen, C.B. (1976). J. Biol. Chem., 252, 1659.
10. Stewart II, W.E., Lin, L.S., Wiranowska-Stewart, M., and Cantell, K. (1977). Proc. Natl. Acad. Sci., 74, 4200.
11. Stewart II, W.E. (1977). "Interferons and Their Actions", pp. 49, CRC Press, Ohio.
12. Törmä, F.T. and K. Paucker (1976). J. Biol. Chem. 251, 4810.

PRODUCTION, PURIFICATION AND PROPERTIES OF HUMAN LYMPHOBLASTOID INTERFERON

K.H. Fantes
C. J. Burman
G. D. Ball
M. D. Johnston
N. B. Finter

Department of Virology
Wellcome Research Laboratories
Beckenham, Kent, England

I. INTRODUCTION

Only those interferons that are obtained by immunologically specific induction of lymphocytes (type II interferons; Youngner and Salvin, 1973; Epstein *et al.*, 1974) are strictly speaking lymphokines as defined by Dumonde *et al.*, (1969). Other more widely studied interferons have been produced by non-specific stimulation not only of lymphocytes but also of non-lymphocytic cells. Thus the three best known types of human interferon are made by fibroblasts (after induction with polyinosinic-polycytidylic acid; Vilcek *et al.*, 1968; Billiau *et al.*, 1973), by primary leukocytes (Gresser, 1961; Strander and Cantell, 1966) and by lymphoblastoid cells (both induced by viruses; Tovey *et al.*, 1974; Strander *et al.*, 1975). Leukocyte and fibroblast interferons have been used clinically with some success in man (reviewed by Dunnick and Galasso, 1979) and it is likely that very large amounts of interferon will be required in the future. The best way to produce the enormous numbers of cells that will be needed for this purpose is to grow them in suspension in large tanks. Of the three cell types only lymphoblastoid cells can be readily cultured in this way and this is the reason why we have developed methods for producing and purifying lymphoblastoid interferon.

ISBN 0-12-213950-X

II. PRODUCTION

Of more than a hundred lymphoblastoid cell lines screened for interferon production, the Namalwa line (Strander *et al.*, 1975) was found to give the highest yields (Christofinis and Finter, 1977) and was therefore selected for large-scale production. The cells are grown in calf serum containing RPMI-1640 medium, in stirred aerated bottles and tanks with capacities ranging from 100 to 1000 L. Temperature, pH and Redox values are automatically controlled. Cell concentration usually reaches 2-3x10^6/ml. Sendai virus is added (final concentration 10-50 HA units/ml) to induce the formation of interferon, the cells are removed 16 to 20 hours later and the crude interferon in the filtrate (titres usually 3,000 to 10,000 reference units/ml) is then subjected to a number of purification steps.

III. PURIFICATION

In developing the finally adopted purification process several methods were investigated, four of them in some detail. These were:

Method 1: Precipitation with trichloroacetic acid, dispersion of the precipitate in acid aqueous ethanol and fractionation of the resulting ethanolic extracts.

Method 2: Chromatography on Sulpho-Propyl-Sephadex.

Method 3: Antibody Affinity Chromatography.

Method 4: Chromatography on Ultrogel AcA54.

A. Method 1

Fantes (1966) found that chick interferon could be reversibly precipitated with trichloroacetic acid (TCA) and that it and human leukocyte interferon (Fantes, 1970) were soluble in acid aqueous ethanol. Crude lymphoblastoid interferon was precipitated with TCA (final concentration 2.5%), the precipitate extracted with aqueous ethanol (94% ethanol, pH 3.5), and the contents of the ethanolic extracts fractionated by a stepwise increase of the pH (Cantell *et al.*, 1974). Interferon purified in this way had an average specific activity of approximately 2x10^5 U/mg protein, sometimes considerably higher.

B. Method 2

Earlier attempts to purify the interferon on CM-Sephadex were not very successful. The more acidic cation exchanger Sulpho-Propyl Sephadex proved much more suitable, especially when the C-25 grade was used where albumin and other macromolecular contaminants were excluded. The interferon was retained by the gel at pH4, washed free from non-bound impurities with 0.15M acetate buffer pH4, and eluted with 0.15M phosphate buffer at pH7-8. Material with a specific activity of 5-10x10^4 U/mg protein was usually obtained.

C. Method 3

Affinity chromatography on immobilised anti-interferon globulins proved a most valuable tool. As the crude interferon contains calf serum (which must be reduced to negligible levels in the purified concentrates), the aim was to use interferon antisera that were free from anti-calf serum protein componenents. This was achieved in three ways: a) by employing antiserum (kindly donated by Dr.K.Cantell) prepared against interferon that contained human instead of calf serum (Mogensen *et al.*, 1975); b) by raising antiserum in rabbits against interferon that contained horse- instead of calf-serum; c) by immunising calves.

Globulins from these sera were prepared by ammonium sulphate precipitation and freed from antibodies to known protein impurities (Namalwa cells, Sendai virus and allantoic fluid) by repeated passage through a Sepharose-4B "scrubber" column, to which these known contaminants had been covalently linked (Anfinsen *et al.*, 1974). The purified globulins were themselves coupled onto Sepharose-4B (by means of cyanogen bromide). Interferon was retained by such columns from neutral solution, it was washed free from non-bound proteins and eluted at pH 2.2. The average specific activity of interferon purified in this way was 2-4x10^6 units per mg protein.

D. Method 4

Interferon samples of varying degree of purity were sometimes subjected to chromatography on Ultrogel AcA54. Best results were achieved when this was done at pH 3.5 and when the volume of the applied interferon solution was not more than about 4% of that of the gel bed volume. Depending on the purity of the input material, considerable further purification of partly purified interferon was achieved.

E. Combination of Methods 1 and 3

A combination of TCA-precipitation, ethanol extraction and antibody affinity chromatography was finally adopted for the small- and large-scale routine purification of the interferon. Nine consecutive batches purified in this way had an average specific activity of $6.0 \pm 3.1 \times 10^7$ U/mg protein which represented an average purification factor of 32,000.

IV. PROPERTIES OF FIBROBLAST-, PRIMARY LEUKOCYTE- AND LYMPHOBLASTOID INTERFERONS

As mentioned in the Introduction human interferon is mainly obtained from three kinds of cells, namely fibroblasts, primary leukocytes and lymphoblastoid cell lines. According to their physicochemical and biological properties the interferons fall into two distinct types, termed respectively Le (leukocyte) and F (fibroblast)[1]. The three kinds of cells all produce both types of interferon, but in very different proportions. The Le- type is the major component of the interferons produced by primary leukocytes and by Namalwa cells, but is present only as a trace in fibroblast interferon. The F-type is by far the largest constituent of fibroblast interferon but only forms small proportions of the other two interferons (see below). Some of the characteristics of the three interferons are presented in the following and their similarities and differences are discussed.

A. Physicochemical Properties

1. Molecular Weight. The molecular weights of Le-, F- and lymphoblastoid (Ly-) interferons have been determined by various authors, either by gel-filtration or by SDS-polyacrylamide electrophoresis. Those of Le- and Ly- interferon were usually found to range between 15,000 and 23,000 daltons (Fantes, 1970; Stewart and Desmyter, 1975; Havell *et al.*, 1977 and 1978a; Bridgen *et al.*, 1977), but both interferons consist of two major components with molecular weights of 15,000-18,000 and 21,000-23.000. F- interferon seems to consist of

[1]Le-, Ly- or F- "interferon" only indicates that the interferon was obtained from Le-, Ly-, or F- cells. Le- or F- "type" refers to the respective physicochemical entity.

only one component with a molecular weight of about 20,000 (Anfinsen *et al.*, 1974; Knight, 1976; Cavalieri *et al.*, 1977; Berthold *et al.*, 1978).

2. *Isoelectric Point.* The IEPs of the three interferons were determined by several authors, mainly by iso-electric focusing. The IEPs of Le- and Ly- interferons were found to be similar, three main peaks ranging between pH values of 5.2 to 6.6 (Fantes, 1970; Havell *et al.*, 1977 and 1978a; Lin and Stewart, 1978). F- interferon, according to Havell *et al.* (1977), exhibits only one broad peak (pH 6.8-7.8), but Morser *et al.*, (1978) found three (pH 5.2, 5.8, 6.3), which were however, reduced to only one (at pH 6.3), after treatment with sialidase.

3. *Carbohydrate Content.* Some authors believe that Le- and Ly- interferons do not contain carbohydrate, (Mogensen *et al.*, 1974; Morser *et al.*, 1978) but others consider them to be glycoproteins (Bose and Hickman, 1977; Stewart *et al.*, 1977). There is, however, general agreement that F- interferon is a glycoprotein (Dorner *et al.*, 1973); Bose *et al.*, 1976; Knight, 1976).

4. *Stability.* Le- and Ly- interferons are considerably more stable than F- interferon under a variety of conditions: heat, low and high pH (Strander *et al.*, 1975), guanidine and surface denaturation (Edy *et al.*, 1974), mechanical stress (Cartwright *et al.*, 1977), contact with various body fluids (Harmon *et al.*, 1976; Cesario, 1977).

5. *Hydrophobic Properties.* F- interferon is much more hydrophobic than the other two interferons, as shown mainly by its chromatographic behaviour on a variety of non-polar or weakly polar matrices. E.g., it binds much more readily to agarose-immobilised Cibacron Blue (Jankowski *et al.*, 1976), carboxy pentane, amino hexane, bovine serum albumin (Jankowski *et al.*, 1975) and to tryptophan, tyrosine and phenylalanine (Sulkowski *et al.*, 1976), and is often only eluted in the presence of ethylene glycol.

6. *Binding to Chelated Metals.* Le- and Ly- interferons are either not bound or bound much less readily than F- interferon to a number of metal-chelates. Immobilised Zn^{++}, Co^{++}, Ni^{++} and Cu^{++} all retained F- interferon, but only the last two weakly bound Le- interferon (Edy *et al.*, 1977; Sulkowski *et al.*, 1978; Chadha *et al.*, 1978).

7. Binding to Lectins. F- interferon is retained by immobilised concanavalin A and lectins obtained from horseshoe crab and lotus, but not by three other lectins. This suggests that this interferon contains N-acetyl-neuraminic acid, L-fucose and D-mannose, but not D-galactose, N-acetyl-glucosamine or N-acetyl-galactosamine. Le-interferon was not bound by any of the lectins (Jankowski *et al.*, 1975). Some of these findings had previously been reported by others (Dorner *et al.*, 1973; Mogensen *et al.*, 1974).

8. Binding to Polynucleotides. F- interferon is readily retained by polymers of cytidylic, uridylic, adenylic and inosinic acid (von Muenchhausen, 1978), but Le-(Chadha *et al.*, 1978) and Ly- interferon (Fantes and Burman, 1978) are bound weakly or not at all by at least polyinosinic acid.

B. Biological Properties

1. Antigenic Characteristics. Le- and Ly- interferons are antigenically identical or at least very similar, but F-interferon seems to be unrelated. Results have not always been unambiguous, as all three interferons (and therefore also the corresponding antisera) contain varying proportions of both Le- and F- type components. Thus, Le- and Ly- interferons contain respectively 1% or less (Berg *et al.*, 1975; Havell *et al.*, 1977) and about 13% (Havell *et al.*, 1978a) of an F- type component and F- interferon a trace of the Le- type (Havell *et al.*, 1978b). In general, antisera raised against F- interferon do not neutralise Le- interferon (Mogensen *et al.*, 1974; Berg *et al.*, 1975) whilst anti Le- interferon sera have some activity against F- interferon (Strander *et al.*, 1975; Paucker *et al.*,1975). Antisera to Le- and Ly- interferons neutralise the two interferons to the same extent (Adams *et al.*, 1975; Cantell, 1979), though slight differences were reported by Pyhälä (1978).

2. Antiviral Dose Response. Antiviral dose response curves of Le- and Ly- interferons are parallel (Johnston, 1978), but F- interferon gives rise to a different slope (Stealey and Fantes, 1975; Edy *et al.*, 1976; Hilfenhaus,1978).

3. Anticellular Activity. Cell growth inhibitory effects of Le- and Ly- interferons are identical (Christofinis and Finter, 1977), but F- interferon shows a different response curve (Edy *et al.*, 1976). Einhorn and Strander (1977) found Le- interferon relatively more effective than F- interferon against lymphoblastoid cells but less so against osteosarcoma cells.

4. Antiviral Activity in Non-Human Cells. Le- and Ly-interferons are much more active than F- interferon in cells of non-human origin. Thus they exhibit very marked activities - sometimes even greater than in human cells - in bovine and porcine cells (Gresser *et al.*, 1974) and in monkey, rabbit, cat and dog cells (Desmyter and Stewart, 1976). F- interferon is either inactive or only weakly active in heterologous cells.

V. CONCLUSION

The reasons why Namalwa cells were chosen for the large-scale production of human interferon have been discussed, purification methods have been presented and the physico-chemical and biological properties of three classes of human interferon have been compared. It has been shown that interferons obtained from primary leukocytes and from Namalwa cells are closely related and that they differ markedly from fibroblast interferon. It is possible that there will be room for both kinds in antiviral and antitumour therapy, especially in view of their tissue specific anticellular action.

REFERENCES

Adams, A., Lidin, B., Strander, H., and Cantell, K. (1975). *J.Gen.Virol. 28*,219.

Anfinsen, C.B., Bose, S., Corley, L., and Gurari-Rotman D. (1974). *Proc.Nat.Acad.Sci.U.S.A. 71*, 3139.

Berg, K., Ogburn, C.A., Paucker, K., Mogenson, K.E. and Cantell, K. (1975). *J.Immunol. 114*, 640.

Berthold, W., Tan, C., and Tan, Y.H. (1978). *J.Biol.Chem. 253*, 5206.

Billiau, A., Joniau, M., and DeSomer, P. (1973). *J.Gen.Virol. 19*, 1.

Bose, S., Gurari-Rotman, D., Rüegg, U.T., Corley, L., and Anfinsen, C.B. (1976). *J.Biol.Chem. 251*,1659.

Bose, S. and Hickman (1977). *J.Biol.Chem. 252*, 8336.

Bridgen, P.J., Anfinsen, C.B., Corley, L., Bose, S., Zoon, K.C., Rüegg, U.T. and Buckler, C.E. (1977). *J.Biol.Chem. 252*, 6585.

Cantell, K., Hirvonen, S., Mogensen, K.E. and Pyhälä, L.(1974). *In* "The Production and Use of Interferon for the Treatment and Prevention of Human Virus Infections" (C.Waymouth, ed.)., P.35. Tissue Culture Association, Rockville, Md.

Cantell (1979). Personal Communication.

Cartwright, T., Senussi, O., and Grady, M.D. (1977). *J.Gen. Virol. 36*,317.

Cavalieri, R.L., Havell, E.A., Vilcek, J., and Pestka, S. (1977). *Fed. Proc. 36*,1992.

Cesario, T.C. (1977). *Proc. Soc.Expl.Biol.Med. 155*, 582.

Chadha, K.C., Armosino, M.E., Kane, C., Grob, P., and Sulkowski, E. (1978). Personal Communication.

Christofinis, G.J., and Finter, N.B. (1977). "Preparation, Standardization and Clinical Use of Interferon". Yugoslav Academy of Science and Art, Zagreb.

Desmyter, J., and Stewart, W.E. (1976). *Virol. 70*, 451.

Dumonde, D.C., Wolstencroft, R.A., Panayi, G.S., Matthew, M., Morley, J., and Howson, W.T. (1969). *Nature, London, 224*, 38.

Dunnick, J.K., and Galasso, G.J. (1979).*J.Inf.Dis. 139*, 109.

Dorner, F., Scriba, M., and Weil, R. (1973). *Proc.Nat.Acad. Sci.U.S.A. 70*, 1981.

Edy, V.G., Billiau, A., Joniau, M., and DeSomer, P. (1974). *Proc.Soc.Exp.Biol.Med. 146*, 249.

Edy, V.G., Billiau, A., and DeSomer, P. (1976). *J.Gen.Virol. 31*, 251.

Edy, V.G., Billiau, A., and DeSomer, P.(1977). *J.Biol.Chem. 252*, 5934.

Einhorn, S., and Strander, H. (1977). *J.Gen.Virol. 35*,573.

Epstein, L.B., Kreth, H.W., and Herzenberg, L.A. (1974). *Cell. Immunol. 12*, 407.

Fantes, K.H. (1966). *In* "Interferons" (N.B.Finter, ed.), p.122, North Holland Publishing Company, Amsterdam.

Fantes, K.H. (1970). *N.Y.Acad.Sci. 173*, 118.

Fantes, K.H., and Burman, C.J. (1978). Unpublished results.

Gresser, I. (1961). *Proc.Soc.Expl.Biol.Med. 108*, 799.

Gresser, I., Bandu, M.T., Brouty-Boye, D., and Tovey, M. (1974). *Nature, London, 251*. 543.

Harmon, M.W., Greenberg, S.B., and Couch, R.B. (1976). *Proc. Soc.Expl.Biol.Med.152*, 598.

Havell, E.A., Yip, Y.K., and Vilcek, J. (1977). *Arch.Virol.55*, 121.

Havell, E.A., Yip, Y.K., and Vilcek, J. (1978a). *J.Gen .Virol. 38*, 51.

Havell, E.A., Hayes, T.G., and Vilcek, J. (1978b). *Virol. 89*, 330.

Hilfenhaus, J. (1978). *J.Biol.Stand. 6*, 159.

Jankowski, W.J., Davey, M.W., O'Malley, J.A., Sulkowski, E., and Carter, W.A. (1975). *J.Virol. 16*, 1124.

Jankowski, W.J., von Muenchhausen, W., Sulkowski, E., and Carter, W.A. (1976). *Biochem. 15*, 5182.

Knight, E. (1976). *Proc.Nat.Acad.Sci.U.S.A. 73*, 520.

Lin, L.S., and Stewart, W.E. (1978). *Fed.Proc. 37,* A953.
Mogensen, K.E., Pyhälä, L., Törmä, E., and Cantell, K. (1974). *Acta.Path.Microbiol.Scand. 82B,* 305.
Mogenson, K.E., Pyhälä, L., and Cantell, K. (1975). *Acta. Path.Microbiol.Scand. 83B,* 443.
Morser, J., Kabayo, J.P., and Hutchinson, D.W. (1978). *J.Gen. Virol. 41,* 175.
Muenchhausen, W.von, Mikulski, A.J., Vastola, K., and Sulkowski, E. (1978). Personal Communication.
Paucker, K., Dalton, B.J., Ogburn, C.A., and Törmä, E. (1975). *Proc.Nat.Acad.Sci.U.S.A.72,* 4587.
Pyhälä, L. (1978). *Acta.Path.Microbiol.Scand.86C,* 291.
Stealey, V.M., and Fantes, K.H.(1975). Unpublished results.
Stewart, W.E., and Desmyter, J. (1975). *Virol.67,*68.
Stewart, W.E., Lin, L.S., Wiranowska-Stewart, M., and Cantell, K. (1977). *Proc.Nat.Acad.Sci.U.S.A.74,* 4200.
Strander, H. and Cantell, K. (1966). *Ann.Med.Expl.Biol.Fenn. 44,* 265.
Strander, H., Mogensen, K.E., and Cantell, K. (1975). *J.Clin. Microbiol. 1,* 116.
Sulkowski, E., Davey, M.W., and Carter, W.A. (1976). *J.Biol. Chem. 251,* 5381.
Sulkowski, E., Vastola, K., Oleszek, D., von Muenchhauses, W. (1978). Personal Communication.
Tovey, M.G., Begon-Lours, J., and Gresser, I. (1974). *Proc.Soc. Expl.Biol.Med. 146,* 809.
Vilcek, J., Ng, H., Friedman-Kien, A.E., and Krawciw, T. (1968). *J.Virol. 2,* 648.
Youngner, J.S., and Salvin, S.B. (1973). *J.Immunol. 111,* 1914.

MEDIATOR INDUCTION IN HUMAN MONONUCLEAR CELLS BY STRAINS OF CORYNEBACTERIUM PARVUM[1]

Lois B. Epstein
Della Goldblatt
Karen Yu

Cancer Research Institute and
Department of Pediatrics
University of California
San Francisco, California

Jack H. Dean

Department of Immunology
Litton Bionetics
Kensington, Maryland

Ronald B. Herberman

National Cancer Institute
National Institutes of Health
Bethesda, Maryland

Joost J. Oppenheim

National Institute of
Dental Research
National Institutes of Health
Bethesda, Maryland

Ross E. Rocklin

Department of Medicine
New England Center Hospital
Boston, Massachusetts

Masao Sugiyama

Department of Otorhinolaryngology
Osaka City Medical School
Osaka, Japan

[1]*Supported by NIH grant AI 12481*

ISBN 0-12-213950-X

C. parvum, strain 6134 induces interferon in human lymphocytes (1,2). Nylon fiber column purified T lymphocytes are competent in this regard (1) and also proliferate in response to this organism (1,3). C. parvum, recently reclassified as Proprionibacterium (4), can be divided into distinct groups and serologic types which differ in their lymphoreticular stimulatory effects *in vivo* (5,6). To determine whether various strains also differ in their ability to induce interferon or stimulate lymphocyte proliferation *in vitro* the following experiments were performed. Microcultures containing either T lymphocytes or T lymphocytes and macrophages were prepared according to the method of Goldblatt *et al.* (7). Heat inactivated, preservative free preparations of various C. parvum strains, prepared especially by Burroughs Wellcome Co., were added at the initiation of the cultures at a final concentration of 140 μg/ml. ^{3}H-thymidine (spec. act. 2.1 C/mmole) was added during the last two hours of the 7 day culture period, and the extent of incorporation of ^{3}H-thymidine into DNA used as a measure of the proliferative response. The results are depicted in Table I.

TABLE 1. Strain differences in the ability of C. parvum to induce proliferation and the production of interferon in human T lymphocytes

Strains	*IF Titer*		*^{3}H-Thymidine Incorporation (cpm)*[a]	
	T[b]	*T+M*[c]	*T*	*T+M*
P. acnes, I-6134	661	267	120	401
6290	183	117	113	640
6276	134	95	73	526
P. acnes, II-5936	78	267	7	35
P. granulosum-5888	6	8	48	678
P. avidum, I-6966	100	45	74	409

[a]*Means of quadruplicate samples from 5 experiments.*
[b]*Cultures containing T lymphocytes.*
[c]*Cultures containing T lymphocytes and macrophages.*

Strain 6134 was by far the most potent interferon inducer. Interferon production and T lymphocyte proliferation were dissociated with 2 strains. Strain 5936 had a greatly reduced ability to stimulate T lymphocyte proliferation. Strain 5888 was unable to induce significant amounts of interferon. Thus, differences in genetic structure and in biochemical and serological properties can be reflected in differences in the ability of these strains to affect 2 different parameters of the cellular immune response, proliferation and mediator production. Also, the excellent ability of strain 6134 to induce interferon in human lymphocytes parallels its marked lymphoreticular stimulatory effects *in vivo* in animal systems. Correspondingly, the poor ability of strain 5888 to induce interferon parallels its minimal lymphoreticular stimulatory effects *in vivo* (5).

Further studies were performed to determine whether C. parvum is also capable of inducing other mediators. Therefore, human T lymphocytes with or without macrophages were cultured in the presence of strain 6134, a potent interferon inducer or strain 5888, a poor interferon inducer. Cultures were also prepared with PHA and PPD (the latter used only with lymphocytes from donors with positive skin test response to PPD). Such cultures served as positive controls for the production of the other mediators. Supernatants were collected after 7 days of culture and aliquots were assayed for interferon (8), MIF (9, 10), LIF (11), MF (12) and LAF (13).

The results are depicted in Table II.

TABLE II. Mediator induction by C. parvum, PHA, and PPD

Components of Culture	*T[a]/T+M[b]*				
Mediators Assayed	*IF*	*MIF*	*LIF*	*MF*	*LAF*
PHA	+/+	+/+	+/+	+/+	-/+
PPD	+/+	-/+	+/+	+/+	-/+
C. parvum-6134 (P. acnes, I)	+/+	-/-	+/+	-/-	-/+
C. parvum-5888 (P. granulosum)	-/-	+/+	+/+	-/-	-/+

[a] *Cultures containing T lymphocytes.*
[b] *Cultures containing T lymphocytes and macrophages.*

Like PHA and PPD, both strains of C. parvum induce the production of LIF and, when macrophages are present, of LAF. By contrast, neither strain of C. parvum induces the production of MF. However, the 2 strains of C. parvum act differently from one another with regard to IF and MIF induction. Whereas strain 6134 is a potent IF inducer, it fails to induce MIF. In a contrary manner strain 5888 induces MIF but fails to induce IF. This dissociation of IF and MIF induction by the 2 strains of C. parvum permits the generation of IF free of MIF (using strain 6134 as inducer) and of MIF free of IF (using strain 5888). This will now permit experiments to be performed in which the effects of human interferon on the immune response can be assessed without the potential complicating effects of MIF in the system. Furthermore, all of these results suggest that the various strains of C. parvum are valuable probes for investigating the mechanisms which control mediator induction.

REFERENCES

1. Sugiyama, M., and Epstein, L.B. *Cancer Res. 38,* 4467 (1978).
2. Hirt, H.M., Schwentek, M., Becker, H., and Kirchner, H. *Clin. Exp. Immunol., 32,* 471 (1978).
3. Godal, T., Klepp, O., and Onsrud, M. *Cancer Immunol. and Immunother. 3,* 69 (1977).
4. Cummins, C.S., and Johnson, J.L. *J. Gen. Microbiol. 80,* 433 (1974).
5. Adlam, C., and Scott, M.T. *J. Med. Microbiol. 6,* 261 (1973).
6. McBride, W.H., Dawes, J., Dunbar, N., Ghaffar, A., and Woodruff, M.F.A. *Immunol. 28,* 49 (1975).
7. Goldblatt, D., McManus, N.H., and Epstein, L.B. *Immunopharm. 1,* 13 (1978).
8. Epstein, L.B. *In* "Manual of Clinical Immunology" (N.R. Rose and H. Friedman, eds.) p. 120. American Society for Microbiology, Washington (1976).
9. Rocklin, R.E. *In* "Manual of Clinical Immunology" (N.R. Rose and H. Friedman, eds.) p. 95. American Society for Microbiology, Washington (1976).
10. Landolfo, S., Herberman, R.B., and Holden, H.T. *J. Immunol. 118,* 1244 (1977).
11. McCoy, J.L., Dean, J.H., and Herberman, R.B. *In* "In Vitro Methods in Cell-Mediated and Tumor Immunity" (B.R. Bloom and J.L. David, eds.) p. 621. Academic Press, New York (1977).

12. Bonnard, G.D., Schendel, D.J., West, W.H. *et al, In* "Human Lymphocyte Differentiation: Its Application to Cancer" (B. Serrou and C. Rosenfeld, eds.), p. 319. Elsevier/North Holland, New York (1978).
13. Meltzer, M.S. and Oppenheim, J.J. *J. Immunol. 118,* 77 (1977).

DISCUSSION

VILCEK: Rather than inducing an "intermediate" form of interferon, *C. parvum* could be sometimes leading to the production of a mixture of *Le* (type I) and *T* (type II) interferon. To me this seems a less complicated interpretation, consistent with Epstein's experimental results.

EPSTEIN: In collaborative studies with O'Malley of Roswell Park we have found that on phenyl-sepharose columns, designed to elucidate the degree of hydrophobicity of the substances tested, C. parvum-induced interferon has 3 peaks, and that these 3 peaks are similar to 3 peaks observed with PHA-induced interferon. Thus although the C. parvum interferon is heterogeneous, it has the same hydrophobicity profile and the same sensitivity to heating as PHA-induced interferon. Yet, C. parvum also shows the same activity on heterologous cells as type I, "classical" leukocyte interferon induced by Sendai virus and is neutralized by antiserum to that "classical" interferon. With regard to sensitivity to acid pH, C. parvum-induced interferon is intermediate between the extremely sensitive PHA-induced interferon and the extremely stable leukocyte interferon. For all of these reasons we feel that C. parvum interferon represents an intermediate form which has some of the properties of both type II, immune interferon and type I, classical interferon.

PICK: It is my feeling that Epstein's treatment of the LIF or MIF results as mean values, obtained by averaging results derived from testing a number of supernatants and comparing mean value to mean value, is not warranted. Rather she should compare MIF, LIF and interferon values of individual supernatants.

EPSTEIN: I have done exactly what Pick is suggesting. MIF, LIF, LAF and MF were assayed on the same supernatant samples in which we assayed for interferon.

NEUMANN: In the mouse system we also induce interferon but no macrophage migration inhibitory factor (MIF) with CN 6134; this was in pure macrophage cultures devoid of T cells. I would like to know, what happened when Epstein added the C. parvum to pure macrophage cultures. It would also be interesting to know, whether, in this situation, she studied the mediator response already after several hours. In the mouse, CN 6134 induces interferon in macrophage cultures within 6 - 10 hr after which levels decrease.

EPSTEIN: CN 6134 did not induce interferon in macrophage cultures (derived from human blood monocytes) at any time after induction.

HOLDEN: Data obtained by Djeu in our laboratory may add to the divergent findings in the matter of the different types of interferon. Tumor cells inoculated into mice induce high serum levels of interferon. This interferon is sensitive to low pH and is neutralized by two different antisera to type I interferon. Since the results could not be accounted for by a mixture of the two types of interferon, perhaps this is also another situation in which this particular interferon has properties that are intermediate between type I and type II interferon.

MAYER, M.: Can the human viral, immune and so called intermediate interferons be distinguished by appropriate antibodies?

EPSTEIN: There is currently available only an antiserum to Sendai virus-induced leukocyte interferon. This antiserum will not neutralize the antiviral activity of interferon generated by the PHA stimulation of human T lymphocytes, but will neutralize the antiviral activity of the interferon induced in those same cells by C. parvum.

EVIDENCE THAT IMMUNE INTERFERON AND MACROPHAGE MIGRATION INHIBITORY FACTOR ARE DISTINCT ENTITIES

Christine Neumann
Clemens Sorg

Department of Experimental Dermatology
University of Münster
Münster, Germany

Recently, interferons(IF) have evoked interest because -besides their anitviral effect- they possibly take part also in the regulation of the immune response (1). The cells of the immune system not only respond to IF but also may produce an IF which is called "immune interferon" (2). This activity is produced in lymphocyte cultures upon stimulation with antigen or mitogen (3) and thus is counted as a lymphokine. Another lymphokine, macrophage migration inhibitory factor (MIF) (4) and IF were found to appear simultaneously in the sera of mice which had been immunized with BCG. On a molecular weight basis they could not be separated and it therefore was concluded, that both activities might be two different functions of the same molecule (5). In humans, T-cells have been claimed to be the source for antigen or mitogen induced IF (6). In mice, we presented evidence that macrophages which were stimulated in vitro by T-cell products can produce an IF which shares some properties with the immune IF found in lymphocyte cultures (7). We concluded that macrophages are at least one source for IF in an immunological situation. The role of T-cells in MIF-production is well established (8). Here, we investigated, whether in the situation of mitogen stimulated lymphocytes in vitro IF and MIF are produced by different

ISBN 0-12-213950-X

cell types.

A dissociation of mediator production was already evident by the differential capacity of thymus, lymph node and spleen cells to produce MIF and IF upon stimulation with Concanavalin A (Con A). Lymphocytes were stimulated with Con A by a pulse exposure method washing the lymphocytes several times after stimulation (9). Lymphocytes from spleens and lymph nodes were further incubated for 45 to 65 hours at a concentration of 4×10^6 cells/ml and from thymus at a concentration of 10×10^6 cells/ml. As can be seen from table 1, considerable MIF was produced by lymphocytes from spleen, lymph nodes and thymus. The migration inhibition was due to a material produced by the stimulated lymphocytes and not to residual Con A (9). IF, however, which was abundantly produced by stimulated spleen cells was only produced in small amounts by lymph node lymphocytes and was never found in supernatants from stimulated thymus cells. In another set of experiments, lymphocytes from spleens or lymph nodes were enriched for T-cells and depleted of macrophages by passage over adherence column s (7). It is also shown in table 1 that the ability to produce MIF and to proliferate upon pulse exposure to Con A is not impaired by this procedure, while the production of IF was largely abolished. These results suggest that MIF is produced by highly purified T-cells while for the production of IF other cells might be responsible.

The addition of certain types of macrophages to the enriched T-cell population restored IF production in vitro (7). As can be seen from table 2 the addition of macrophages which were grown from bone marrow in the presence of colony stimulating activity (10) were able to restore IF production in combination with spleen T-cells. These macrophages produced <2 units IF when cultured alone. Macrophages grown from proteose peptone or casein induced peritoneal exudates however, did not restore IF production. MIF on the other hand was readily produced by these cultures. Similar results were obtained with lymph node T-cells (not shown).

From these results it was clear, that macrophages played an important role in the induction of lymphocyte IF, possibly being producers of IF under these conditions. When macrophages from bone marrow or spleen were incubated with supernatants from Con A-stimulated T-cells containing no IF activity, 12-48 units IF were produced in cultures containing 5 x 10^5 pure macrophages. This IF was sensitive to treatment at pH2 and at 56°C and therefore exhibited properties of Type II interferon (5). It was investigated whether macrophages induced for IF production also produce MIF. Macrophages from bone marrow were exposed to various IF-inducers including supernatants from ConA stimulated T-cells. The macrophage cultures were washed after several hours of induction, reconstituted with fresh medium and the supernatants were assayed after 30 h incubation. In macrophage cultures IF was also induced by ds RNA Poly rI: rC (64-256 units/ml) and by C.-parvum, strain CN 6134 (16-64 units /ml). Another strain of C.-parvum, CN 5888 did not induce IF in macrophage cultures. The IF induced by Poly rI:rC and CN 6134 were relatively stable at pH2 and therefore exhibited properties of Type I interferon. MIF on the other hand was induced by neither of these agents in macrophage cultures derived from bone marrow.(11).

TABLE I. Differential production of interferon (IF) and macrophage mirgration inhibitory factor (MIF) by different lymphocyte populations[1]

	IF (units)	Migration inhib. (%)	^{3}H dThd (cpm)[2]
Whole spleen	80 (32-128)[3]	49 (40-62)[4]	26.139
Spleen T	2 (0-4)	45 (30-56)	23.057
Lymph node	4 (0-8)	46 (38-58)	32.518
Lymph n. T	O	30 (19-38)	43.272
Thymus	O	55 (47-62)	29.039

1) Spleen, lymph node (4 x 10^6 cells/ml) and thymus (10 x 10^6 cells/ml) stimulated with 10 ug Con A/ml (2h pulse)
2) 1 u Ci tritiated thymidine (5 h pulse). Mean of three experiments.
3) IF units based on reference IF G 002-904-511. Mean and range of 4 experiments.
4) Percent inhibition of macrophage migration. Mean and range of 4 experiments.

TABLE II. Restoration of Interferon production by macrophages (MØ)

	spleen-T alone[1]	+ MØ (b.m.)[2]	+MØ (prot.p.)[3]	+MØ (cas.)[4]
IF (u)	1	128	O	O
MIF (%inhib.)	40	44	31	28

1) 4 x 10^6/ml (column purified), stimulated with 10 ug Con A (2 h pulse).
2) bone marrow derived MØ, IF negative when cultured alone (not shown).
3) proteose peptone
4) casein-induced peritoneal exudate.

A similar dissociation for MIF and IF production by macrophages could be demonstrated by the in vitro culture of pure spleen macrophages (98 % phagocytic for IgG-coated SRBC) which derived from animals injected with either CN 6134 or CN 5888 7 days before. These macrophages produced considerable amounts of IF when they were derived from animals which had been injected with CN 6134. No MIF activity was detected in these cultures. The injection of CN 5888 did not lead to significant production of either mediator.

In summary, we describe situations where MIF but no IF was produced by T-cells as well as situations where IF but no MIF was produced by macrophages. As the cellular requirements for both mediators clearly were different, it is concluded that they are distinct molecules.

REFERENCES

1. Gresser, I., (1977). Cell.Immunol. 34, 406.
2. Falcoff, R.J., (1972). J.Gen.Virol. 16, 251.
3. Wheelock, E.F., (1965). Science 149, 310.

4. Bloom, B.R., (1971). Adv. Immunol. 13, 101.
5. Salvin, S.B., Youngner, J.S., and Lederer, W.H. (1973) Infect. Immun. 7, 68.
6. Epstein, L.B., Kreth, H.W., and Herzenberg, L.A. (1974) Cell.Immunol. 12, 407.
7. Neumann, Ch., and Sorg, C., (1977). Eur.J.Immunol. 7, 719.
8. Morita, C., and Soekawa, M., (1972). Poult.Sci. 51, 433.
9. Manheimer, S., and Pick, E., (1973). Immunology 24, 1027.
10. Austin, P.E., Mc Culloch, E.A., and Till, J.E., (1971). J.Cell.Physiol. 77, 121.
11. Neumann, Ch., and Sorg, C. (1978) Eur.J.Immunol. 8, 582.

DISCUSSION

COHEN, S.: Some years ago we showed that virus infection of non-lymphoid cells leads to the production of an MIF that is antigenically like lymphocyte-derived MIF. We demonstrated that this MIF war distinct from interferons by means of the kinds of "mirror image" experiments I mentioned previously. The data that Neumann and Epstein have presented tend to support this finding. Epstein is studying either a mixture of interferons or an intermediate type. Is the interferon Neumann is studying type I or type II?

NEUMANN: In the situation of Con A-induced spleen cell interferon we are dealing by definition with type II. In the situation of T supernatant-induced macrophage interferon we do not know. It is labile at pH 2, but it may very well be a mixture.

SALVIN: When Youngner and I first described type II interferon and MIF in the serum of sensitized mice, we stated that we were then unable to separate the two lymphokines. However, type I (viral) interferon was readily separable from MIF. We prefer the term "type II" interferon to "immune" interferon, since this interferon can be produced in mice that are "sensitized" but not necessarily "immune".

EPSTEIN: Would Neumann comment on why she finds mouse macrophages sensitive to the interferon induction at a very limited step of their maturation or differentiation pathway.

NEUMANN: Using in vitro cultures of mouse bone-marrow and studying various functional capacities of mononuclear phagocytes along their maturation pathway from progenitor cells to mature macrophages, we found that the cells were only susceptible to interferon induction over a very limited stage of their differentiation, while they expressed other functions over a broad phase of maturation. Further evidence comes also from studies using peritoneal exudate macrophages. The inducibility of interferon depends not only on the irritant used in inducing peritoneal exudates but also on the time elapsed in culture before induction is performed. For example, macrophages in exudates induced by protease peptone or thioglycollate become susceptible to interferon induction by LPS only after several days of culture. So the capability to activate the interferon gene may be critically related to the actual state of differentiation or activation of the macrophage.

LOHMANN-MATTHES: Promonocytes cultured from mouse bone-marrow have characteristics in common with "Null-cells". We have shown that promonocytes have high NK activity. Kirchner and I have evidence that purified populations of bone-marrow promonocytes produce interferon *spontaneously*. This capacity is lost when the promonocyte has matured to an adherent mature bone-marrow macrophage; it then produces interferon only upon induction.

STUDIES OF THE PRODUCER CELL OF INTERFERON IN HUMAN LYMPHOCYTE CULTURES

Holger Kirchner
Rainer Zawatzky

German Cancer Research Center
Heidelberg, FRG

Hans-Hartmut Peter
Helga Dalügge

Medical School of Hannover
Hannover, FRG

Interferon production in human lymphocyte cultures induced by mitogens has been studied for some years and it has been shown that both T cells and B cells may respond to these stimuli albeit with different kinetics (1). More recently, the cell producing interferon in response to Sendai Virus or Herpes Simplex Virus (HSV) has appeared to be a non-T cell, since it was found in the cell fraction which did not form rosettes with sheep erythrocytes (SRBC) - (2,3). In contrast, Sugiyama and Epstein have reported that the cell producing interferon in response to *C. parvum* was a T cell since it did not adhere to nylon wool (4). In this report we want to present some experiments in which we have used the techniques of SRBC rosetting *and* of the nylon wool columns, as well as a variety of additional separation procedures. We have found that the cells producing interferon in response to HSV and *C. parvum* were similar in that they did *not* form rosettes with SRBC and were *not* adherent to nylon wool, suggesting that these cells were neither typical B cells nor typical T cells. A full account of this work is given elsewhere (5). All techniques used in the two collaborating laboratories have been described in previous papers (6,7).

In Table I an experiment is shown in which the titers of interferon were measured in human lymphocyte cultures after a

ISBN 0-12-213950-X

TABLE I. Effects of Multi-Step Treatment Schedules on Interferon Production by Human Lymphocytes

	Stimulant Added			Markers	
Type of Culture	None	HSV	C. parvum	Ig	Latex-Phag.
Fraction F[1]	10[3]	537	243	15	21
Fraction FFF[2]	10	482	257	4	5
FFF plus Nylon Wool	10	432	321	2	2
FFF Nylon plus Ig-anti Ig	10	495	335	<1	<1

[1] Obtained after treatment by a Ficoll-Hypaque gradient
[2] FFF = treatment by Ficoll-Hypaque plus plastic adherence plus iron files/magnet
[3] Interferon titer (IU/ml)

multi-step treatment schedule. The cells were consecutively treated by a Ficoll-Hypaque gradient, by iron filings plus a magnet, by plastic adherence, by a nylon wool column, and by an Ig-anti-Ig column. The cell population which was obtained after all these treatments was fully capable of producing interferon in response to HSV or C. parvum. Since this population contained considerably less than 1% of cells staining for surface immunoglobulins and less than 1% of phagocytic cells, we conclude that the producer cell of interferon in response to both stimuli is not a typical B cell nor a macrophage.

In Table II it is seen that the population in human peripheral lymphocytes which forms rosettes with SRBC does not produce interferon in response to HSV or C. parvum (it does, however, produce interferon in response to phytohemagglutinin). Furthermore, when the population which was obtained after the multi-step procedure described above was treated with SRBC, again only the non-rosetting population produced interferon in response to C. parvum or HSV. The latter population was also highly active in an assay for natural killer (NK) cell activity (7).

In conclusion, our data show that interferon in response to C. parvum or HSV is produced by a cell, which is non-phagocytic, negative for Ig surface markers and does not form rosettes with SRBC. Such characteristics of a "non-rosetting T cell" are typical for the cell type mediating NK activity. Indeed, we have found such activity in the cell population which was active for interferon production and which was obtained after the complete sequence of depletion techniques. Previously, it has been shown that NK cell activity may be augmented by interferon (8). Our data show that the interferon producing

TABLE II. Effect of Rosetting with SRBC on Interferon Production in Human Lymphocyte Cultures

Exp.	Type of Culture	Stimulant Added		
		None	HSV	C. parvum
I	Fraction F[1]	10[2]	730	450
	F, Rosetting with SRBC	10	20	25
	F, Nonrosetting with SRBC	10	850	530
II	FFF Nylon Ig-Anti Ig	10	470	320
	Same,Rosetting with SRBC	10	10	20
	Same,Nonrosetting with SRBC	45[3]	420	370

[1] See Table I
[2] Interferon titer (IU/ml)
[3] Moderate titers of interferon were consistently found in this fraction

cell is found in the same pool of cells highly depleted of typical T cells, B cells or macrophages that is able to mediate NK cell activity. In more recent experiments we have also found that the cell producing interferon in response to tumor cells is found in the same fraction (Peter, Leibold, Dalügge and Kirchner, unpublished observation).

REFERENCES

1. Epstein, L.B., Kreth, W., and Herzenberg, L.A., Cell. Immunol. 12, 407 (1974).
2. Yamaguchi, T., Handa, K., Shimizu, Y., Abo, T., and Kumagai, K., J. Immunol. 118, 1931 (1977).
3. Rasmussen, L., and Merigan, T., Proc. Natl. Acad. Sci. USA 75, 3957 (1978).
4. Sugiyama, M., and Epstein, L.B., Cancer Res. 38, 4467 (1978).
5. Kirchner, H., Peter, H.H., Hirt, H.M., Zawatzky, R., Dalügge, H., and Bradstreet, P.,Immunobiology,in press 1979.
6. Hirt, H.M., Schwenteck, M., Becker, H., and Kirchner, H., Clin. Exp. Immunol. 32, 471 (1978).
7. Peter, H.H., Eife, R.F., and Kalden, J.R., J. Immunol. 116, 342 (1976).
8. Gidlund, N., Örn, A., Wigzell, H., Senik, A., and Gresser, I., Nature 273, 759 (1978).

REGULATION OF THE ACTIVITY OF NATURAL KILLER CELLS BY INTERFERON AND PROSTAGLANDINS

Howard T. Holden
Michael J. Brunda
Ronald B. Herberman

Laboratory of Immunodiagnosis
National Cancer Institute
Bethesda, Maryland

Julie Y. Djeu

Division of Virology
Bureau of Biologics
Bethesda, Maryland

Natural killer (NK) cells are a subpopulation of lymphocytes that have spontaneous anti-tumor activity (reviewed in Herberman and Holden, 1978). In mice this reactivity peaks between 5-8 weeks and declines to baseline levels after 12 weeks. However, this pattern can be altered under a variety of environmental and experimental conditions, with NK activity either increased or decreased in relation to the usual spontaneous levels.

As summarized here, we have found that at least two different mediators, interferon (IF) and prostaglandins (PG), play a role in the regulation of this cytotoxic reactivity.

NK activity can be augmented *in vivo* and *in vitro* by a variety of IF inducers (Herberman *et al.*, 1977) and by IF itself (Gidlund *et al.*, 1978: Djeu *et al.*, 1979a). For stimulation of NK activity by poly I:C, macrophages are required for boosting both *in vivo* and *in vitro*, while augmentation of NK activity directly by IF does not require macrophages (Djeu *et al.*, 1979b).

ISBN 0-12-213950-X

Although NK activity is usually labile in culture (Herberman *et al.*, 1975a), we have devised culture conditions that maintain this reactivity for up to 48 hours (Djeu *et al.*, 1979a). This allowed us to examine the metabolic events required for the expression of both spontaneous and boosted NK activity. Inhibitors of DNA synthesis, such as mitomycin C, had no effect on either spontaneous or boosted NK activity. Although an inhibitor of RNA synthesis, actinomycin D, also had no effect on the spontaneous activity, it inhibited boosting by IF (Table I). There was a correlation between the percent inhibition of ^{3}H-uridine incorporation and the inhibition of boosting by IF. Recently Dr. John Ortaldo in our laboratory has found that RNA synthesis was required only during the first five hours after treatment with IF; treatment thereafter with inhibitors of RNA synthesis had no effect on the levels of NK activity. Boosting of NK activity by IF was inhibited by pretreatment with inhibitors of protein synthesis (data not shown) or at early (1 hr after IF treatment, Table II) and intermediate times (4-6 hr) (data not shown). There was still a slight inhibition of boosting at 18 hr after IF treatment (Table II). NK activity from cells that had been boosted for longer periods of time and also spontaneous NK activity were not affected by these agents (data not shown).

Decreases in NK activity have been observed during the growth of murine sarcoma virus (MSV)-induced tumors (Herberman *et al.*, 1975b, Becker and Klein, 1976). Since it has been reported that PG production was associated with these tumors (Humes and Strausser, 1974), we decided to investigate the regulatory role of PG on NK activity. PGE_1 and PGE_2 reduced

TABLE I. Effect of Actinomycin D on Boosting of Mouse NK Activity by Interferon

Treatment[a] *actinomycin D (μg/ml)*	*IF*	*Cytotoxicity LU*[b]*/10*^{7} *cells*	*Incorporation of* ^{3}H*-UdR: % of untreated cells*
----	-	14.8	100
----	+	77.0	110
50.0	+	17.0	6
5.0	+	55.6	23
0.5	+	80.4	99

[a]*Spleen cells from 7 week old CBA/N mice were incubated for 1 hour with actinomycin D and then for 1 hour with IF.*
[b]*Lytic units/10*^{7} *cells; target cell was RL♂1.*

TABLE II. Effect of Protein Synthesis Inhibition after in vitro Boosting of Mouse NK Activity with IF

Drug treatment (M)		Boosting for 1 hr -IF	Boosting for 1 hr +IF	Boosting for 18 hr -IF	Boosting for 18 hr +IF
----		4.0[a]	21.6	12.1	40.8
Emetine	10^{-5}	6.1	7.1	8.9	21.8
	10^{-6}	5.6	9.9	9.9	35.8
	10^{-7}	5.8	20.4	10.6	36.0
Pactamycin	10^{-5}	5.4	10.1	9.5	10.2
	10^{-6}	5.1	7.4	9l8	24.6
	10^{-7}	5.0	8.0	10.1	39.2

[a]Percent cytotoxicity vs RLδ1 targets at 200/1 A/T ratio.

NK activity about 50% when added to the 4 hr ^{51}Cr release assay at 10^{-6}M while PGA_1 and PGA_2 were less effective, and $PGF_{1\alpha}$ and $PGF_{2\alpha}$ had no effect (data not shown). For maximal inhibitory effects, PG had to be present in the assay since pretreatment of the effector population produced only slight depression of NK activity. PG's exerted similar effects on spontaneous and boosted NK activity (Table III).

We then examined whether PG might play a role in inhibition of NK activity *in vivo* in tumor-bearing animals. Mice inoculated with MSV on day 0 were given indomethacin, an inhibitor of PG synthesis, in their drinking water on days 7-14 and then tested for NK activity (Table IV). The depressed NK activity of tumor-bearing animals was partially or

TABLE III. Effect of PG on Spontaneous and Boosted NK Activity

	IF	Prostaglandin added to assay: None	Prostaglandin added to assay: PGE_1[a]	% Inhibition of the response by PGE_1[b]
CBA, 6 weeks	-	33.6[c]	19.0	49.0
CBA, 12 weeks	-	13.5	-	-
CBA, 12 weeks	+	25.6	15.5	44.2

[a]10^{-6}M.
[b]Based on lytic unit calculations.
[c]Percent cytotoxicity; target cell was RLδ1.

TABLE IV. Effect of Indomethacin on NK Cytotoxicity of Spleen Cells from Tumor-Bearing Mice

	CBA		Swiss nude
Treatment	Exp. 1	Exp. 2	Exp. 3
None	18.9[a]	12.0	34.0
Indomethacin[b]	27.3	9.2	33.8
MSV, day 14	9.8	7.0	17.4
MSV, day 14 + indomethacin	24.9	11.5	26.1

[a]*Percent cytotoxicity.*
[b]*Mice were given indomethacin in their drinking water (20μg/ml) from day 7 until day 14.*

completely reversed by treatment with indomethacin, or aspirin, inoculated one day before the test (data not shown). The depressed activity in animals that have had a tumor for two weeks or longer could not be reversed by these inhibitors of PG synthesis. This suggests that either prolonged exposure to PG had an irreversible effect on NK activity or that there is another mechanism for suppression during the later phases of tumor growth.

From the above data we have formulated a model for the regulation of mouse NK activity (Figure I). Inactive NK cells can, in the absence of experimental manipulation, differentiate *in vivo* into active NK cells by a mechanism that is not clear at this time, but which may involve IF. IF can augment the level of NK activity but it is not known whether IF is acting on both inactive and active populations or only on one of them. In any event, boosting by IF is dependent on RNA and protein synthesis and there appears to be an intermediate boosted state during which the activity can be decreased by inhibitors of RNA synthesis (first 5 hrs after IF) or of protein synthesis (approximately 18 hrs). Thereafter the boosted activity of NK cells becomes stable and is no longer sensitive to either of these inhibitors. The spontaneous activity of NK cells, and the augmented activity of IF-treated NK cells, appear to be equally susceptible to PG mediated inhibition. PG may regulate NK activity *in vivo* and may partially account for the reduced NK activity in tumor bearing animals.

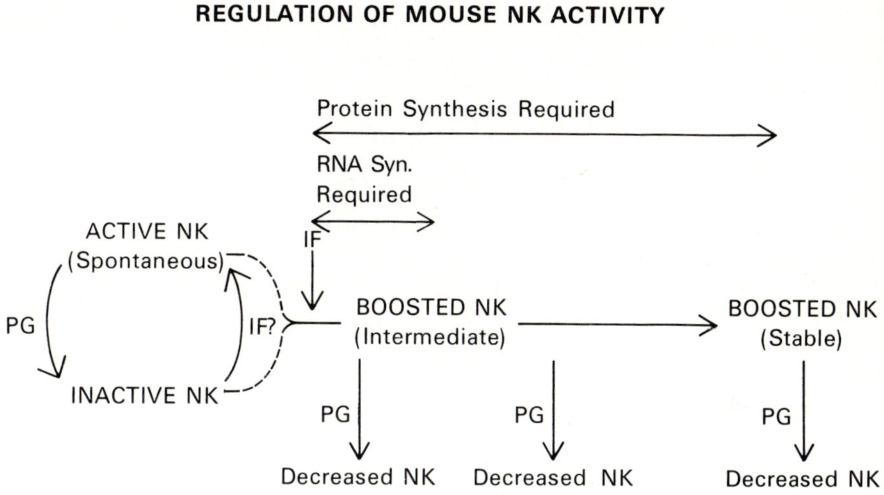

FIGURE 1. A model for the regulation of mouse NK activity.

REFERENCES

Becker, S., and Klein, E. (1976). *Eur. J. Immunol. 6*, 892.

Djeu, J.Y., Heinbaugh, J.A., Holden, H.T., and Herberman, R.B. (1979a). *J. Immunol. 122*, 175.

Djeu, J.Y., Heinbaugh, J.A., Holden, H.T., and Herberman, R.B. (1979b). *J. Immunol. 122*, 182.

Gidlund, M., Orn, A., Wigzell, H., Senik, A., and Gresser, I. (1978). *Nature 273*, 759.

Herberman, R.B., and Holden, H.T. (1978). *Adv. Cancer Res. 27*, 305.

Herberman, R.B., Nunn, M.E., Holden, H.T., and Lavrin, D.H. (1975a). *Int. J. Cancer 16*, 230.

Herberman, R.B., Nunn, M.E., Holden, H.T., and Lavrin, D.H. (1975b). *Int. J. Cancer 16*, 216.

Herberman, R.B., Nunn, M.E., Holden, H.T., Staal, S., and Djeu, J.Y. (1977). *Int. J. Cancer 19*, 555.

Humes, J.L., and Strausser, H.R. (1974). *Prostaglandins 5*, 183.

INTERFERON AUGMENTS HUMAN NK-CELL ACTIVITY THROUGH RECRUITMENT OF "PRE-NK" CELLS

E. Saksela
T. Timonen
Departments of Obstetrics and Gynaecology
University Central Hospital, Helsinki,
Department of Pathology
Helsinki University, Finland

K. Cantell
Central Public Health Laboratory
Helsinki, Finland

I. INTRODUCTION

Blood mononuclear cells produce interferon as a result of contact with virus-infected or tumor cells (1). Interferon strongly augments human natural killer (NK) cell activity (1, 2). It is not known, whether interferon enhances the activity of initially active circulating NK cells, or recruits an entirely new population of effector cells to NK activity.
The purpose of the present study was to characterize NK cells responsive to interferon.

II. MATERIALS AND METHODS

A. Effector cells

100 ml samples of citrate venous blood was collected from healthy male volunteers. Mononuclear cells were purified with Ficoll-Isopaque gradient centrifugation, depletion of adherent cells on glass surfaces, and finally nonadherent cells were run through nylon wool columns.

B. Purification of natural killer cells

Natural killer cells cytotoxic against fetal fibroblasts were isolated by adsorption and elution of effector cells

ISBN 0-12-213950-X

from target cells as previously described (3).

C. Cytotoxicity experiments

A ^{51}chromium-release assay for cell-mediated cytotoxicity against fetal fibroblasts grown on Degalan beads has been described before (4). Effector:target cell ratio varied between 8:1-15:1, and exposure time was 20 h.

D. Human leukocyte interferon

Human leukocyte interferon was produced and partially purified as described previously (5). The preparation used contained 6×10^6 units/ml, and 1.5 mg protein/ml.

E. Interferon assay

The interferon activity in blood mononuclear cell-target cell co-culture supernatans was assayed by the reduction of vesicular stomatitis virus plaques on U (human amnion) cells and expressed in terms of units assaigned to the British research standard 69/19 (6).

III. RESULTS

A. Production of interferon as a result of blood mononuclear cell-target cell contact

To study the effect of exogenous interferon on human NK cells, such NK sensitive target cells have to be used, which do not themselves induce the interferon release. Fetal fibroblasts were suitable targets in this respect, whereas K 562 induced the interferon synthesis (Table I).

Table I. Interferon production by blood mononuclear cells in contact with fetal fibroblasts (FF) or K 562

INCUBATION CONDITIONS[a]	IF TITER IU/ml
Medium only	<20
FF	<20
K 562	350

[a]5×10^6 purified lymphocytes co-cultured for 24 h with 1×10^6 K 562 cells or fetal fibroblasts (FF)

B. The effect of exogenous interferon and K 562 contact on the cytotoxicity of different fractions obtained after the adsorption and elution of NK cells from fetal fibroblasts

In Figure 1, the effect of 6000 IU of human leukocyte interferon and preincubation in contact with K 562 cells on the cytotoxicity of NK cell enriched (AE), NK cell depleted (NA) and control populations is demonstrated. Interferon and K 562 contact did not augment the NK activity of effector cells initially cytotoxic against fetal fibroblasts, whereas a strong enrichment of cytotoxicity was detected in the nonadherent fraction as well as in the input population.

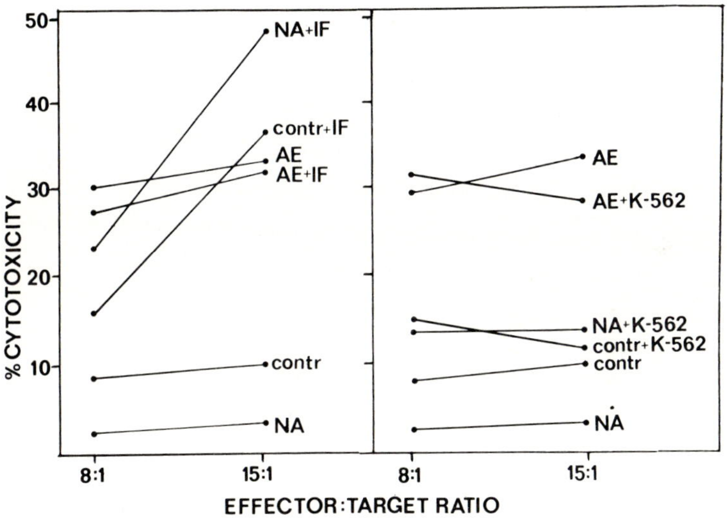

FIGURE 1. The effect of interferon on the natural killer cell activity against fetal fibroblasts of different fractions after the adsorption and elution of natural killer cells from fetal fibroblast-coated beads. AE= adsorbed and eluted cells, NA= fetal fibroblasts nonadherent cells; cont= cells absorbed with cell-free beads; IF= fractions tested for cytotoxicity in the presence of 6000 IU of purified leukocyte interferon; K 562= fractions tested for cytotoxicity in the presence of K 562 at the ratio of 10 lymphocytes/K 562.

The results indicate that NK cells cytotoxic against interferon-noninducing target cells represent an initially active killer cell population, whereas those NK cells nonadherent to fetal fibroblasts are effectors recruitable to NK activity with exogenously added interferon or interferon produced at the contact of interferon inducing target cells.

IV. SUMMARY AND CONCLUSIONS

The present results demonstrated that interferon induced cytotoxic activity of a dormant NK cell population in human peripheral blood. On the other hand, it had no effect on effector cells initially cytotoxic against fetal fibroblasts. Thus, NK cells in human peripheral blood can be divided in "mature" and "pre-NK" cells. We do not know, whether these effector cells belong to a same subgroup of lymphocytes. We have shown elsewhere that "pre-NK" and "mature" NK cells are morphologically similar (7) suggesting that they may represent the same subgroup at different activation levels.

ACKNOWLEDGEMENTS

This work has been supported by grants from the Sigrid Jusélius Foundation, National Research Council for Medical Sciences, Finland, and by grant No 1 R01 CA 23809-01 from the National Cancer Institute, NIH, USA.

REFERENCES

1. Trinchieri, G., and Santoli, D., J. Exp. Med. 147, 1314, (1978).
2. Herberman, R.R., Ortaldo, J.R., and Bonnard, G.D. Nature 227, 221, (1979).
3. Timonen, T., and Saksela, E., Cell. Immunol. 40, 69, (1978).
4. Timonen, T., and Saksela, E., J. Immunol. Methods 18, 123, (1977).

5. Cantell, K., and Hirvonen, S., J. Gen. Virol. 39, 541, (1978).
6. Mogensen, K.E., Cantell, K., J. Gen. Virol. 22, 95, (1974).
7. Saksela, E., Timonen, T., Ranki, A., and Häyry, P., Immunol. Rev. 44, 71 (1979).

DISCUSSION

LANDY: It was recently reported by Senik, Gresser et al. that interferon administered to neonatal mice 15 days of age, a time at which NK activity is normally never manifested (it begins to appear spontaneously at day 23 - 25), leads to the prompt appearance of NK activity in these immunologic "prematures". Admittedly this finding could be interpreted as evidence for an effect by IF on precursors of NK cells presumed to be present in meonates. But it seems to me that this could equally involve an effect of IF on natural suppressor cells against NK, a category of non-induced regulatory cells described by Cudkowicz.

FRIDMAN: Concerning the possibility that interferon enhances NK cell activity in young mice by inhibiting suppressor cells rather than by inducing NK cells, Senik in collaboration with Gresser have since shown that interferon does not interfere with suppressor cells for NK cell activity although enhancing the response. Therefore, even in these very young mice, interferon seems to be acting directly on pre-NK cells.

HENNEY: Have the cells in the non-adherent compartment which kill after exposure to IF really been characterized as NK cells? Is the increase due to an expansion of the population of NK cells or to an increased activity at the level of individual NK cells? It appears to me that the data Timonen has presented are discordant with those of Roder and Wigzell (Proc. Nat. Acad. Sci., 1978).

TIMONEN: We have performed contact analyses from the total fibroblast-nonadherent populations mixed with K 562 target cells. In this system, most of the lymphoid cells conjugating with K 562 were morphologically NK cells. As IF-induced NK cells are cross-reactive against total fibroblasts and K 562, we take this as evidence that the cells boosted by IF are NK cells. Thus IF expands the NK cell clone size. As for Roder's data, our results in the total fibroblast system differ from his in the YAC lymphoma system. The difference is most probably due to the target cells used. In our hands, "pre-NK" cells adhere to interferon inducing K 562 cells; this is in accord with Roder's data. One could speculate that the target cell structures recognized by the "pre-NK" cells for activation differ from the target structures recognized by the active NK cells for target cell lysis. I think it probable that total fibroblasts possess only the latter target structures.

KIRCHNER: I believe that the model Timonen is proposing (pre-NK cells → IF → NK cells) is intriguing. Does he consider that this sequence of events is happening in vivo? In that case it would be especially interesting to know, which cell is producing the interferon that drives this reaction.

TIMONEN: We have been studying the producer cells of the K 562 induced interferon. It seems that most of the activity is derived from macrophages, or is dependent on the presence of macrophages. However, there is always residual interferon production in mononuclear blood cells exhaustively depleted of macrophages. We have some evidence that this interferon is derived from NK cells themselves.

FRIDMAN: I would like to comment on the possibility that there exist different stages (pre-NK to mature NK cells) at which NK cells may or not respond to interferon. Testing the effect of fibroblast and leukocyte interferon, on induction of NK cell activity in vitro on peripheral lymphocytes from patients with cancer disease, Lucero in our laboratory, in collaboration with Falcoff, has shown that there may be three patterns:

(1) Patients with normal NK cell activity whose lymphocytes can be enhanced by interferon

(2) Patients with low NK cell activity, such as those with CLL, whose NK activity could be normalized by treatment with interferon. These patients presumably have "pre-NK" cells, induced by interferon

(3) Finally, patients such as those treated with BCG, who exhibit high NK cell activity not further enhanced by interferon.

These data suggest that in man there may be pathologic states which mimic the different physiological stages of NK cells.

HOLDEN: I have two comments to add to this discussion. First, our laboratory has examined NK cells extensively before and after boosting, both in mouse and in man. We have found that these cells are similar with respect to specificity of reactivity and in their identifying characteristics. Second, there are several experimental conditions in which NK activity can be depressed. However, the ability to counteract the depression by interferon or interferon inducers varies depending on the methods that had been used to depress NK activity. Depressed NK activity in tumor bearing animals can be reversed by interferon or interferon inducers. However, when it has been depressed by intravenous injection of *C. parvum*, NK activity in mice does not appear to be stimulated by IF or IF inducers, as we have found or, for that matter, when it has been depressed by ^{89}Sr, as shown by Kumar.

EFFECTS OF INTERFERON ON SENSITIZATION AND EXPRESSION OF DELAYED HYPERSENSITIVITY IN THE MOUSE

Edward De Maeyer
Jaqueline De Maeyer-Guignard

Institut Curie - Biologie
Université de Paris-Sud
Orsay, France

In addition to its antiviral activity, type I interferon has many other biologic effects, among which the antitumor effect and the various effects on the immune system have received most attention (1,2). We have been interested for some time in the effect of type I mouse interferon on cell-mediated immunity, and this paper more specifically deals with some of our work on delayed hypersensitivity (DH).

I. EFFECT OF INTERFERON ON DH IN THE MOUSE

A. *Effect of interferon on expression of DH*

1. Exogenous interferon. Animals sensitized to either picryl chloride, sheep red blood cells (SRBC) or Newcastle disease virus (NDV) do not react upon challenge with the same antigen if they have been treated with 10^6 units of interferon at some time during the 24 hours preceding the challenge. When less than 10^6 units of interferon are given, some reaction occurs, but to a significantly lesser extent than in control animals. To act, interferon can be administered systemically and does not have to be injected into the organ

Supported by the INSERM (ATP N° 28-76-60) and the Ligue Nationale Française contre le Cancer

ISBN 0-12-213950-X

receiving the challenge dose of antigen (ear or footpad). Histological examination of ears or footpads fully confirms the results as measured macroscopically by calipers (3,4).

2. *Endogenous interferon.* The use of If-1 congenic mice has unequivocally demonstrated that interferon produced by the mouse during viral infection can, like exogenous interferon, cause a decreased expression of DH. If-1 congenic mice differ from C57BL/6 mice by their levels of NDV-induced circulating interferon (5) and cell-mediated immune reactions, after inoculating of NDV, are more depressed in high than in low interferon producers (3). Since circulating interferon production is a common denominator of many virus infections, these results strongly suggest that interferon contributes to the decreased intensity of cell-mediated immune reactions, sometimes observed during and immediately after viral infections. This phenomenon was first reported by von Pirquet (6), who described a decreased skin reactivity to tuberculin in children with measles, and has been repeatedly confirmed for many other virus infections in animals and in man (7).

B. *Effect of interferon on sensitization*

Experiments using either SRBC or NDV as antigen indicate that interferon can decrease and even completely inhibit sensitization. In order to obtain this effect, interferon has to be administered to the mice 24 hours before the antigen (4,8). This timing of interferon administration is crucial, because when interferon is given at the same time or after the antigen, there is no effect, or even enhancement of DH. Administration of about 10^6 units of mouse interferon by the intravenous route to C57BL/6 mice, two to three hours after immunization with a suboptimal dose of SRBC, significantly enhances the reaction of the animals when challenged in their footpads four days later. This indicates that interferon can have opposite effects, and either decrease or enhance sensitization, depending on the time it acts.

II. RESULTS OBTAINED WITH ELECTROPHORETICALLY PURE MOUSE INTERFERON

Until very recently, mouse and also human type I interferon had not been purified to homogeneity, and in spite of careful controls with mock interferons and interferon preparations of different cellular and species origins, there remained some legitimate doubt as to whether the non antiviral effects -including those on the immune system- were due to interferon or to some other substance(s) contaminating the interferon preparations.

We have recently achieved purification of mouse interferon by two-step affinity chromatography, first on a poly(U) agarose column (9), and then on a column of sheep anti-mouse interferon globulin, coupled to affigel-10 (10). The purity of the eluted material can be assessed by electrophoresis on polyacrylamide slab gels in the presence of SDS. Electrophoretically pure (EP) mouse interferon shows two bands upon staining with Coomassie brilliant blue, one having a MW 35,000 dalton and the other having a MW of 22,000 dalton. Both molecular forms have antiviral activity. The specific activity of pure mouse interferon is 2.4×10^9 reference units/mg (11).

In collaboration with I. Gresser and M. Tovey, we have examined EP mouse interferon for a number of biological effects previously ascribed to crude or partially purified interferon preparations, and we have been able to establish that the same molecules responsible for the antiviral action of interferon are also responsible for these varied biologic effects, including the effect on sensitization and expression of delayed hypersensitivity in the mouse (Table I and Fig. 1).

TABLE I. Some biological effects obtained in vitro and in the animal with electrophoretically pure mouse interferon[a]

ANTICELLULAR EFFECT

Inhibition of cell multiplication of mouse tumor cells (L1210) in vitro.

ANTITUMORAL EFFECT

Inhibition of the growth of a transplantable tumor (Ehrlich ascites cells) in mice.

EFFECTS ON CELLS OF THE IMMUNE SYSTEM

- *inhibition of antibody formation in vitro*
- *delayed type hypersensitivity in vivo*
  - . *inhibition or enhancement of sensitization*
  - . *inhibition of expression*
- *enhancement of NK cell activity in vivo and in vitro*

[a]*(I. Gresser, J. De Maeyer-Guignard, M. Tovey and E. De Maeyer), submitted for publication.*

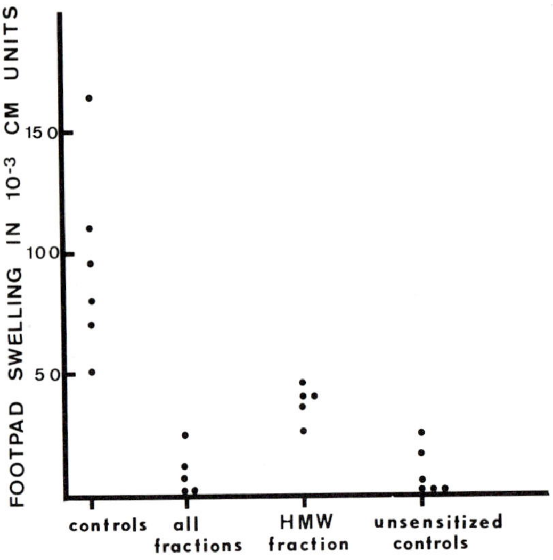

FIGURE 1. Effect of pure IF on expression of DTH to SRBC. 3 groups of 5 BALB/c mice were sensitized to SRBC by iv inoculation of 10^6 cells. 4 days later, prior to footpad challenge (with 10^8 cells in 40 μl) : one group received ip 5 X 10^6 units of EP interferon, containing both 35,000 and 22,000 MW forms (all fractions), the 2nd group received ip 5 X 10^5 units of interferon of the 35,000 MW form only (eluted from a gel (HMW fraction)) and the 3rd group served as control. 24 hours after footpad challenge, footpad swelling was measured in all animals. Each point on the figure represents the footpad swelling of one mouse.

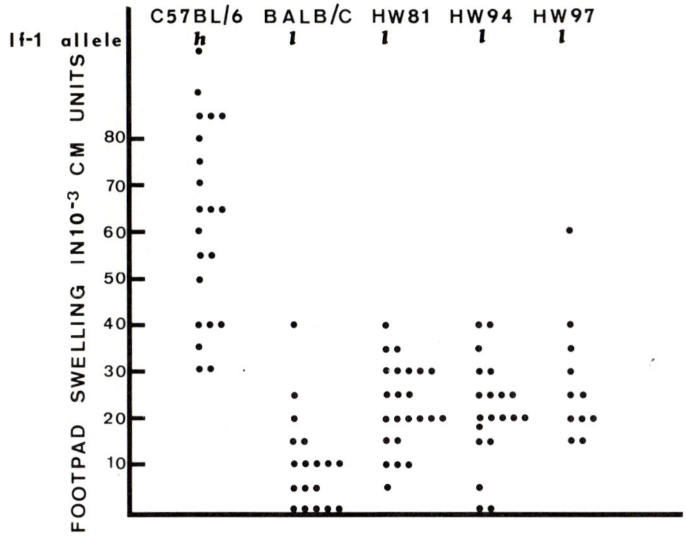

FIGURE 2. DTH to NDV in congenic strains.

Extent of DH to NDV in C57BL/6, BALB/c and in 3 B6.C-H-28^{c}-If-1^{l} congenic lines (HW 81, 94 and 97). All mice had been immunized with 5 X 10^{6} plaque forming units (pfu) of NDV, and were challenged in their left footpad with 4 X 10^{7} pfu, 5 days later. Each point represents the footpad swelling of an individual mouse, measured 48 hrs after footpad challenge.

III. DH TO NDV IS INFLUENCED BY THE LEVEL OF INTERFERON PRODUCTION AS DETERMINED BY THE ALLELE AT If-1

Since interferon can influence the afferent and efferent pathways of DH to a variety of antigens, a relevant question is the possible influence of virally induced interferon on the establishment of DH to the inducing virus. The congenic If-1^{l} mice have been instrumental in providing an experimental approach to this question. Studies in BALB/c and C57BL/6 mice have revealed that the expression of DH is more pronounced, and especially of longer duration, in the high interferon producing C57BL/6 strain than in the low interferon producing

BALB/c. This could theoretically be explained by the high interferon production of C57BL/6, since interferon enhances sensitization when administered after the antigen, and this is of course the sequence of events after inoculation of a non-replicating virus like NDV. This explanation receives further experimental support from the results obtained in B6.C-H-28^{c}-If-1^{l} congenic mice (Fig. 2). The DH reaction of these animals is much closer to that of BALB/c than to that of C57BL/6. This indicates that, on a C57BL/6 background, the intensity of DH to NDV is influenced by the allele at If-1, in that the reaction is stronger in If-1^{h} than If-1^{l} mice. The possibility however that enhanced DH and enhanced interferon production are just two expressions of the same gene -i.o.w. and "enhanced reaction to NDV locus"- is ruled out by results obtained in recombinant inbred lines (12), in that the 3 If-1^{h} RI strains do not have enhanced DH to NDV, but respond more like BALB/c . This finding shows that in addition to the If-1^{h} allele, a combination of other genes, present in the C56BL/6 background, are necessary for the high interferon production to stimulate DH to NDV (13).

CONCLUSION

Experiments using pure mouse interferon have confirmed earlier results obtained with partially purified interferon preparations, and demonstrated unequivocally that interferon can influence both the afferent and the efferent pathways of the delayed hypersensitivity reaction in the mouse. We believe that this effect is one of the mechanisms by which cell-mediated immune reactions are altered during viral infections.

Furthermore, type I interferon produced as a result of virus inoculation can influence the establishment of DH to the inducing virus, as shown by the effect of the alleles at the If-1 locus on DH to NDV. In this respect the If-1 locus acts as an NDV-specific immune response locus, since it affects cell-mediated immunity to this virus through interferon production.

REFERENCES

1. Gresser, I. (1977). *In* "Cancer-a comprehensive treatise", Vol. 5 Chemotherapy (F. Becker, ed.), p. 521. Plenum Press, New-York.
2. Epstein, L.B. (1977). *In* "Interferon and their actions", (W. Stewart II, ed.), p. 92. C.R.C. Press, Cleveland.
3. De Maeyer, E., De Maeyer-Guignard, J. and Vandeputte, M. (1975). *Proc. Nat. Acad. Sci. USA 72,* 1753.
4. De Maeyer, E. (1976). *J. Infect. Dis. 133,* A63.
5. De Maeyer, E., De Maeyer-Guignard, J. and Bailey, D.W. (1975). *Immunogenetics 1,* 438.
6. Von Pirquet, C. (1908). *Deut. Med. Wochenschrift 34,* 1297.
7. Notkins, A.L., Mergenhagen, S.E. and Howard, R.J. (1970). *Ann. Rev. Microbiol. 24,* 525.
8. De Maeyer-Guignard, J., Cachard, A. and De Maeyer, E. (1975). *Science 190,* 574.
9. De Maeyer-Guignard, J., Thang, M.N. and De Maeyer, E. (1977). *Proc. Natl. Acad. Sci. 74,* 3787.
10. Sipe, J.D., De Maeyer-Guignard, J., Fauconnier, B. and De Maeyer, E. (1973). *Proc. Soc. Acad. Sci. USA 70,* 1037.
11. De Maeyer-Guignard, J., Tovey, M.G., Gresser, I. and De Maeyer, E. (1978). *Nature 271,* 622.
12. Bailey, D.W. (1971). *Transplantation 11,* 325.
13. De Maeyer, E., De Maeyer-Guignard, J. (1979). *Interferon 1979,* in press.

DISCUSSION

YOSHIDA: Does de Maeyer have any idea of the mechanism by which exogenous interferon can suppress the expression of DTH?

DE MAEYER: I do not.

YOSHIDA: Did de Maeyer examine the effect of interferon on the production of lymphokines in vitro?

DE MAEYER: No, but I believe it would be very worth while to do so.

ALTMAN: Does the genetic susceptibility to the induction of type I IF correlate with susceptibility to induction of type II IF?

DE MAEYER: There is no correlation between the alleles of IF-1 and high or low production of type II IF; IF-1 specifically influences interferon production induced by NDV.

ROCKLIN: I would like to suggest one possible mechanism to explain part of the immunosuppressive effect of interferon on delayed hypersensitivity. It was shown by Notkins that interferon enhances histamine release. Furthermore recent evidence from many laboratories indicates that suppressor cells bear histamine receptors and are activated by histamine in vitro. Therefore, it is possible that interferon-induced histamine release in vivo could activate suppressor cells which would either inhibit the sensitization process or the elicitation of a response in a sensitized animal.

MAYER, M.: Do all preparations of highly purified interferon have precisely the same ratio of antiviral activity to these other *in vitro* activities? Does the antiviral activity of pure interferon co-chromatograph in constant ratio to these other *in vitro* activities?

DE MAEYER: The three different preparations of electrophoretically pure interferon that were examined by us *did* have comparable ratios of antiviral to the non-antiviral effects that were studied in vitro. Of course the accuracy of most of these tests is such that I cannot claim that it was "precisely" the same.

In many tests, non-interferon containing fractions or gel-slices were examined together with the active fractions. They were found to be devoid not only of anti-viral activity but also of all the non-antiviral activities that were examined. When the anticellular and antiviral effect of pure interferon eluted from 2 mm gel-slices were measured, constant ratios were obtained.

DE WECK: Has this highly purified IF been tested on macrophages? What effects does it have?

DE MAEYER: We are presently engaged in a collaborative study with Rabinovitch of N. Y. U., using electrophoretically pure mouse interferon. He is examining the effects of pure interferon on macrophages. Preliminary results indicate that this product elicits activation.

SALVIN: What types of antibody synthesis have been affected by type I interferon? I understand that the plaque assay has been used primarily.

FRIDMAN: Mouse type I interferon, both crude and purified, inhibits 19S PFC to SRBC in a primary response and 19S + 7S PFC in a secondary response. Inhibition was observed when interferon was added at the beginning of the culture and not at the later phases.

DAVID: Would De Maeyer tell us what were some of the decisive steps that proved crucial for increasing the purity and specific activity of IF by five logs between 1958 and 1979.

DE MAEYER: One of the most decisive steps was certainly the improvements made in the production of interferon. This increased efficiency of interferon production was the result of the effort of many people in many different laboratories. Mainly, it was the combination of high interferon producing cell lines, superinduction and priming of interferon production. The high interferon producing cell lines were found as a result of trial and error since a blueprint for a high interferon producing cell line does not exist even now. For example the cell line which was used for the production of our mouse interferon was the high producing C-243 line, as described by Baron and collaborators.

DAVID: IF can either augment or depress delayed hypersensitivity. What are the conditions for augmentation or depression?

DE MAEYER: When interferon is administered prior to antigen, sensitization is inhibited; if interferon is given a few hours after the antigen, sensitization is enhanced.

DI SABATO: It was reported a few years ago that viral interferon enhances the expression of the H-2 antigens on the surface of normal murine thymocytes. Has this finding been reproduced with the purest preparations of interferon?

DE MAEYER: Electrophoretically pure interferon does augment the expression of H-2 antigen on mouse L1210 cells cultivated in the presence of interferon. We have not yet repeated these experiments with normal thymocytes.

INCREASED SENSITIVITY TO INTERFERON IN MOUSE CELLS CARRYING THE RESISTANCE ALLELE MX IS SELECTIVE FOR MYXOVIRUSES

Otto Haller
Heinz Arnheiter
Jean Lindenmann

Division of Experimental Microbiology
Institute for Medical Microbiology
University of Zürich
8028 Zürich, Switzerland

Ion Gresser

Institut de Recherches Scientifiques sur le Cancer
94800 Villejuif, France

Mice bearing the allele Mx are resistant to challenge by orthomyxoviruses in vivo. This resistance can be abrogated by treatment with anti-interferon serum (1). To explain the role of interferon in this system one has to postulate that orthomyxoviruses are more sensitive to interferon in Mx-bearing cells than in control cells, and that this sensitizing effect of the Mx allele is limited to orthomyxoviruses and leaves the interferon sensitivity of other viruses untouched.

These postulates were tested in peritoneal macrophage cultures from resistant and susceptible mice. Immediately after withdrawal from the peritoneal cavity, macrophages exhibit the resistance phenotype of the donor animal (2). However, after 3 weeks in culture, macrophages become uniformely susceptible to infection by M-TUR, a macrophage-adapted strain of influenza A virus, while retaining their initial susceptibility to vesicular stomatitis virus (VSV). It thus becomes possible to compare the effect of graded doses of interferon on the growth of M-TUR and VSV in both Mx-carrying and in control macropha-

ISBN 0-12-213950-X

TABLE I. Growth inhibition by interferon of M-TUR or VSV virus in cultured macrophages from backcross mice segregating for the allele Mx

Virus	genotype of cells	Interferon units	Mean LOG_{10} $TCID_{50}$/ml				
			6	12	24	36	48 h p.i.
M-TUR	+/+	0	3.5	4.5	6.7	7.7	n.d.
	Mx/+	0	3.3	4.3	7.0	7.2	n.d.
	+/+	20	n.d.	3.3	3.7	4.7	8.0
	Mx/+	20	n.d.	3.0	2.0	1.7	1.5
VSV	+/+	0	3.0	3.7	4.0	3.3	n.d.
	Mx/+	0	3.0	3.5	4.0	3.5	n.d.
	+/+	10	n.d.	1.0	1.8	1.2	1.0
	Mx/+	10	n.d.	1.0	2.0	1.0	1.0

Macrophage cultures were established from individual mice classified as resistant or susceptible to M-TUR. After 3 weeks in culture, 10^6 cells were exposed for 18 h to various NIH units of mouse C-243 cell interferon prior to infection at a multiplicity of 10 with either M-TUR or VSV. After incubation for 60 min at 37°C the virus inoculum was removed by repeated washings. Supernates from individual cultures were assayed for infectivity at the times after infection indicated. Titers represent mean values from 3 cultures.

TABLE II. Degree of protection by graded doses of interferon against M-TUR depends on macrophage genotype

Interferon units	LOG_{10} $TCID_{50}$/ml of 24 h supernates			
	M-TUR		VSV	
	A/J	A2G	A/J	A2G
0	6.2	6.5	4.0	4.0
2.5	5.5	4.5	3.5	3.3
10	5.0	3.5	1.5	1.8
20	4.5	3.0	1.0	1.3
40	4.0	2.0	1.0	1.0

ges. Table I shows the growth of M-TUR and VSV in macrophages taken from backcross mice previously classified as carriers or non-carriers of the allele Mx. 20 units of interferon severely impede the growth of M-TUR in Mx-bearing cells (5 logs difference at 24 h, 5.5 logs at 36 h), but affect the same virus much less in control cells (3 logs difference at both 24 and 36 h). By contrast, 10 units of interferon have the same inhibitory power against VSV in both Mx-carrying cells and in controls.

In Table II, the effects of graded doses of interferon on virus yield at 24 h in macrophages from A2G mice (homozygous for the allele Mx) and from A/J mice are compared. For instance, 10 units of interferon reduce M-TUR yield by 1.2 logs in A/J macrophages, but by 3.0 logs in A2G macrophages. VSV yield under the same circumstances are reduced by 2.5 and 2.2 logs.

We conclude that the antiviral state induced by interferon is more inhibitory to orthomyxoviruses in the presence of the allele Mx than in its absence. The antiviral state towards other viruses is not affected by Mx.

ACKNOWLEDGMENTS

This work was supported by the Swiss National Science Foundation, grants No. 3.139-0.77 and 3.393-0.78.

REFERENCES

Haller, O., Arnheiter, H., Gresser, I., and Lindenmann, J. J. Exp. Med. 149, 601, 1979.

Lindenmann, J., Deuel, E., Fanconi, S., and Haller, O. J. Exp. Med. 147, 531, 1978.

DISCUSSION

VILCEK: I assume that Haller has analysed the statistical significance of the difference between virus yields from macrophages of the two mouse strains he employed.

HALLER: Yes. The differences in M-TUR (but not VSV) reduced yield, induced by interferon, are significant.

ZSCHIESCKE: Does Haller have any information whether tumor-bearing mice carrying the MX gene respond differently to the anticellular effect of interferon than do normal mice?

HALLER: Such studies have not been performed thus far.

INTRODUCTORY STATEMENT ON MONOKINES

OPPENHEIM: There are a number of monokines, i. e. macromolecular factors with enhancing or stimulating activities made by macrophages:

(1) Lymphocyte-activating factor (LAF), originally described by Waksman and co-workers, classically found to stimulate thymocytes to proliferate, having two effects: (a) direct mitogenic effect, (b) augmenting effect on lectin-stimulated thymocytes. Most studies have not succeeded in separating these two effects chromatographically, also the quantitative effect of augmenting lectin-induced proliferation is greater than direct mitogenicity.

(2) T cell-activating factor (TAF), also described by Waksman, which is assayed on rat lymph node cells and has only augmenting activity and no direct mitogenic effect.

(3) B cell-activating factor (BAF), described by Wood, increasing the antibody response of human or mouse peripheral B cells. It appears increasingly that BAF and LAF are not separable by various purification techniques and are probably the same substance.

(4) Thymocyte-differentiation factor (TDF), described by Beller and Unanue, inducing a decrease in the expression of TL and an increase in H-2 antigens in thymocytes, as well as a change in the distribution of Ly 1,2 in these cells. TDF may be chromatographically distinct from LAF, either as a larger molecule or as an aggregate containing LAF.

Activated lymphocytes (by lectin or antigens) are capable of stimulating macrophages to produce LAF and other monokines; it is therefore at times very difficult in a mixed population to assert whether the proliferating effect observed on lymphocytes is due to a lymphocyte- or to a macrophage-derived product. Some conditions such as high serum concentration, higher cell concentrations and lymphocyte stimulants favor the production of a lymphocyte-derived mitogenic factor (LMF). The mitogenic factor also stimulates thymocytes and the peaks of activity overlap those of LAF, a low (15,000) and a high molecular weight (50 - 70,000) serum-associated form. Both forms stimulate human T-lymphocytes but as a distinctive characteristic, the human LMF can also stimulate human B-cell proliferation.

A large number of stimulants induce macrophages to produce increased amounts of LAF [1]. Almost anything that perturbs

ISBN 0-12-213950-X

the macrophage membrane appears to stimulate and increase LAF production to some extent. It is difficult to find a common denominator for all the substances reported to stimulate LAF production; Diamantstein has argued that an increase in C-GMP is responsible. In fact, we found that a number of compounds known to increase C-GMP, viz. vitamin C, serotonin, PMA and transfer factor also increase LAF production. Adjuvants may also act partly by increasing LAF production, which may act as second signal in the immune system.

[1] Editor's comment: *The statements that many agents may stimulate LAF release has to be considered with great caution in view of the experiments reported by Lachman. Not only commercially available sera but also many lots of tissue culture media in fluid or powder form, amino acids, Ficoll-Hypaque solutions etc. are contaminated with endotoxin in amounts sufficient to insure near optimal LAF release! According to Lachman, provided all culture medium components are carefully screened as being endotoxin-free, only LPS is found to induce LAF production from macrophages. Human monocytes are extremely sensitive to LPS and 10 pg/ml is sufficient to insure maximum LAF release. It may be suspected that most lymphocyte culture supernatants, even from so called control non-stimulated cells, do contain appreciable amounts of LAF.*

PROPERTIES OF HUMAN MONOCYTE DERIVED LYMPHOCYTE ACTIVATING FACTOR (LAF) AND LYMPHOCYTE DERIVED MITOGENIC FACTOR (LMF)

J.J. Oppenheim
H. Northoff
A. Greenhill
B.J. Mathieson

NIDR and NIAID
Bethesda, Maryland

K. Smith
S. Gillis

Dartmouth Medical School
Hanover, New Hampshire

I. INTRODUCTION

LMF is produced by antigen-activated thymic derived (T) lymphocytes, but the process of activation is macrophage dependent (1). Conversely LAF is produced by monocytes, but activated T lymphocytes can potentiate its production (2). We routinely use unfractionated peripheral blood mononuclear cells (MNL), obtained by Ficoll hypaque gradients to obtain optimal LAF and LMF production. Although MNL can be stimulated to produce both mediators, LPS stimulates MNL to produce only LAF (3) whereas antigen (3) or lectin (4) stimulated MNL produce LMF. However it remains to be established whether the supernatants containing LMF also contain LAF. In this paper four different approaches designed to differentiate between LAF and LMF will be briefly presented.

ISBN 0-12-213950-X

II. RESULTS AND DISCUSSION

A. *Gel Filtration of LAF and LMF*

Both human LAF and LMF induce mouse thymocyte proliferation. These two mediators are biochemically similar in that they both elute from Biogel P100 in two regions with molecular weights (MW) of 12-22,000 and 50-70,000. When LAF is chromatographed on Sephadex G150, the two peaks of activity elute in the 12-26,000 and 50-150,000 MW range (Table 1). With both types of gel, the higher MW activity cochromatographs in the region of the serum proteins. We have demonstrated that the low MW LAF is in part converted to the high MW form of LAF following the addition of human serum, reconcentration and rechromatography (5). These data suggest that LAF can bind to a protein component of human serum. Nevertheless the high MW LAF exhibits functional distinctions from the low MW LAF (6). Only the high MW LAF induced the proliferation of human E rosette + (T enriched) human lymphocytes (Table 1). Only low MW LAF can substitute for macrophages in pokeweed mitogen stimulated T helper dependent polyclonal immunoglobulin production by human B cells(6). In contrast, both the high and low MW pools of streptolysin-O (SLO) induced LMF stimulate human T cell proliferation (6). The low MW LMF was also mitonic for E rosette - (B cell enriched) lymphocytes (Table I).

B. *Thymocyte Target Cells of LAF and LMF*

LAF has been reported to activate cortisone resistant thymocytes (CRT) to a greater extent than normal thymocytes (7). We observed that both LAF and LMF stimulated CRT more than thymocytes from untreated mice (Table 2). The majority of thymocytes are agglutinated by peanut agglutinin (PNA^+) and can be separated from PNA^- thymocytes (8). PNA^- thymocytes have all the characteristics of CRT (8,9). It has been reported that supernatants of lectin activated lymphocytes stimulate PNA^- thymocytes to proliferate, but can activate PNA^+ thymocytes only in conjunction with concanavalin A (Con A) (9). We observed that PNA^- rather than PNA^+ thymocytes were the target subpopulation of both LAF and LMF (Table 2). Thus, these mediators actually activate only the small subpopulation of medullary thymocytes. This complements the data that factors in supernatants of thymic epithelial cells activate predominantly PNA^+ thymocytes (10).

TABLE I. PROLIFERATIVE RESPONSE OF MOUSE THYMOCYTES AND HUMAN LYMPHOCYTES TO PARTIALLY PURIFIED HUMAN LAF AND LMF

Stimulant	C3H/HeJ Thymocytes	Human Mononuclear Cells		
		Unfractionated	E-rosette +	E-rosette -
None	482[c]	340	61	315
LAF Pool II[a]	12,349	1790	284	715
IV	4963	215	32	307
None	374	212	35	131
LMF Pool II[b]	1685	1281	283	252
IV	2960	1823	544	2504

[a]LAF containing supernatants of human MNL incubated with 50 μg/ml LPS for 48 hrs were fractionated on Sephadex G150. The fractions were pooled, concentrated 20 fold and their proliferative activity tested at 1:20 dil. on thymocytes and 1:4 dil. on lymphocytes. The MW range of the pooled fractions in Pool II was 52-150,000, and in Pool IV 12-26,000.

[b]LMF containing supernatants of human MNL incubated with 1:20 dil. of Streptolysin-O (SLO) for 48 hrs were chromatographed on Biogel P100. Active fractions were pooled, concentrated 30 fold and tested as above. The MW range of the pooled fractions in Pool II was 50-70,000 and in Pool IV 12-22,000.

[c]Mean cmp of 3HTdR incorporated by triplicate cultures. The SEM varied by <20% from the mean.

C. *Inhibition of LAF and LMF by Sugars*

A number of simple sugars can competitively inhibit antigen induced (macrophage dependent) lymphocyte transformation (11). We therefore tested the effect of nontoxic doses of a battery of sugars on mediator induced thymocyte proliferation (kindly provided by Dr. A Muchmore NCI, NIH). Allose at a concentration of 25 mM consistently inhibited the thymocyte proliferative response to both LAF and antigen-induced LMF but not to Con A, PHA or Con A induced LMF. It is therefore possible that Con A-LMF differs significantly from SLO-LMF. However, allose fails to differentiate SLO-LMF from LPS-LAF.

TABLE II. IDENTITY OF THYMOCYTE SUBPOPULATION THAT PROLIFERATES IN RESPONSE TO HUMAN LAF AND LMF

	Mean 3HTdr uptake by C3H/HeJ thymocytes			
Stimulant	1.5×10^6 Untreated	1.5×10^6 PNA +	0.5×10^6 PNA -	0.5×10^6 cortisone resistant
None	426	268	575	815
LPS-LAF Pool II[a]	854	342	7421	10,351
IV	2220	2050	24,585	8500
SLO-LMF Pool II	536	172	2964	1856
IV	318	590	31,326	4427
Concanavalin-A[b]	18,986	58,180	28,841	N.D.

[a]See footnote to Table I. LAF and LMF were tested at a 1:20 dil.
[b]Con A was used at 5 μg/ml

TABLE III. INHIBITION OF HUMAN LAF AND LMF INDUCED THYMOCYTE PROLIFERATION BY SUGARS

	Mean 3HTdR uptake by C3H/HeJ thymocytes		
Stimulant	None	Allose	L-Arabinose
LPS-LAF Pool II	4115[a]	115	1025
LPS-LAF Pool IV	8002	470	4200
SLO-LMF Pool IV	3900	530	1849
Con A-LMF + MAM[b]	54,326	43,165	34,981
Con A(2.5 μg/ml)	48,403	50,000	47,000
PHA (2 μg/ml)	2220	1761	1322

[a]Cultures stimulated by 1:10 dil. of partially purified mediators. Unstimulated thymocyte cultures incorporated <300cpm of 3HTdR.
[b]Unfractionated sups. of Con A stimulated MNL assayed at 1:4 dil. in presense of 0.05 methyl α-D-mannose.

D. *T Cell Growth Factor (TCGF) Activity of Mediators*

Supernatants of lectin stimulated lymphocyte cultures contain TCGF which is essential to support the continued growth of normal cytotoxic T lymphocyte lines (CTLL) (12). It was observed that only the low MW SLO-LMF but not the high MW SLO-LMF nor high and low MW LAF were able to support the proliferation of CTLL (Fig. 1A). In addition, the LMF activity, as has been shown for TCGF (12), can be absorbed by human CTLL cells (Fig. 1B). This observation provides a clearcut functional distinction between LAF and LMF.

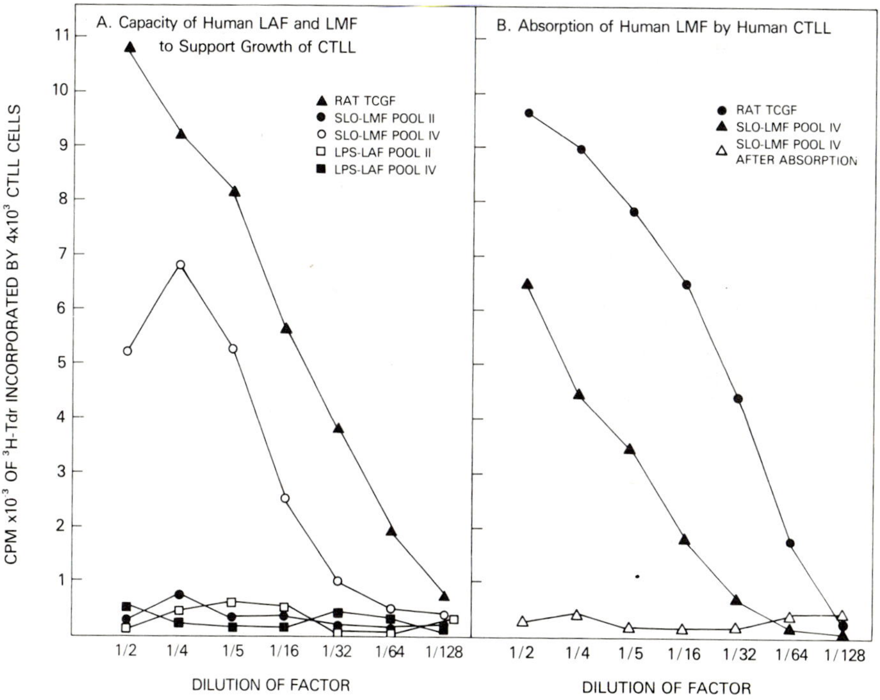

FIGURE 1. Capacity of murine (C57Bl6) cytotoxic T lymphocyte lines (CTLL) to proliferate for 24 hrs in the presence of various mediators. A) A comparison of the capacity to support the growth of CTLL cells by 48 hr supernatants (1) of rat spleen cells cultured with 5 μg/ml concanavalin A (RAT TCGF) (2) 1:20 dil. of partially purified human SLO-LMF or (3) with LPS-LAF. B) The capacity of low MW SLO-LMF to support growth of CTLL before and after absorption with 0.5 ml of 5 x 10^7 human CTLL cells for 4 hrs at $37^{o}C$.

III. SUMMARY

The thymocyte stimulating activities of LAF and antigen induced LMF both have similar high and low MW forms. Both LAF and LMF stimulate PNA$^-$ rather than PNA$^+$ subpopulations of thymocytes to proliferate. Both LAF and LMF but not lectin induced thymocyte proliferation are inhibited by allose. However, a low MW form of antigen-induced LMF exhibits several unique functional properties. This LMF unlike LAF supports the growth of normal cytotoxic T cell lines and induces B cell proliferation. The possibility that some LAF is present in partially purified LMF can still not be ruled out.

REFERENCES

1. Littman, B.H. and David, J.R. (1978). *Cell. Immunol. 39,* 374.
2. Mizel, S.B., Oppenheim, J.J., and Rosenstreich, D.L. (1978) *J. Immunol. 120,* 1497.
3. Oppenheim, J.J., Togawa, A. and Wahl, S. (]979). In "Cell Biology and Immunology of Leukocytes. Ed. M. Quastel Acad. Press N.Y. (In Press).
4. Northoff, H. and Oppenheim, J.J. (1979). In Proc. of 13th LCC Ed. G. Kaplan Acad. Press (In Press).
5. Togawa, A., Oppenheim, J.H. and Mizel, S.B. (1979). *J. Immunol. 122,* 2112.
6. Oppenheim, J.J., Moore, R., Gmelig-meyling, F., Togawa, A., Wahl, S., Mathieson, B.J., Dougherty, S. and Carter, C. (1979). In Regulatory Role of Macrophages in Immunity Eds. E.R. Unanue and A.S. Rosenthal. Pub. Acad. Press (In Press).
7. Blyden, G., and Handschumacher, R.E. (1977). *J. Immunol. 118,* 1631.
8. Reisner, Y. Linker-Israeli, M., and Sharon, N. (1976). *Cell Immunol 25,* 129.
9. Irle, C., Piguet, P-F., and Vassali, P. (1978). *J. Exp. Med. 148,* 32.
10. Kruisbeek, A.M. and Astaldi, G.C.B. (1979). *J. Immunol.* (In Press).
11. Muchmore, A.V., and Blaese, R.M. (1979). In Regulatory Role of macrophages in Immunity Eds. E.R. Unanue and A.S. Rosenthal Pub. Acad. Press (In Press).
12. Gillis, S., Ferm, M.M. Ou, V. and Smith K.A. (1978). *J. Immunol. 120,* 2027.

PURIFICATION AND CHARACTERIZATION OF HUMAN LYMPHOCYTE ACTIVATING FACTOR[1]

Lawrence B. Lachman
Richard S. Metzgar

Department of Immunology and Microbiology
Duke University Medical Center
Durham, North Carolina

I. PRODUCTION OF HUMAN LYMPHOCYTE ACTIVATING FACTOR

Lymphocyte Activating Factor (LAF) is released from human monocytes (Blyden and Handschumacher, 1977) and monocytic leukemia cells (Lachman et al., 1978) cultured for twenty-four hours in tissue culture medium containing 5% human serum and 10^{-7} to 10^{-9} gms/ml of E. coli lippopolysaccharide (LPS). The assay for LAF is stimulation of {^{3}H}thymidine incorporation into DNA by mouse thymocytes. Most commercially available tissue culture medium and serum contains sufficient quantities of endotoxin to stimulate maximum LAF release from monocytes (Lachman and Metzgar, 1979). LPS is the only macrophage stimulant we have found which stimulates LAF release. Phorbol Myristic Acetate (PMA) and $NaIO_4$ solutions, which were demonstrated by the lymulus amebocyte lysate assay to be negative for the presence of endotoxin, did not stimulate LAF release. LAF is released only from mononuclear cells cultured in the presence of serum, and the release of LAF is blocked by the presence of cycloheximide. Polymyxin B inhibits the release of LAF in cultures containing LPS, but does not reduce the mitogenic properties of LAF upon mouse thymocytes. Attempts to incorporate radioactive amino acids and sugars into LAF de novo have been unsuccessful, and no human cell lines have been demonstrated to release LAF.

[1]This work was supported by grants by the American Cancer Society (IM-117) and National Institutes of Health (AM08054).

ISBN 0-12-213950-X

II. PURIFICATION OF HUMAN LYMPHOCYTE ACTIVATING FACTOR

Lymphocyte Activating Factor is purified from the serum proteins contained in the conditioned medium by a three step procedure of hollow fiber diafiltration, hollow fiber ultrafiltration and isoelectricfocusing. In the first step, the conditioned medium is diafiltered using a 50,000 MW cut-off hollow fiber cartridge and six liters of buffer per liter of medium (Lachman et al., 1978). In the second step the diafiltrate is concentrated by ultrafiltration to forty mls using a second hollow fiber cartridge of 5,000 MW cut-off. The third step of purification is pH 8-4 sucrose gradient isoelectricfocusing (IEF) of the 5,000 MW fraction.

Hollow fiber diafiltration readily separates the low MW (∿14,000 daltons) LAF activity from serum proteins and high MW (∿86,000 daltons) LAF. Diafiltration of the conditioned medium, as compared to ultrafiltration using a 50,000 MW cut-off cartridge, results in increased yield of low MW LAF activity. The negative feature of diafiltration is the large volume of diafiltration (six liters per liter of conditioned medium) which must be concentrated prior to IEF. Ultrafiltration of the diafiltrate using a 5,000 MW cut-off hollow fiber cartridge is very rapid, but results in an 80% loss in activity. This poor recovery of LAF activity is probably due to adsorption of the serum-free LAF to the membrane of the hollow fiber cartridge. LAF is non-specifically adsorbed to cellulose sterile filters, most membranes used for ultrafiltration, and various chromatographic media. Alternative techniques for concentration of the <50,000 MW diafiltrate are being investigated.

IEF of the 5-50,000 MW fraction results in purification of the LAF activity from all demonstrable proteins. LAF is recovered from IEF in a single sharp peak with an average isoelectric point of pH 7.0 (Lachman et al., 1977). The yield of LAF activity following IEF is only 20% of the 5-50,000 MW fraction, but the increase in purity is of >1,000 fold. Although, no protein bands are visible following polyacrylamide gel electrophoresis (PAGE) of the IEF purified sample, LAF may be further purified by preparative PAGE. LAF activity is found as a single peak of activity in 7.5% and 12% gels (Lachman et al., 1977). All experiments involving biochemical characterization of LAF or evaluation of biological activity have been performed with IEF purified LAF.

TABLE I. Effect of Chemical Hydrolysis Upon LAF Activity

Chemical	Conditions	Decrease in LAF Activity	
		Experiment 1	Experiment 2
$NaIO_4$	10 mM, 37°, 4 hr.	98%	91%
BrCN	0.07 M in 3NHCl, 25°, 2 hr.	85%	100%
2-Mercaptoethanol	1%, 37°, 4 hr.	-3%	-18%

III. BIOCHEMICAL CHARACTERIZATION OF HUMAN LYMPHOCYTE ACTIVATING FACTOR

The MW of LAF has been estimated as ∿14,000 daltons from Sephadex gel filtration chromatography (Blyden and Handschumacher, 1977). Enzymatic digestion of purified LAF using insolubilized enzymes resulted in the finding that LAF activity adsorbed to the insolubilizing agent (CM-cellulose, agarose). Chemical hydrolysis of LAF activity with cyanogen bromide or $NaIO_4$ resulted in complete loss of LAF activity (Table I). Reduction of LAF with 2-mercaptoethanol did not reduce LAF activity. These results indicate that LAF is a glycoprotein and that cysteine dimers are not essential for biological activity. LAF is inactivated following heat treatment of 100° for 10 mins., but loses only 50% activity when heated to 56° for 30 mins.

REFERENCES

Blyden, G., and Handschumacher, R. E. (1977). J. Immunol. 118, 1631.

Lachman, L. B., Hacker, M. P., and Handschumacher, R. E. (1977). J. Immunol. 119, 2019.

Lachman, L. B., Metzgar, R. S. (1979). Fed. Proc. 28, 932.

Lachman, L. B., Moore J. O., and Metzgar, R. S. (1978). Cell. Immunol. 41, 199.

DISCUSSION

PAPERMASTER: McEntire and Smith in our laboratories have demonstrated binding of smaller MW (15 - 35,000 daltons) lymphokine moieties, labelled biosynthetically in culture with ^3H amino acids, to human and mouse serum proteins such as albumin and α-2 macroglobulin used to supplement RPMI 1640 culture medium and labelled with 125 I.

MORELL: I have two questions for Oppenheim concerning the B-cell proliferation induced by low molecular weight LAF/LMF:

(1) Are human B-lymphocytes hit directly by these factors or is some T-helper cell function involved?

(2) Is the B cell response polyclonal with intercellular synthesis and secretion of IgM, IgG and IgA - thus comparable to PWM-induced B cell activation - or is there a preferential synthesis of one or the other Ig class?

OPPENHEIM:

(1) The B-cells contain the usual 3 - 5 % contaminating T cells. Therefore the B cell mitogenic effect of LMF may be T-dependent.

(2) We do not know as yet whether our LMF induces B cell immunoglobulin production. However, LAF can substitute for the macrophages needed to enable PWM to induce PWM-induced polyclonal immunoglobulin production.

LANDY: The lymphokine community is indebted to Lachman for his perception of the magnitude of the threat represented by endotoxin to orderly, meaningful LAF research. The fact is that endotoxin is ubiquitous. Unless one takes extraordinary precautions this microbial component insinuates itself into any and all materials and operations. It is a reasonably safe conclusion that a great deal of the work in the lymphokine field, indeed in immunology generally, has inadvertently involved the participation by this ubiquitous biologically potent microbial entity. Particularly vulnerable are column processing maneuvers, actually just about all standard protein fractionation procedures. Simple bacteriological examination of such "exposed" materials will promptly reveal the magnitude of bacterial contamination involved. Once elaborated, there is no acceptable way of removing endotoxin; it is far more realistic to *avoid* its introduction. The most useful means involves baking all glassware at 170° C and careful screening of all biologic materials used.

DVORAK: Lachman's remarks regarding endotoxin are well taken and are reminiscent of data by Hibbs (Science, *1977*) indicating the ubiquity of endotoxin in many culture media. I have two questions for him:

(1) How confident can one be that a weakly positive Limulus assay ("cloudy", rather than a firm clot) in fact indicates the presence of endotoxin?

(2) Is it possible to obtain commercially endotoxin-free tissue culture medium and serum?

LACHMAN:

(1) I have found that a firm clot (lpg/ml endotoxin) always indicates that the medium will produce spontaneous LAF release. The "cloudy" result in Limulus assay sometimes results in LAF release. I think a "cloudy" result is best considered a negative test for endotoxin. There are some spectrophotometric techniques which measure turbidity of the Limulus assay solution; this may increase the sensitivity of the assay and offer a more scientific approach than the descriptive results.

(2) Endotoxin-free tissue culture medium (be certain to specify with glutamine) can be obtained from Microbiological Associates, Bethesda, Maryland. Endotoxin-free serum can be obtained from Sterile Systems Inc., West Bethesda, Maryland; they plan to have endotoxin-free medium as well as serum in the near future.

PICK: I would like to mention that it is unwarranted to assume that cyclic GMP is the intracellular mediator responsible for mediating of the stimulus-inducing LAF formation. Although it has been reported in the literature, we have not found any cyclic GMP elevation to be induced by PMA, acetylcholine, carbamylcholine, serotonin and only a moderate cyclic GMP elevation to be induced by ascorbic acid. I would like also to stress the need of using controls for all tests with PMA. Phorbol or other non-cocarcinogenic derivates of phorbolmyristic acid should be shown not to induce the biological effect.

CHARACTERIZATION OF LYMPHOCYTE ACTIVATING FACTOR OBTAINED FROM THE MURINE MACROPHAGE CELL LINE, $P388D_1$

Steven B. Mizel

Laboratory of Microbiology and Immunology
National Institute of Dental Research
National Institutes of Health

I. BIOCHEMICAL STUDIES ON LAF

The $P388D_1$ murine macrophage cell line has been used as a cell source for the production of lymphocyte activating factor (LAF) (Lachman, et al., 1976; Mizel, et al., 1978a). The LAF produced by $P388D_1$ cells appears to be both biologically and biochemically indistinguishable from the LAF produced by normal murine macrophages (Mizel, et al., 1978 a,b; Mizel, 1979 a,b). Although absolute purity has not yet been demonstrated, $P388D_1$-derived LAF has been purified approximately 20,000-fold by ammonium sulfate fractionation, sequential chromatography on DEAE cellulose, Sephacryl S200, and phenyl Sepharose, and polyacrylamide gel electrophoresis (Mizel, manuscript in preparation).

Chemical characterization studies on the partially purified LAF have revealed that this factor is a single polypeptide chain of 12,000-16,000 m.w. which is relatively resistant to attack by proteolytic enzymes and irreversible denaturation by agents such as urea and sodium dodecyl sulfate (SDS) (Table I). The biologically active form of LAF is not dependent on disulfide linkages as evidenced by the insensitivity of LAF activity to incubation with 2-mercaptoenthanol and iodoacetamide. However, LAF activity was almost completely destroyed during a 4 hr incubation with 1% phenylglyoxal, a compound which covalently attaches to arginine residues. In contrast, the histidine-modifying reagent, diethylpyrocarbonate, did not significantly impair the functional activity of

ISBN 0-12-213950-X

TABLE I. CHEMICAL CHARACTERIZATION OF LAF OBTAINED FROM THE P388D$_1$ MACROPHAGE CELL LINE

Property	Comments
12,000-16,000 m.w.[a,b]	LAF single polypeptide chain
pI = 5.0-5.6[b]	LAF exhibits charge heterogeneity
Proteolytic enzyme sensitivity:[b]	
Trypsin	LAF relatively insensitive
Chymotrypsin	LAF relatively insensitive
Papain	LAF relatively insensitive (native state); LAF sensitive in 8M urea
Streptomyces griseus Protease	LAF sensitive
Sodium Periodate[c]	LAF insensitive
Neuraminidase[c]	LAF insensitive
con A Sepharose[b]	Does not bind LAF: No accessible mannosyl or glycosyl residues on LAF
2ME + Iodocetamide[b]	LAF insensitive; No essential disulfide linkages
SDS (0.1-0.5%)[b]	LAF relatively insensitive
Urea (8M)[b]	LAF relatively insensitive
Cyanogen Bromide	No active fragments of LAF
Phenylglyoxal[c]	LAF sensitive to arginine modification
Diethylpyrocarbonate[c]	LAF relatively insensitive to histidine modification
Zn^{++}-Sepharose[c]	Does not bind LAF; No accessible cysteine or histidine residues on LAF

[a] Mizel, et. al., 1978b
[b] Mizel, 1979a
[c] Mizel, unpublished observations

LAF. Treatment of LAF with cyanogen bromide (100-fold excess, 0.1 N HCl, 24 hrs, 25°C) did not result in the production of any biologically active fragments.

II. BIOLOGICAL STUDIES ON LAF

Biological studies with the relatively pure P388D$_1$-derived LAF have revealed that LAF plays a key role in the macrophage-dependent activation of thymus-derived lymphocytes (Table II). In some activation events, e.g., thymocyte proliferation and the developemnt of stable E rosette-forming capacity by human peripheral blood T cells, LAF is apparently the only macrophage-associated signal that is required. In contrast, LAF-mediated enhancement of in vitro antibody responses, lymph node T cell proliferation, and alloantigen specific cytotoxic T cell activity also require the presence of the specific antigen used to prime the T cells. It is not known whether LAF and antigen act directly on the same cell or on separate, but interacting T cell subpopulations. It should be mentioned that not all LAF-initiated T cell activation processes are associated with T cell proliferation. For example, LAF markedly increases the number of stable E rosette-forming human T cells, but has little if any effect on the proliferation of these cells.

Dayer, et.al., (1978) have recently reported that human monocytes produce a soluble factor, termed mononuclear cell factor (MCF), which markedly enhances the production of collagenase and prostaglandins by human synovial cells obtained from patients with rheumatoid arthritis. The target cell of MCF is not a lymphocyte or monocyte, but a distinct class of nonlymphoid cells. MCF exhibits a number of biochemical properties in common with LAF, e.g., m.w. and behavior on DEAE cellulose and hydroxyapatite. In collaboration with Drs. Jean-Michel Dayer and Stephan Krane, we therefore investigated the possibility that MCF and LAF were related or identical macrophage products. Our results indicate that 1)partially purified MCF exhibits thymocyte mitogenic activity and 2)LAF (purified 20,000-fold; specific activity = 3.5×10^5 units/mg protein) markedly enhances the production of collagenase and prostaglandin by human synovial cells. Thus we have concluded that MCF is LAF. These studies also demonstrate that LAF has a cell target spectrum of activity which extends beyond the lymphocyte class of cells. This cellular spectrum of LAF activity may be one means by which the macrophage can regulate the immune responsiveness of a number of cell types involved in humoral, cell-mediated, and localized inflamatory responses.

TABLE II. BIOLOGICAL ACTIVITIES OF $P388D_1$-DERIVED LAF

1)	Stimulates thymocyte proliferation	Lachman, et al., 1976; Mizel, et al., 1978a
2)	Enhances antigen-induced T cell proliferation	Mizel, S.B. and A. Ben-Zvi, unpublished data
3)	Enhances the in vitro antibody response to T-cell dependent antigens	Farrar, J.J. and S.B. Mizel, unpublished data
4)	Protects against the immunosuppressive effect of steroids on the in vitro antibody response to a T cell-dependent antigen (GRMF activity)	Mishell, R.I., S.B. Mizel, S.M. Shiigi, and K.H. Grabstein, unpublished data
5)	Enhances the generation of alloantigen specific cytotoxic T cells	Farrar, et al., 1979
6)	Increases the number of stable E rosette-forming human peripheral blood T cells	Ben-Zvi, A., S.B. Mizel, and J.J. Oppenheim, unpublished data
7)	Stimulates collagenase and prostaglandin production by human synovial cells cultured in vitro	Mizel, S.B. J.M. Dayer, and S.M. Krane, unpublished data

REFERENCES

Dayer, J.M., Goldring, S.R., and Krane, S.M. (1978). In "Proceedings, Mechanisms of Localized Bone Loss" (Horton, Tarplay and Davis, eds.) pp. 305-318.

Farrar, W.F., Mizel, S.B., and Farrar, J.J. (1979). *Fed. Proc. 38*, 1006.

Lachman, L.B., Blyden, G.T., Hacker, M., and Handschumacher, R.E. (1976). *Cell. Immunol. 34*, 416.

Mizel, S.B. (1979a). *J. Immunol.* In Press.

Mizel, S.B. (1979b). In "Molecular Mediators of Cellular Immunity: Characterizations and Actions" (J.W. Hadden and W.E. Stewart II, eds.) Humana Press, New Jersey, In Press.

Mizel, S.B., Oppenheim, J.J., and Rosenstreich, D.L. (1978a). *J. Immunol. 120*, 1497.

Mizel, S.B., Oppenheim, J.J., and Rosenstreich, D.L. (1978b). *J. Immunol. 120*, 1504.

DISCUSSION

WOOD: Does phenylglyoxal inhibit the activities of high molecular weight LAF? If so, does phenylglyoxal inhibit the activities of high LAF not shared by low molecular weight LAF?

MIZEL: We have not examined the effect of phenylglyoxal on high molecular weight LAF.

DE WECK: Have all the biological activities Mizel has listed for LAF been tested with the purest material available?

MIZEL: Stimulation of thymocyte mitogenesis, antibody synthesis, T cell-mediated cytotoxicity, synovial cell collagenase and prostaglandin production have been examined with our purest preparation of LAF.

FARRAR: A point of interest regarding the accessory cell required for LAF-mediated enhancement of the PFC response. We also have demonstrated the requirement for an accessory cell during the induction of the response and have found this cell to be present in the spleens of nude mice. By means of the fluorescent activated cell sorter these all prove to be approximately 80 % low density theta positive. I think this finding may provide further evidence for the idea that LAF enhances PFC responses indirectly through T cells, or in this instance through pre-T cells.

MüHLRADT: Bretz has shown that proteases activate quite a number of lymphoid cell populations. Is LAF a protease?

MIZEL: We have not fully explored this possibility. LAF is not affected by the inhibitor phenylmethyl sulfonyl fluoride (PMSF), which inhibits trypsin and chymotrypsin-like enzymes.

GODFREY: Are there proleolytic or other enzymatic activities associated with any of these activating factors?

MIZEL: There are insufficient data presently available on LAF.

DI SABATO: It seems to me that, owing to the fact that lymphokines are present in very minute amounts, we have to distinguish between "biochemical" purity and "functional" purity. In other words, there is no certainty that all the various activities that Mizel has listed are really due to LAF, despite the fact that he has been working with a highly purified preparation of this factor.

MIZEL: I quite agree. These activities are associated with LAF at its present state of purity.

MAYER: It is not necessary to wait for pure material before testing for enzymatic activity. I suggest that co-chromatography be employed, i. e. an attempt to separate any possible enzymatic activity from LAF activity.

LACHMAN: Human and mouse LAF share a common MW of 12 - 15,000 but differ in several other properties:

(1) Human LAF is a glycoprotein sensitive to $NaIO_4$ and cyanogen bromide hydrolysis.

(2) Human LAF does *not* exhibit the charge heterogeneity manifested by mouse LAF. The pI of human LAF is a very sharp pH 7.0 and when IEF purified LAF is run on preparative gels, LAF activity is recovered as a *single* sharp peak of activity.

Both human and mouse LAF are very stable factors (this is contrary to initial beliefs concerning LAF).

MIZEL: Handschumacher and co-workers initially reported the human LAF to be periodate insensitive. What is the difference between their work and Lachman's finding that human LAF is periodate sensitive?

LACHMAN: Handschumacher did not use a high enough concentration of $NaIO_4$ I used 10m M $NaIO_4$ for 4 hours at 37°C. The LAF sample was dialyzed against PBS prior to the experiment. Handschumacher used only 1m M $NaIO_4$ and the chemical may have decomposed in solution before the LAF was hydrolyzed.

DAVID: I do not think one needs to have a factor purified to apparent homogeneity before determining whether it (or a contaminant present) has enzymatic activity. Also the many functions now attributed to 12 - 16,000 LAF could ultimately be due to more than a single material. There is nothing peculiar about enzymatic assays that they should require more pure material than other biologic systems. In both situations it could be the activity of contaminants that is being perceived. In both one could miss an activity because of the presence of an unknown inhibitor.

WAKSMAN: This is an opportune time to respond to Oppenheim's gentle dig about "lumpers" and "splitters". What one splits depends on one's orientation. These last reports have given us elegant examples of fine splitting of the mediators from a chemical standpoint and heavy lumping of the cell populations being tested. One cannot help feeling that it is just as important to define the real target of the agent as the actual agent. The use of whole thymocytes as an assay population is a particularly vivid example of this problem especially when one assays ^{3}HTdR incorporation at 72 hours. One can confuse the effects of TMP (LAF) as a mitogen with TAF as a potentiator and with TDF, which changes nonresponsive cells to responsive cells. The fine chemistry loses a significant part of its value with such messy assay systems.

EDITOR'S COMMENT: During the meeting, the group of workers dealing with antigen-non specific T cell proliferation and helper factors agreed that the monokine variously denominated lymphocyte-activating factor (LAF), macrophage-derived T cell replacing factor (TRF_M), B cell-activating factor (BAF), mitogenic protein (MP) and B cell differentiation factor (BDF) probably represent the same molecule for which the new generic name of interleukin 1 (IL_1) *has been proposed.*

Similarly the murine thymocyte stimulating factor (TSF) has been considered to be identical with thymocyte mitogenic factor (TMF), T cell growth factor (TCGF), costimulator, killer cell helper factor (KHF) and secondary cytotoxic T cell inducing factor (SCIF). This factor has now been newly denominated interleukin 2 (IL_2).

PURIFICATION, PHYSICOCHEMICAL CHARACTERIZATION AND A BIOLOGICAL ROLE OF LYMPHOCYTE ACTIVATING FACTOR (LAF)[1]

James S. Economou
Hyun S. Shin

Department of Microbiology
The Johns Hopkins University
School of Medicine
Baltimore, Maryland

Lymphocyte activating factor (LAF) is a relatively thermolabile protein elaborated by activated macrophages (MØ) that is mitogenic for mouse thymocytes (ThC). LAF generated in 24 hour, LPS-activated MØ cultures is heterogeneous with respect to molecular weight and isoelectric point. Supernatants from short-term (2 hr.), serum-free MØ cultures contained a single dominant species of LAF with an isoelectric point of 4.8. This pI 4.8 LAF was partially purified using a three step protocol employing isoelectric focusing, gel filtration and polyacrylamide disc gel electrophoresis. The final product was enriched at least 631-fold from serum-free MØ culture supernatants (Table I). This pI 4.8 LAF activity has a Stokes radius of 22 Å with a calculated diffusion coefficient ($D_{20,w}$) of 9.7 X 10^{-7} cm^2/sec as determined by gel filtration on Sephadex G-75. The apparent sedimentation coefficient was determined to be 2.0 S by sucrose gradient ultracentrifugation. The buoyant density of LAF is 1.30 g/cm^3 as determined by CsCl isopycnic ultracentrifugation; the partial specific volume was estimated to be 0.72. Using the Svedberg equation, the molecular weight of LAF was calculated to be 18,000 daltons. The frictional ratio was calculated to be 1.25 (1).

[1] *Supported by U.S.P.H.S. N.I.H. Grants 2 RO1 CA-14113 and 9 RO1 CA 24442-04 and contract N00014-75-C-0142 from the Office of Naval Research.*

ISBN 0-12-213950-X

TABLE I. Summary of the Partial Purification of Lymphocyte Activating Factor (LAF).

Purification Stage	*Activity (Units)*	*Protein (μg)*	*Specific Activity (Units/μg)*	*Purification (-fold)*	*Cumulative Per Cent Recovery*
Starting Supernatant	*43,500*	*45,675*	*0.95*	*1*	*100*
Isoelectric Focusing	*14,200*	*207*	*68.5*	*72*	*32*
Gel Filtration	*10,650*	*25*	*426*	*448*	*24*
Polyacrylamide Disc Gel Electrophoresis	*6,000*	*$<$10*	*$>$600*	*$>$631*	*14*

Many groups have demonstrated the MØ dependence of lectin-driven proliferation of T lymphocytes (2-4). In some systems, the MØ requirement could be replaced by supernatants from activated MØ cultures (2,4,5). In general, however, these supernatant activities have not been physicochemically characterized. Paetkau and coworkers demonstrated that the Con A-driven proliferative response of mouse ThC is MØ dependent, and could be replaced by supernatants from Con A-stimulated spleen cells. This supernatant activity, termed "costimulator", has a molecular weight of 30,000 daltons (5). We have confirmed the MØ requirement for the mitogenic response of ThC to Con A, and have shown that MØ function can be completely replaced by partially purified LAF (Figure 1). It is interesting that our LAF and "costimulator" share a biological property but are obtained from different cell sources and are physicochemically distinct. This finding underlines the importance of using chemically defined lymphokines and monokines in cellular immunology research.

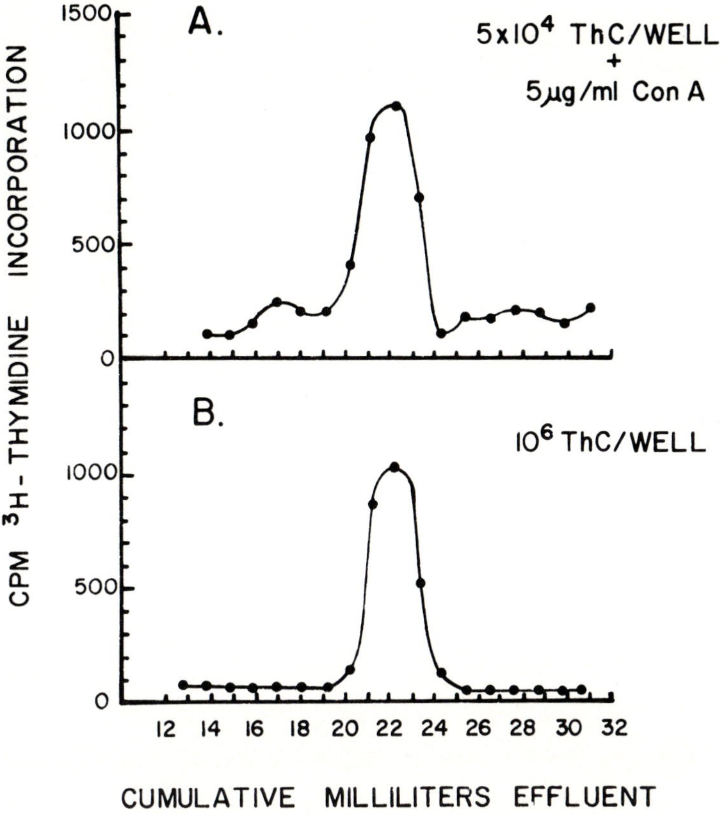

FIG. 1. Activity on thymocytes of Sephadex G-75 LAF fractions. An activated MØ culture supernatant was electrofocused on a preparative sucrose gradient and a single LAF peak with an isoelectric point of 4.8 was obtained. This activity was gel filtered on a Sephadex G-75 column. Column fractions assayed against ThC cultured at 10^6 cells/well (panel B) demonstrated the LAF peak. ThC cultured at 5×10^4 cells/well are completely unresponsive to Con A. This LAF peak permitted ThC cultured at 5×10^4 cells/well to proliferate in the presence of 5 µg/ml Con A (panel A). This LAF peak by itself was not mitogenic for ThC cultured at this low cell density (not shown).

REFERENCES

(1) Economou, J. S., and Shin, H. S. (1978). *J. Immunol.* *121*, 1446.
(2) Mills, G., et al. (1976). *J. Immunol.* *117*, 1325.
(3) Rosenstreich, D. L., et al. (1976) *J. Immunol.* *116*, 131.
(4) Katz, S. P., et al. (1978). *J. Immunol.* *121*, 2386.
(5) Shaw, J., et al. (1978). *J. Immunol.* *120*, 1967.

BIOCHEMICAL PROPERTIES AND CELLULAR REQUIREMENTS OF BAF

David D. Wood
Mary-Jo Staruch

Department of Immunology
Merck Institute for Therapeutic Research
Rahway, New Jersey

Human monocytes when incubated with bacterial endotoxin (LPS) at concentrations as low as 1 ng/ml release significant quantities of a factor (BAF) which stimulates the IgM plaque response of T cell deficient murine splenocytes to heterologous erythrocytes (1). Since muramyl dipeptide (MDP, a derivative of peptidoglycan) has been shown to stimulate the release of a thymocyte mitogen from human monocytes, BAF release in the presence of MDP was assessed (2). In Figure 1 the activity of BAF released by monocytes from four different donors has been plotted relative to the maximal BAF activity released in the presence of LPS by the same monocytes. Concentrations of MDP as low as 10 ng/ml yielded near maximal stimulation; however, regardless of the dose tested, MDP never induced as much BAF activity as did LPS.

Upon chromatography of LPS stimulated monocyte supernatants on Sephadex, the elution profiles of the thymocyte mitogen, PHA comitogen, and BAF differ significantly from each other (Figure 2). Nevertheless, the fractions eluting near 15,000 daltons contain all three activities. Upon chromatography of these fractions on Sephadex or isoelectric focusing, the three activities continue to coelute (3). Therefore, although much of the thymocyte stimulatory activity of these supernatants is resolvable from BAF, these procedures do not completely separate the three activities.

In addition to B cells, the response to BAF depends upon an irradiation insensitive splenocyte which can be removed by filtration of nude splenocytes over Sephadex G10 at 37°C in Eagles minimal essential medium buffered with 10mM HEPES and

ISBN 0-12-213950-X

TABLE 1. Accessory Cell Requirement for BAF Response

Dilution of BAF	Anti-HRBC PFC/culture of nude splenocytes: 10^6 unfractionated	10^6 G-10 filtered	10^6 G-10 filtered + $4x10^5$ X-GR[a]
0	10	0	6
1:40	544 (1.7)	0	308 (2.4)
1:10	1,585 (1.5)	0	1,644 (1.7)

[a]1000 R irradiated G10 retained cells alone give 0 PFC.

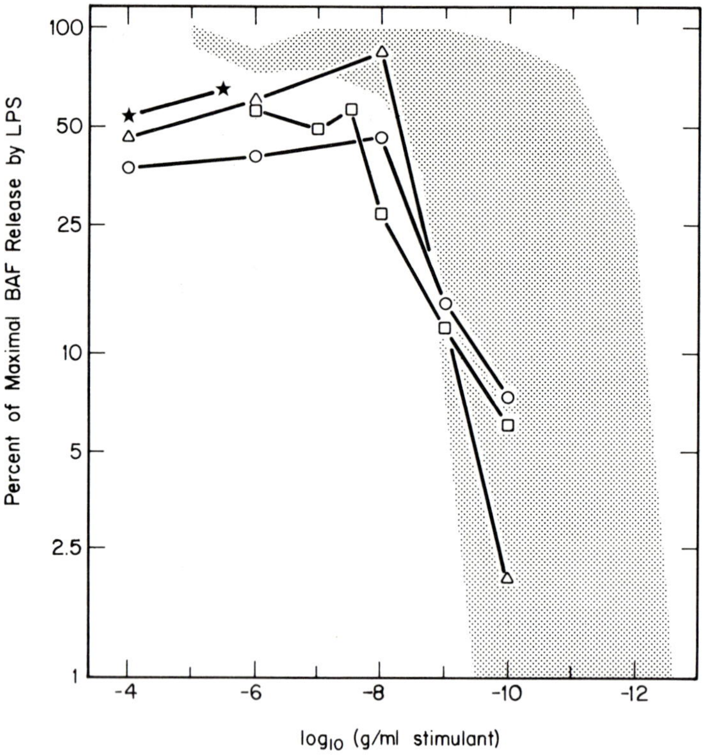

FIGURE 1. MDP stimulates BAF release. 10^6 human monocytes/ml were cultured for 48 hours with MDP (lines) or bacterial endotoxin. The shaded area envelopes the BAF activity observed in endotoxin stimulated cultures from 8 different donors.

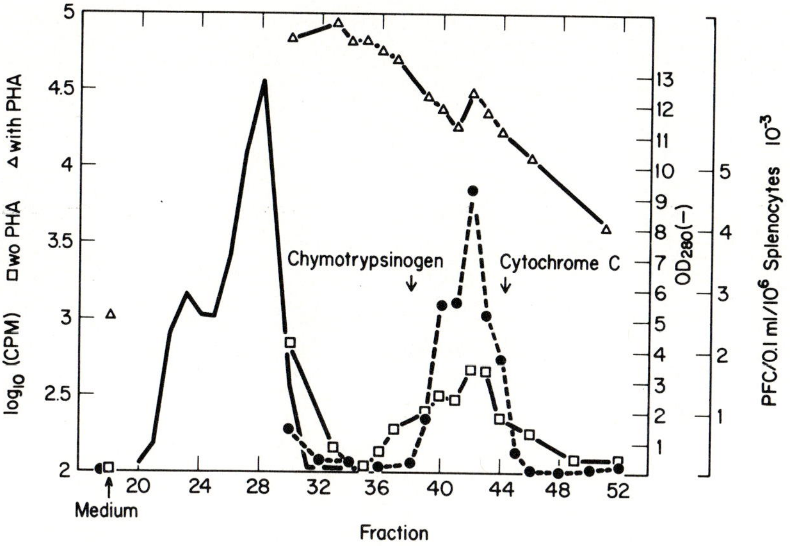

FIGURE 2. Elution of monokines on Sephadex G75. BAF activity was measured on T depleted C57B1/6J splenocytes (●). LAF activity was measured on CBA/J thymocytes in the presence (△) or absence (□) of 1.25 ul/ml PHA-P.

supplemented with 5% fetal calf serum (Table 1). In contrast, filtration in balanced salt solution - 5% fetal calf serum failed to adequately remove this accessory cell. Greater than 95% depletion is consistently seen with Balb/c nude, while the responses of normal Balb/c and C3H mice are typically reduced by 80% or more. It is not yet clear whether this accessory cell is a macrophage. It is resistant to killing with anti-mouse-μ, sensitive to lysis with anti-Ia serum (ATH anti-ATL), and poorly adherent to plastic. Attempts to reconstitute the response with splenic or peritoneal macrophages have given variable results.

REFERENCES

1. Wood, D. D., and Cameron, P. M. J. Immunol. 121, 53 (1978).
2. Oppenheim, J. J., Togawa, A., Chedid, L., and Mizel, S. B. Cell. Immunol. In press.
3. Wood, D. D. J. Immunol. In press.

THYMOCYTE RESPONSE TO A GROWTH-PROMOTING ACTIVITY FROM MACROPHAGES: A DUAL-SIGNAL MODEL

David I. Beller and Emil R. Unanue

Department of Pathology
Harvard Medical School
Boston, Massachusetts

Recent studies on the mechanism of action of growth-promoting factors indicate that at least two stimuli are required to initiate and maintain proliferation in growth-arrested fibroblasts (1). There is evidence that optimal proliferation of antigen- or mitogen-stimulated lymphocytes may also involve multiple inductive signals (2 - 4).

Since macrophage culture fluid (MCF) contains a 15,000-dalton protein, sometimes referred to as lymphocyte-activating factor, which preferentially stimulates thymocyte proliferation (5, 6), we evaluated the possibility that a multiple-signal mechanism might also characterize the mode of action of the macrophage mitogen. We have found that the growth-promoting activity of MCF is exerted on thymocytes only during a limited period after initiation of culture when the recently harvested thymocytes are still spontaneously proliferating. The response of the *resting* thymocyte to MCF requires that this cell receive an additional activating signal which can be conferred by a brief, essentially non-mitogenic lectin pulse. Thus, induction of proliferation in the resting lymphocyte seems to require the sequential exposure to two stimuli.

KINETICS OF SPONTANEOUS AND STIMULATED THYMOCYTE PROLIFERATION

In these experiments, thymocytes were initially resuspended at 10^7 cells per ml in 1 ml of RPMI 1640 medium supplemented with 10% FCS, 1% L-glutamine, 3 mM HEPES, antibiotics, and with or without MCF or Con A in 17-x-100 mm test

ISBN 0-12-213950-X

tubes. From these tubes 10^6 *viable* cells were subcultured daily into multi-well tissue culture trays containing 200 μl per well. At the time of subculture, cells were pulsed with 0.4 μCi of ^{3}H-thymidine; the cells were harvested twenty-four hours later, and the trichloroacetic acid-precipitable radioactivity determined by standard procedures. The macrophage culture fluid used in these experiments was a twenty-four-hour supernatant conditioned by peritoneal macrophages which had been activated *in vivo* by infection of A/St mice with live *Listeria monocytogenes*. The macrophages were cultured in 150 cm^2 tissue culture flasks at 4 x 10^6 cells per ml in 20 ml of medium (6).

The time course of basal ^{3}H-thymidine incorporation by A/St thymocytes, measured during successive twenty-four-hour periods after initiation of culture, indicates that significant cell cycling occurs only on the first day (Figure 1a). We attempted to correlate this loss of cycling activity with the mitogenic response to MCF by introducing MCF at different times after the onset of culture. It is clear from Figure 1a that the addition of MCF at the initiation of culture permitted the thymocytes to continue in DNA synthesis for three to four more days. However, delaying exposure to MCF by twenty-four to forty-eight hours caused a substantial (70 to 80%) reduction in the stimulated proliferation. This result was not attributable to a shift in the time of peak response, since ^{3}H-thymidine uptake was assayed on three successive days. Nor can this phenomenon be attributed to loss of viability, since, in these experiments, 10^6 viable cells were subcultured daily for ^{3}H-thymidine incorporation. The validity of this phenomenon is further supported by following the kinetics of response to a different mitogen, Con A. In Figure 1b, it can be seen that, in contrast to the results obtained with MCF, delaying exposure to Con A delays the time but not the magnitude of the proliferative response. Thus, it appears that the ability of thymocytes to respond to the mitogenic stimulus in MCF is preferentially lost in a temporal pattern which coincides with decline in spontaneous proliferation.

RESTORATION OF RESPONSIVENESS TO MCF BY CON A PRETREATMENT

We then sought means to restore to cultured thymocytes their original level of responsiveness to MCF. Experiments of Toyoshima, *et al.* (4), which revealed that lectins might provide an early, activating stimulus (not itself mitogenic) in addition to a later stimulus to proliferate suggested that

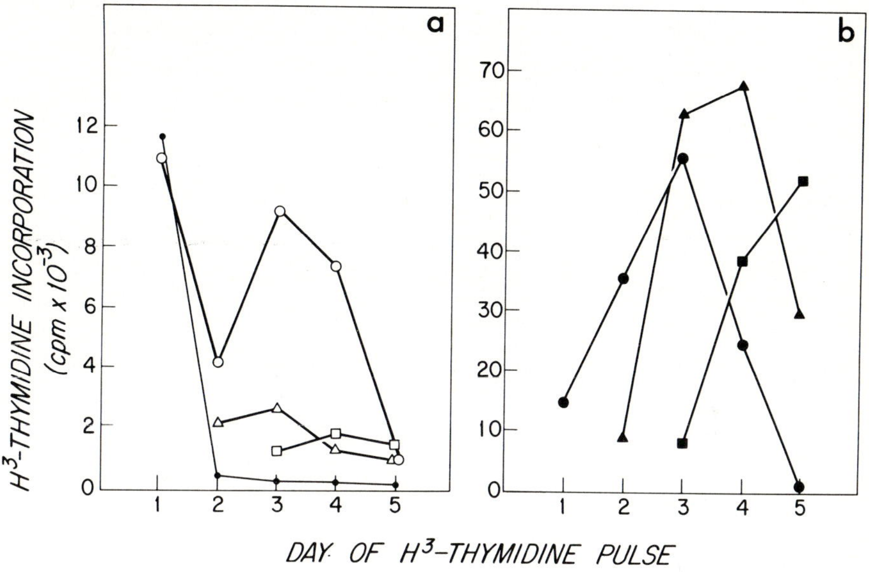

FIGURE 1. Kinetics of spontaneous and stimulated proliferation of A/St thymocytes. Figure 1a shows basal proliferation (•—•) and effects of 25% (v/v) conditioned medium from macrophages (MCF) added at the initiation (o—o) of culture (Day 1) or at Day 2 (Δ—Δ) or Day 3 (□—□). Figure 1b shows the effects of continuous exposure to 5 μg per ml of Con A added at Day 1 (●—●), Day 2 (▲—▲), or Day 3 (■—■).

presenting lectin and MCF in sequence might provide a means to restore the MCF response. Thus, thymocytes were first cultured in medium or MCF as in the previous experiment. On Day 3, aliquots of cells previously maintained in medium were pulsed with Con A, 5 μg per ml, for varying periods of time. All pulses were terminated simultaneously by washing cells twice and then resuspending them in medium with 0.05 M α-methyl mannoside. Cells were incubated for one hour at 37°C, then resuspended in fresh α-methyl mannoside without (middle panel) or with (right panel) 25% MCF. From each group, 10^6 viable cells were then aliquoted in triplicate into each of three multi-well trays. One tray was pulsed with ^{3}H-thymidine on each of three successive days. Figure 2 shows that, when thymocytes were cultured for two days in medium alone, then given MCF on Day 3, they did not display substantial proliferation. A two-hour pulse of Con A, although itself not mitogenic, enhanced the subsequent response to MCF; a six-hour pulse completely restored the response. While the longer pulse showed some direct mitogenic

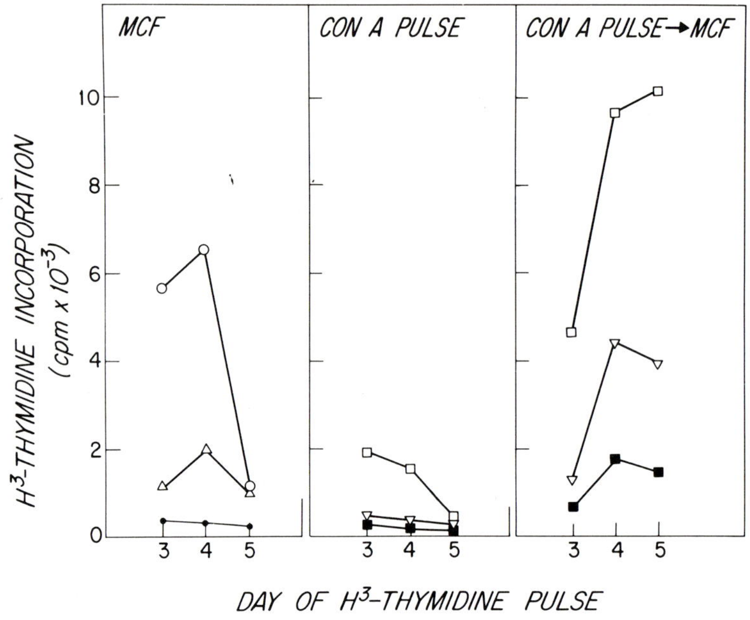

FIGURE 2. Restoration of responsiveness to MCF by brief pretreatment with Con A. The left panel shows the diminished proliferation when cells were first given MCF on Day 3 of culture (Δ) relative to those given MCF on Day 1 (o); spontaneous proliferation is also shown (•). The second panel indicates the response of thymocytes to a Con A pulse of ten minutes (■), two hours (∇), or six hours (□) in duration. The third panel reveals the effect of these lectin pulses on the subsequent response to MCF initiated on Day 3.

stimulation on Days 3 and 4, this returned to background levels by Day 5, the time when synergy with MCF was most striking. Thus, the ability of Con A to restore the thymocyte response to MCF can be distinguished from its potential to induce proliferation.

These data indicate that MCF provides a qualitatively distinct signal which requires an activated target cell but *not* the continuous presence of the presumptive "first signal". This activated state appears to be an inherent quality of spontaneously cycling thymocytes. It is lost when thymocytes stop cycling in culture but may be reinstated by a brief lectin pulse (first signal).

Since the mitogenic stimulation of lymphoid cells by PHA requires the presence of macrophages (or exogenous MCF, 7), as does stimulation of antigen-primed lymphocytes by specific antigen (3) or of responder lymphocytes by allogenic cells in the mixed lymphocyte reaction (8), it is possible that all these proliferative events also require two signals. It seems a reasonable speculation that mechanistically they may be similar to events discussed here: activation of the cell (by mitogen or antigen) which induces receptivity to stimulation by a macrophage mitogen.

ACKNOWLEDGMENTS

Supported by Grants from the National Institutes of Health and from the Council for Tobacco Research—U.S.A., Inc.

REFERENCES

1. Pledger, V. J., Stiles, C. D., Antoniades, H. N., and Scher, C. D. (1977). *Proc. Natl. Acad. Sci. USA 74*, 4481.
2. Greenberg, P., and Bluestein, H. (1978). *J. Immunol. 121*, 239.
3. Rosenwasser, L., and Rosenthal, A. (1978). *J. Immunol. 120*, 1991.
4. Toyoshima, S., Iwata, M., and Osawa, T. (1976). *Nature 264*, 447.
5. Gery, I., and Waksman, B. H. (1972). *J. Exp. Med. 136* 143.
6. Calderon, J., Kiely, J.-M., Lefko, J., and Unanue, E. R. (1975). *J. Exp. Med. 142*, 151.
7. Rosenstreich, D. L., Farrar, J. J., and Dogherty, S. (1976). *J. Immunol. 116*, 131.
8. Alter, B. J., and Bach, F. H. (1970). *Cell Immunol. 1*, 207.

DISCUSSION

BELLER: I have a few further comments on the relation of proliferation to thymocyte maturation. We have found that macrophage culture fluid, generated from PEC previously activated *in vivo* by injection of *Listeria* i. p., can stimulate thymocyte differentiation. When immature thymocytes, isolated by BSA gradient fractionation, are cultured in the macrophage culture fluid for 2 - 3 days, they show a quantitative physiological increase in surface H-2 and decrease in sensitivity to lysis with anti-TL and complement. We fractionated this material to see if the activity was due to the "classical" 15 K dalton LAF. We found that although the 15 K material had no effect in the differentiation assays an approximately 35 K material was active (we refer to this material as thymocyte differentiating factor TDF). The lack of effect of LAF, which is the predominant mitogenic activity found in the culture fluid, suggested that proliferation *per se* was not sufficient to induce maturation. The presence of mitomycin C during the culture of thymocytes with TDF was subsequently shown not to affect the induced maturation, and thus it became clear that, in our system, proliferation was neither *necessary* nor *sufficient* to direct maturation.

OPPENHEIM: I would like to supplement Beller's information on the effect of a monokine on thymocyte differentiation. In collaboration with Matthieson, we are finding that partially purified LAF-containing supernatant of human mononuclear cells significantly increases the expression of Ly-t-1 and decreases Ly-t-2 expression on mouse thymocytes. We have provided Matthieson with pools of sephadex GT 150 fractions and she has used fluorescent antibodies and the cell sorter to establish that overnight incubation of mouse thymocytes with a factor eluted in the void volume produces a significant shift in the population of fluorescent cells. The viability and size of the thymocytes does not change, but many more thymocytes become stained brightly with αLy 1.1. These data suggest that a factor, which may be similar to the TDF activity described by Beller, is produced by activated monocytes. Controls using supernatants of unstimulated monocytes had no effect.

PICK: I think it is essential for all people working on macrophage-derived factors, such as LAF, to eliminate the possibility that the effect is due to a protease. This could be done by the use of more or less specific protease inhibitors such as SBTI, Trasylol, EACA or TLCK. This can be controlled whether or not one's material is pure. I would also like to know the kinetics of the membrane marker changes induced by Beller's factor.

BELLER: I agree that the possible enzymatic nature of monokines is certainly worth evaluating and should be explored. However, I do not see how an enzymatic mode of action would in any way diminish the importance of these findings, as I think Pick implies when he suggests that it is essential to eliminate the possibility of a protease. Rather, this idea should be evaluated like any other potential mechanism.

As for the kinetics of the TDF induced membrane alterations, little or no H-2 is seen before 24 hours, while the increase is nearly complete by 48 hours. The loss of sensitivity to anti-TL and complement does not begin until 48 hours and is complete by 72 hours. These reciprocal changes are thus sequential.

SMITH: Would Oppenheim tell us which LAF fraction caused the change in Lyl antigen. We have looked at the effect of proteolytic enzyme inhibition on the activity of T-cell growth factor and there was no effect.

OPPENHEIM: The factor affecting the Ly-t-1 phenotype was located in the void volume. This pool contained only a little of the thymocyte mitogenic activity. Therefore TDF activity may turn out to be biochemically distinct from the proliferative stimulant, but this requires confirmation with better purification.

MüHLRADT: I believe that Shortman and his collaborators have shown that immature thymocytes die faster than mature ones. If one adds something to help them die even faster, one would relatively enrich the mature cells. Is this the effect Beller is seeing? Or does he find an increase in the *absolute* number of mature thymocytes under the influence of TDF?

BELLER: That TDF actually induces maturation is based on the following data.

(1) TDF has no discernable effect on the viability of any of the thymocyte subpopulations.

(2) By using the gradient-fractionated thymocytes we are working with a relatively homogenous population of cells. Thus, any potential selection would be less likely to be of consequence.

(3) Most importantly, when we evaluate surface antigens by immune fluorescence, it is clear that a significant increase in H-2 has been induced in individual cells after TDF treatment.

DI SABATO: We have recently shown in supernatants of murine MLC the presence of an activity that enhances the expression of the H-2 antigens and decreases the expression of the TL antigens ($INTL^+$ strains) on the surface of murine thymocytes. The expression of the thy. antigen is unchanged. It is interesting and possibly significant that, some years ago, Gresser found that purified preparations of interferon evoked a similar effect.

GILLIS: Has Beller tested the effects of his thymic macrophage supernatant on other lymphocyte populations such as nude mouse spleen or bone-marrow? Would it be appropriate now to consider previously detailed effects of thymic epithelial cell culture supernatants as due to contaminant macrophages present in these crude cultures?

BELLER: First let me re-state that this activity was derived from PEC, not thymic macrophages. The work with thymic macrophages has consisted almost entirely of direct stimulation of thymocytes with intact macrophages. Our initial evaluations do indicate that substantial LAF activity is released by thymic macrophages, however we have not evaluated different target cell populations, other than to show that TDF does *not* modulate the surface antigens of already mature thymocytes. Thus its activity appears to be directed towards the immature thymocyte.

As for macrophage contamination in thymic epithelial cell cultures, it is perfectly clear that, at least in the mouse, this can represent a substantial source of activity. We have found that primary cultures grown from either explants of thymic stroma or from collagenase-dissociated tissue contain up to 50 % FCR^+, $C3R^+$, later phagocytic and $esterase^+$ cells with typical macrophage morphology.

PROTEOLYSIS, CALCIUM, AND CYCLIC NUCLEOTIDES IN MACROPHAGE T-LYMPHOCYTE INTERACTION

Byron H. Waksman[1]
Jean-Paul Dessaint[2]
Stephen P. Katz[3]

Departments of Pathology and Biology
Yale University
New Haven, Connecticut

TAF (T-cell activating factor) in crude rat macrophage supernatants acts on PHA or ConA-stimulated rat LNC (lymph node cells) or on purified T-cells obtained by passing LNC through glass bead or nylon wool columns in late G_1 (12-24 hr) (1,2,3). TAF alone is completely non-mitogenic for peripheral T-cells, but serves as the quantitative equivalent of whole macrophages in mitogen stimulation.

TAF activity was shown to parallel closely the catheptic carboxypeptidase (CPB) content of individual supernatants, and TAF action could be reproduced by commercial preparations of porcine pancreatic CPB (Fig. 1). TAF activity was partially absorbed by T-lymphocytes stimulated by mitogen, apparently without restriction to a particular phase of the cell cycle.

In the presence of TAF, there was increased and persistant entry of exogenous Ca^{++} into stimulated lymphocytes (Table I). This was followed by a massive Ca^{++}-dependent rise of cyclic GMP, beginning in late G_1 (Fig. 2). Elevation of cGMP in late G_1 by other means (dibutyryl cGMP, carbamyl choline, imidazole) mimicked the action of TAF on mitogen-stimulated cells and gave maximal later DNA synthesis.

[1] *Present address: National Multiple Sclerosis Society, New York, New York.*
[2] *Present address: Institut Pasteur, Lille, France.*
[3] *Present address: Tulane University, New Orleans, Louisiana.*

ISBN 0-12-213950-X

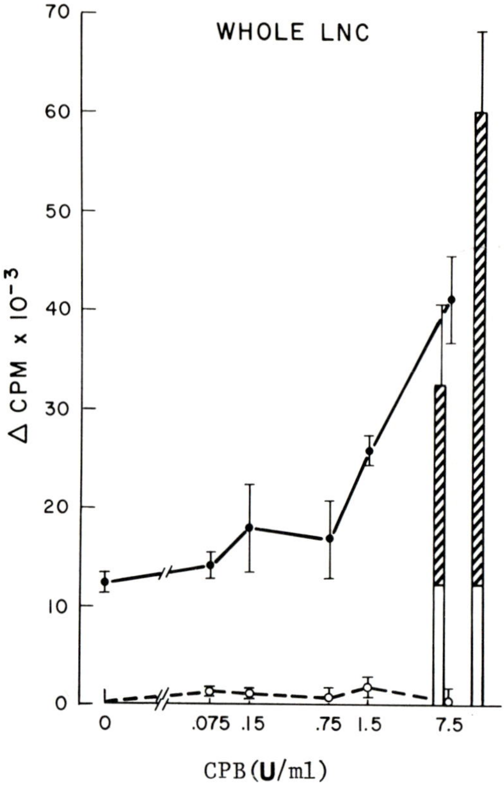

FIGURE 1. DNA synthesis (^{3}HTdR uptake) induced in LNC by PHA (0.5 μl/ml) plus commercial pancreatic CPB (●——) or by CPB alone (○-----). Values obtained with PHA (□) or PHA + TAF (▨) are also plotted according to catheptic CPB content of TAF used. (From 3.)

TABLE I. Calcium Uptake in LNC Exposed to PHA and/or TAF

Time of sampling	$^{45}Ca^{++}$ uptake (Δ cpm x 10^{-3}) PHA	TAF	PHA + TAF
10 min	-3.8	37.7	25.7
1 hr	-4.9	27.6	17.8
6 hr	4.0	-1.5	3.1
12 hr	-5.3	23.3	13.2
18 hr	1.0	2.7	3.2

PHA and/or TAF added at 0 time.
^{45}Ca (1μCi/tube) added 10 min before harvesting.

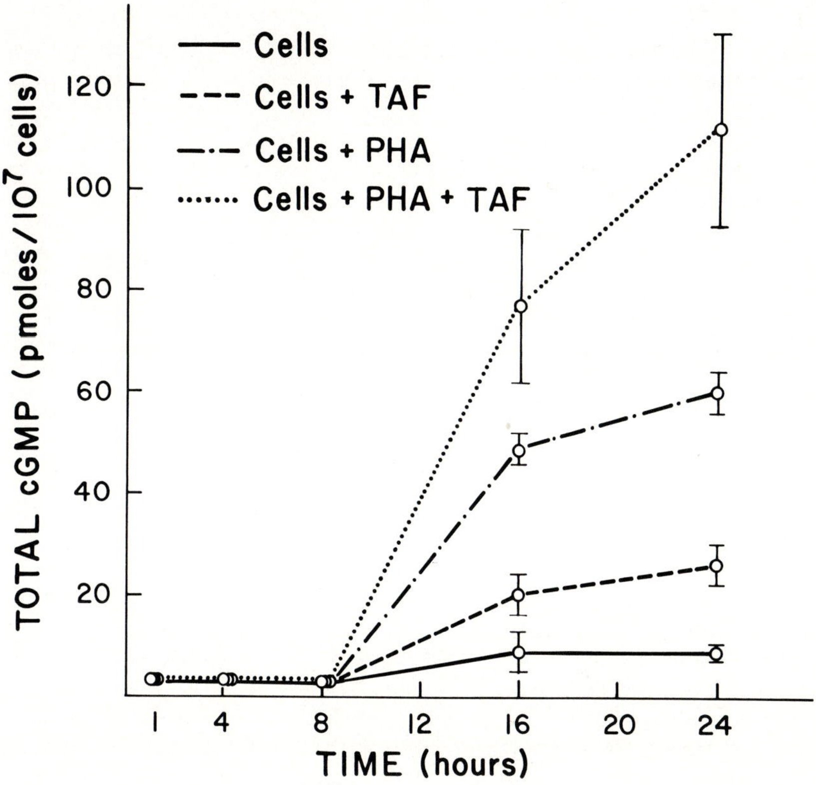

FIGURE 2. Cyclic GMP in LNC stimulated with PHA (2µ/ml) and/or crude TAF. (From 2.)

Macrophage "helper" action on stimulated T-cells *via* CPB stands in contrast to the action of serine proteases (plasmin, thrombin, trypsin) as direct B-lymphocyte stimulants.

REFERENCES

1. Kierszenbaum, F., and Waksman, B. H., *Immunology 33,* 663 (1977).
2. Katz, S. P., Kierszenbaum, F., and Waksman, B. H., *J. Immunol. 121,* 2386 (1978).
3. Dessaint, J.-P., Katz, S. P., and Waksman, B. H., *J. Immunol.* submitted (1979).

DISCUSSION

BELLER: Waksman suggests that the phenotypic changes accompanying maturation, such as those I have evaluated, occur during the G_2 phase of the cell cycle. However, both the increase in surface H-2, and decrease in sensitivity to lysis by anti-TL and complement, occur in the presence of mitomycin-C, which we know inhibits more than 99 % of stimulated ^{3}H thymidine incorporation. Would Waksman comment on this paradox?

WAKSMAN: G_2 was set dowm simply because in one well-studied system, synchronized melanoma cells in culture, the signal to transformation must be applied in G_2 to be effective and it is only in G_2 that the cell has a receptor for the mediator (MSH). In lymphocyte systems, the receptive phase still remains to be identified.

HADDEN: Some years ago we found that an increase in C-AMP lymphocytes synthesizing DNA enhanced rather than inhibited thymidine incorporation. Similar observations have been made concerning the ability of C-AMP to promote the progression of cells through the cell cycle. I wonder whether Waksman has found C-AMP to play an antagonistic role to C-GMP at the G_1-S boundary control point he discussed? The reason I ask is that Whitfield, McManus et al. have presented a series of observations in thymocytes which indicate that, depending on the cationic environment, C-AMP or C-GMP plays a positive role in moving these cells to mitosis. I consider it likely that positive regulation by both, C-AMP and C-GMP under these circumstances could be important in selecting daughter populations. In this case the cycle nucleotide might be linked more to differentiation than to control of the cell cycle.

WAKSMAN: Hadden is quite right in referring to this important area. There are several well studied systems in which increase of C-AMP at a very precise time of the cell cycle determines differentiation (phenotypic change). Thymosin is an example, and it would be fascinating to learn if Beller's TDF acts by raising C-AMP.

A MONONUCLEAR CELL FACTOR MODULATES COLLAGENASE AND PGE_2 PRODUCTION BY RHEUMATOID SYNOVIAL CELLS[1]

Stephen M. Krane
Jean-Michel Dayer

Harvard Medical School
Massachusetts General Hospital
Boston, Massachusetts

I. INTRODUCTION

Cultures of fragments of rheumatoid synovium produce high levels of collagenase and prostaglandins (predominantly PGE_2) (Krane, 1975; Robinson et al., 1975). When cells in such fragments are dispersed with proteolytic enzymes, the adherent cells produce the collagenase and PGE_2 (Dayer et al., 1976). These synovial cell cultures are heterogeneous. During the first 7-10 days, two types of adherent cells predominate: (1) small phagocytic cells with EA and EAC receptors consistent with macrophages; (2) larger non-phagocytic cells often containing multiple stellate processes which lack conventional macrophage markers. After ∿10 days in culture the small cells (macrophages) disappear but the large (stellate) cells persist and the cultures continue to produce collagenase and PGE_2. The levels of collagenase and PGE_2 do gradually decrease with time in culture (weeks to months) and passage by trypsinization. Since the synovium in vivo contains abundant mononuclear cells, we asked whether their products could affect function of the non-macrophage stellate adherent synovial cells (ASC). In the following studies peripheral blood mononuclear cells were examined for the presence of modulating factors.

[1]*Supported by USPHS grants AM-03564, AM-04501 and AM-07258, and grants from the Arthritis Foundation (National and Massachusetts Chapter).*

ISBN 0-12-213950-X

II. RESULTS AND DISCUSSION

In most studies to be described, peripheral blood from normal humans was used as a source of mononuclear cells. Mononuclear cells, obtained from Ficoll-Diatrozoate gradients, were cultured in MEM or RPMI, 5% FCS (heat inactivated), at $\sim 2 \times 10^6$ cells/ml usually for 3 days (Dayer et al., 1977a, 1977b, 1978). Cell-free supernatants were diluted and added to medium for incubation with ASC (the latter usually in the first or second passage) for 3 days. Cell free supernatant media are first treated with TPCK trypsin followed by soybean trypsin inhibitor. Collagenase is assayed by solubilization of reconstituted [^{14}C]glycine-labeled guinea pig skin collagen fibrils.

Table I. Response of ASC to Mononuclear Cell Medium

Mononuclear cell medium (dilution)	*ASC Collagenase units/10^6 cells/3 days*
0	0.60 ± 0.05*
1:40	1.70 ± 0.17
1:20	4.80 ± 1.45
1:10	11.60 ± 2.25

**Mean ± standard error for 3 wells.*

The responses shown in Table I are obtained from mononuclear cells incubated in the absence of any mitogen. The factor present in mononuclear cell medium (MCF) has a mol wt of $\sim$14,000 daltons by gel filtration, is eluted with 0.08-0.12 M phosphate from hydroxyapatite columns and 0.01-0.20 M NaCl from DEAE cellulose (DE52) columns at pH 7.4. Collagenase- and PGE_2-stimulating activities are present in the same fractions at all stages of purification.

In order to interpret further studies to be described, we emphasize that the target ASC divide slowly and different strains must be used since no one culture provides sufficient cells for all experiments. The pattern for the responses to partially purified MCF (gel filtration) of cultures of ASC from different patients is shown in Table II. With age in culture and passage the basal levels of collagenase and PGE_2 decrease, but the magnitude of stimulation with MCF increases.

Table II. Pattern of Response to MCF of ASC as a Function of Age in Culture and Passage

Passage number	*Number of synovial cell strains tested*	*Collagenase (-) MCF units/10^6 cells*	*Collagenase (+) MCF units/10^6 cells*
Zero	*6*	*7 - 30*	*20 - 51*
I	*11*	*2 - 20*	*8 - 43*
II	*15*	*0.1 - 6*	*1 - 32*
III	*12*	*0.1 - 2*	*0.1 - 16*
>III	*10*	*<0.1 - 1*	*0.1 - 16*

Although MCF is present in supernatants from mononuclear cell(MC) cultures incubated alone, addition of polyclonal mitogens increases MCF production (Table III).

In order to determine which mononuclear cell is responsible for production of MCF, in collaboration with L. Chess and J. Bréard, monocyte-macrophages were separated by adherence properties and lymphocytes separated into Ig-(T) and Ig+ (B) populations using antihuman $F(ab)_2$-Sepharose columns. The adherent cells (M) alone produce MCF which in contrast to unfractionated cells (U) does not increase with PWM Isolated Ig-(T) lymphocytes alone produce little MCF with or without PWM. Ig+(B) lymphocytes (not shown) produce MCF but these Ig+ populations are not completely depleted of M since lysozyme (an M marker) is still present. Addition of 5% M to 95% T produces little augmentation of MCF production unless PWM is added.

The increased PGE_2 levels in the cultured ASC produced in response to MCF affect ASC in several ways, including proliferation rate, collagen and other protein synthesis, cell shape and to a variable extent, collagenase production. MCF alone decreases proliferation whereas indomethacin plus MCF increases proliferation greater than indomethacin alone (Dayer et al., 1979). Thus, the mitogenic properties of MCF are revealed only if PGE_2 production is blocked (Table III).At dilutions of MCF used, mononuclear cell PGE_2 levels are sufficiently low as to not affect results.

*Table III. Effect of MCF on Replication of ASC**

Comparison	Mitotic Index Cell number	Mitotic Index $[^3H]$thymidine uptake
Control/control	1.0	1.0
MCF/control	0.90 ± 0.03	0.90 ± 0.08
MCF + indomethacin/control	1.36 ± 0.14	2.57 ± 0.57
Indomethacin/control	1.25 ± 0.28	1.71 ± 0.32

**Average of experiments modified from Dayer et al. (1979).*

Although MCF does not directly affect cAMP content in ASC, the higher PGE_2 levels resulting from MCF stimulation indirectly increase cAMP content. In ASC cultures exposed to MCF or added exogenous PGE_2, the increased cAMP levels return to baseline despite continuous presence of increased PGE_2 in the culture media. When these cells are exposed to exogenous PGE_2 and cAMP levels measured 10 min later, the cAMP response is blunted compared to control ASC. Preincubation with indomethacin prevents the development of the refractory state by inhibition of endogenous PGE_2 production and augments the cAMP response of the ASC to exogenous PGE_2. Preincubation with the mononuclear cell factor plus indomethacin results in an even greater acute cAMP response to further challenge with exogenous PGE_2 than that observed in cells preincubated with indomethacin alone (Dayer et al., 1979).

III. SUMMARY

These studies indicate that the MCF is secreted by monocyte-macrophages but the levels produced are modified by interactions with other mononuclear cells, particularly T lymphocytes. The MCF affects several functions of cultured rheumatoid synovial cells (ASC) which do not have macrophage markers. MCF has chromatographic properties similar to lymphocyte-activating factor (LAF) (Mizel et al., 1978); in collaboration with S. B. Mizel, we have shown in preliminary studies that the most highly purified preparations of murine macrophage LAF stimulate collagenase and PGE_2 production by ASC. Stimulation of ASC collagenase and PGE_2 by MCF may be particularly important in modulating degradative functions in inflammatory joint disease.

ACKNOWLEDGMENTS

Performance of many of the experiments described here was possible only with the collaboration of J. Bréard, L. Chess, S.R. Goldring and D.R. Robinson and the technical assistance of D. Bastian, W. Karge, M. Roelke, P. Rogers, L. Servello and E. Schmidt.

REFERENCES

Dayer, J.-M., Krane, S.M., Russell, R.G.G., and Robinson, D.R. (1976). *Proc. Natl. Acad. Sci. U.S.A. 73,* 945.

Dayer, J.-M., Russell, R.G.G., and Krane, S.M. (1977a). *Science (Wash. D.C.) 195,* 181.

Dayer, J.-M., Robinson, D.R., and Krane, S.M. (1977b). *J. Exp. Med. 145,* 1399.

Dayer, J.-M., Goldring, S.R., and Krane, S.M. (1978). *In* "Proceedings, Mechanisms of Localized Bone Loss" (J.E. Horton, T. M Tarpley, W. F. Davis, eds). Special Suppl. to Calcified Tissue Abstracts, p. 305.

Dayer, J.-M., Goldring, S.R., Robinson, D.R., and Krane, S.M. (1979). *Biochim. Biophys. Acta (Amst.), in press*

Krane, S.M. (1975). *Ann. N. Y. Acad. Sci. 256,* 289.

Mizel, S.B., Oppenheim, J.J., and Rosenstreich, D.L. (1978). *J. Immunol. 120,* 1504.

Robinson, D.R., Dayer, J.-M., and Krane, S.M. (1979). *Ann. N. Y. Acad. Sci., in press.*

DISCUSSION

LITTMAN: As Krane knows Harris has considered plasmin an important activator of collagenase in inflammatory joint disease. Plasminogen activator is produced by monocytes-macrophages. Has anyone looked to see whether LAF also stimulates plasminogen activator production?

We have also been interested in lymphokines in inflammatory joint desease and found that monocytes-macrophages from synovial fluid produce up to 30 times more C_2 than blood monocytes from the same patient. We are seeking to determine whether this is due to the monocyte complement stimulator, a T lymphocyte product.

KRANE: We have preliminary experiments on the levels of plasminogen activator produced by synovial cells in response to the mononuclear cell factor. Despite very large increments in collagenase and PGE_2 levels we see no plateau in plasminogen activator activity. We do not know if C_2 production correlates with the stimulating factor. Production of lysozyme, another constitutive macrophage secretory protein, can under some circumstances be dissociated from production of collagenase- and PGE_2-stimulating factor.

BENDIXEN: As I understand it, the mononuclear cell factor examined in Krane's experiments was produced by normal human peripheral blood monocytes. Did he have the opportunity to examine MCF production in patients with rheumatoid arthritis and to compare production by peripheral blood monocytes and synovial monocytes? Can his assay quantitate the collagenase- and PGE_2-production increase in terms of number of factor-producing monocytes?.

KRANE: We detect stimulating factor in peripheral blood mononuclear cell cultures from normal subjects as well as patients with rheumatoid arthritis. In view of the variation in distribution of mononuclear cells and the endotoxin problem by Lachman, we have not systematically compared these two groups. We are just beginning to look at synovial mononuclear cells as a source of the stimulating factor.

EPSTEIN: Would Krane care to speculate on how his observations *in vitro* relate to actual disease processes *in vivo* that involve joint pathology. I have always regarded the presence of lymphocytes and monocytes in joint fluid as a positive manifestation of host defense mechanisms. Yet according to

Krane's in vitro system, the infiltration of joint fluid with monocytes, by virtue of their ability to liberate a factor that stimulates collagenase, would cause dissolution and destruction of collagen containing structures.

KRANE: For some reason, the presence and persistence of these mononuclear cells and the target collagenase-producing cells result in damage to tissues. The ultimate questions therefore are why the cells are there to begin with and why they increase in number.

BIOCHEMICAL PROPERTIES OF MURINE T HELPER CELL REPLACING FACTOR[1]

Lothar Hübner
Gunhild Müller
Anneliese Schimpl
Eberhard Wecker

Institut für Virologie
und Immunbiologie
Universität Würzburg
Fed. Rep. Germany

Supernatants of murine spleen cells activated with either Con A, alloantigens or - in the case of pre-immunized spleens - the relevant antigen, contain a non-antigen specific T cell replacing factor (TRF) (1-3). TRF has been shown to act late in the response of B cells to T-dependent antigens by providing a differentiation signal to proliferating intermediary B cells (4). It does not contain antigens coded for by the H-2 complex and it is not H-2 restricted in its action (5, 6). The biological activity is mediated by glycoprotein(s) with a predominant MW of about 30,000 D. The polysaccharide side chains seem to be heterogeneous since only a portion of the biological activity can be bound to and eluted from matrix coupled limulus polyphemus hemagglutinin, specific for N-acetyl-neuraminic acid. After removal of the terminal sialic acid residues, TRF activity is retained on Ricinus communis agglutinin-Sepharose from which it can be eluted by galactose. The addition of tunicamycin, an inhibitor of protein

[1] *This work was supported by the SFB 105 and the BCT 108*

ISBN 0-12-213950-X

glycosylation (7), to Con A stimulated spleen cell cultures reduces the amount of TRF detectable in the supernatant without totally obliterating its appearance.

TRF prepared under serum free conditions can be partially purified by means of either of the four consecutive steps shown in Tables I and II. Starting from 650 ml of crude TRF half of which was labelled biosynthetically with ^{3}H-leucine, the material recovered in step D of Table II reveals a single stainable spot after 2D-electrophoresis (1st dimension: IEF at 8 M urea, pH gradient from 3.2-7.85; 2nd dimension: SDS-PAGE in 8 M urea) which is also present in biologically inactive control supernatants derived from unstimulated spleen cell cultures. By virtue of its P_i and MW this spot can be assigned to actin. Actin is, however, by far not the only contaminant. TRF, biosynthetically labelled with ^{3}H-leucine (325 ml) and subjected to the purification steps given in Table 1, upon fluorography, reveals 13 bands in SDS-PAGE and approximately 50 spots in 2D electrophoresis. The following 8 spots are absent in biologically inactive control supernatants:

1)	Pi	6,0	MW	35-37KD	5)	Pi	4,6	MW	34-35KD
2)	"	5,0	"	35-37KD	6)	"	5,2	"	25-30KD
3)	"	5,3	"	34-35KD	7)	"	4,5	"	15-18KD
4)	"	4,7	"	34-35KD	8)	"	5,4		

Spot 6 shows the best agreement with respect to MW and P_i previously described for TRF (9) and is therefore tentatively assigned to TRF. However, spot 3, 4 and 5 cannot as yet be excluded.

On the basis of MW and the maximal concentration of protein in the partially purified biologically active material, the maximally required concentration of TRF is estimated at $< 10^{-10}$ M.

Despite the undoubted presence of contaminating proteins in partially purified TRF, an attempt was made to raise an antiserum against TRF in goats. After three immunizations an antiserum was obtained which bound TRF but did not inhibit its biological activity when added to the indicator cultures together with TRF.

TABLE I. Purification of Radioactively Labelled TRF in 4 Consecutive Steps (Procedure A (8))

Purification step	total volume (ml)	µl tested on nu/nu (day 2)	SRBC PFC/10^6 day 5	% removal of protein in OD	% removal of protein in cpm
A) Original supernatant	200	200	3390		
B) PEG concentration and dialysis	10	10	4790	67	n. d.[a]
C) G-75 gel filtration	30	200	1820	96	99,7
D) Glycin-AH Sepharose + AH-Sepharose	7,5	200	2750	80[b]	83[b]

[a]The removal of radioactive contaminants could not be determined because of the presence of unincorporated ^{3}H-leucine in the original supernatant.

[b]Overall removal of protein: OD = 99,77 %; cpm = 99,9983 %.

TABLE II. *Purification of Radioactively Labelled TRF (Procedure B)*

Purification steps	total volume (ml)	μl tested on nu/nu (day 2)	SRBC PFC/10^6 day 5	total CPM	% of original
Original	650	200	680	–[a]	100[a]
A) After dialysis against PEG	50	50	1265	$6,5 \times 10^7$	30
B) After dialysis against 2 M $(NH_4)_2SO_4$	30	200	n. d.	$1,5 \times 10^7$	7.6
C) After passage over Phenyl-Sepharose	40	200	1517	3×10^6	1.5
D) After Sephadex gel filtration[b]	12	200	450	5×10^4	0.02

[a] The loss of protein was determined by OD. Original total CPM are not given because of unincorporated ^{3}H-leucine in the original preparation.

[b] The 40 ml recovered from Phenyl-Sepharose were concentrated by dialysis against PEG to 3 ml and applied to a Sephadex G 75 column.

Further booster injections led to the production of anitbodies which did inhibit TRF activity and were thus presumably directed against its active center (Table III).

TABLE III. Inhibition of TRF Activity by Goat Anti Mouse TRF

			SRBC PFC/10^6 day 5
BSS			0
TRF	100 µl +	-	2000
TRF	100 µl + anti-TRF	150 ul	3
"	" +	100 ul	60
"	" +	50 ul	245
TRF	100 µl + Control Serum	150 ul	1126
"	" + "	100 ul	1870
"	" + "	50 ul	2200

TRF activity was tested on nu/nu cultures by addition on day 2.

This antiserum also inhibits the immune response to SRBC in spleen cell cultures derived from normal mice where TRF supposedly is produced in situ (Table IV).

TABLE IV. Inhibition of Plaque Formation in C3D2 Spleen Cell Cultures (5 x 10^6/culture) by Goat Anti-TRF IgG

Additions on day 2		Anti-SRBC PFC/culture day 5
Medium		3047 ± 270
Pre-immune IgG	1:5[a]	4140
"	1:20	3960
Anti-TRF IgG	1:5	325
"	1:20	1170

[a]*Final dilutions in culture.*

Two observations suggest that the inhibitory activity of the antiserum is specific for TRF and does not reflect a general adverse effect on B lymphocytes: The effect in nu/nu spleen cultures restored by TRF depends on the amount of TRF added and can be overcome by higher TRF doses. Also, LPS induced plaque formation is not significantly inhibited by the antiserum.

The use of this antiserum ought to help in distinguishing TRF from other factors contained in Con A supernatants and may provide additional means of purification and to assess the physiological role of TRF.

REFERENCES

1) Schimpl, A. and Wecker, E. (1972) Nature 237, 15.
2) Wecker, E., Schimpl, A., Hünig, Th. and Kühn, L. (1975), Annal. N.Y. Acad. Sci. 249, 258.
3) Hünig, Th., Schimpl, A. and Wecker, E. (1977), J. Exp. Med. 145, 1228
4) Hünig, Th., Schimpl, A. and Wecker, E. (1973), J. Exp. Med. 139, 754.
5) Schimpl, A. and Wecker, E. (1975), Transpl. Rev. 23, 176.
6) Hünig, Th. and Schimpl, A. (1979), submitted to Eur. J. Immunol.
7) Takatsuki, A. and Tamura, G. (1971), J. Antibiot. 24, 232.
8) Müller, G., Hübner, L., Schimpl, A. and Wecker, E. (1978), Immunochem. 15, 27.
9) Hübner, L., Müller, G., Schimpl, A. and Wecker, E. (1978), Immunochem. 15, 33.

DISCUSSION

LEON: Would Schimpl tell us whether aggregates of Fc are better competitors of the action of TRF than monomers. If that is so, are irrelevant immune complexes responsible for the action of her anti-TRF, which is certainly not mono-specific?

SCHIMPL: The inhibitory action of the anti-TRF serum is retained in the $(Fab)_2$ anti-TRF fractions. Therefore the Fc receptor does not seem to be involved in inhibition.

ERB: Do anti-TRF antibodies also contain antibodies to C-type particles which might be responsible for the suppression of the primary anti-SRBC response?

SCHIMPL: We think we can exclude the possibility that the anti-TRF antibodies inhibit TRF-induced SRBC responses in nu/nu mice or in normal culture via antibodies to C-type virus. LPS-induced plaque development is not affected by the anti-TRF antiserum, while being highly sensitive to anti-viral 6T71 antibodies.

ARE ALL HELPER FACTORS FOR ANTIBODY SYNTHESIS ALSO MITOGENIC FOR T CELLS?

John J. Farrar
Mary L. Hilfiker
Steven B. Mizel
Janet Fuller-Bonar

National Institutes of Health
Bethesda, Maryland

In 1974, Hunter (Marrack) and Kettman demonstrated the existence of two functionally distinct types of soluble helper activities which served to "initiate" and "expand" the antibody response of antigen-stimulated B cells (1). The concept of two classes of helper factors has emerged from these and similar studies. The first class of helper factors directly or indirectly enhances the activation and proliferation of the antigen-stimulated B cells. Accordingly, this class of factors is maximally effective when added to the cultures at the beginning of the incubation period. The second class of helper factors is presumably involved in the induction of terminal differentiation of the B cells and is most effective when added to the cultures on the second or third day of the incubation period. The late-acting factor described by Schimpl and colleagues and designated T cell replacing factor (TRF) is the most well characterized example of this second class of helper factors (2). Thus, although functionally different helper factors have been described, it is unclear whether these activities are associated with biochemically distinct factors.

During the past three years our laboratory has been involved in the characterization of two helper factors which enhance antibody production and have been shown to be maximally effective when added to the B cell cultures at the beginning of the incubation period. One factor has a molecular weight of 15,000 and exhibits charge heterogeneity on DEAE cellulose and/or PAGE. The factor has been shown to be macrophage-derived and identical to the previously described thymocyte

ISBN 0-12-213950-X

TABLE I. SUMMARY OF THE ROLE OF LYMPHOCYTE ACTIVATING FACTOR AND THYMOCYTE MITOGENIC FACTOR ON THE INDUCTION OF HUMORAL AND CELL MEDIATED IMMUNE RESPONSES.

Source of Enhancing Activity	Early-Acting Antibody Synthesis Helper Activity	Killer Cell Helper Activity	Evidence for the Identity of the Factor
Human mixed leukocyte culture supernatant	15,000 daltons	N.D.	Co-purified with LAF during gel filtration, ion exchange, and gel electrophoresis (3).
Human adherent leukocyte supernatant	15,000 daltons	N.D.	Co-eluted with LAF on Sephadex G-75 (4).
$P388D_1$ macrophage cell line supernatant	15,000 daltons	15,000 daltons	Both activities co-purified with LAF during gel filtration, ion exchange, and gel electrophoresis (5, unpublished data).
Serum from BCG and LPS-treated mice	15,000 daltons	N.D.	Co-eluted with LAF on Sephacryl S-200 (6).
Con A-activated mouse spleen cell culture supernatant	35,000 daltons	35,000 daltons	Co-purified with TMF during $(NH_4)_2SO_4$ precipitation, gel filtration, hydroxylapatite, and hydrophobic chromatography (7).
Mouse mixed lymphocyte culture supernatant	35,000 daltons	35,000 daltons	Co-eluted with TMF on Sephadex G-100 (8, unpublished data).

proliferative monokine designated lymphocyte activating factor (LAF). The second factor has a molecular weight of 35,000 and exhibits heterogeneity as determined by hydrophobic chromatography. This latter factor has recently been shown to be T cell-derived, although macrophage-dependent, and to be identical to a thymocyte proliferative lymphokine designated thymocyte mitogenic factor (TMF). A summary of the chromatographic studies conducted on these two early-acting helper factors from a number of sources is shown in Table I. Also shown in the table is a summary of the data which support the idea that these early-acting helper factors are also capable of serving as helper factors in the induction of alloantigen-specific cytotoxic T cell responses. The data, therefore, support the conclusion that the thymocyte proliferative factors (regardless of whether they are macrophage- or T cell-derived) are early-acting helper factors for antibody synthesis.

The question remains as to whether the thymocyte proliferative early-acting helper factors (LAF and TMF) are biochemically distinct from the class of late-acting helper factors (TRF). Clearly, LAF and TRF are separable on the basis of a difference in molecular weight and cell-of-origin. However, TMF and the late-acting TRF exhibit similar molecular weights and are both T cell-derived and thus are not as readily distinguished. In our studies, a pool of gel filtration fractions (m.w. 25-45,000 from a Con A-induced mouse spleen cell culture supernatant), containing TMF, exhibit *late-acting* T cell replacing activity only when LAF is added at the beginning of the culture period (Table II). We have therefore used this assay system, which measures the synergism between LAF and late-acting T cell replacing activity, in the analysis of the biochemical relationship between TMF and T cell replacing activity.

Recently, we have achieved a partial separation of TMF from the late-acting T cell replacing activity using phenyl sepharose chromatography (Figure 1). In this experiment the principal TMF eluted in the fractions corresponding to Fraction Pool E whereas Fraction Pool F contained the maximal amount of late-acting activity capable of synergizing with LAF. Based on these results we suggest that LAF is capable of synergizing with a factor other than the principal TMF although the failure to achieve complete separation does not allow us to rule out the possibility that LAF may also synergize with TMF. Complete separation of TMF and the late-acting synergizing factor will obviously require further purification of the two activities. However, recent results indicate that TMF is resistant to pH 2.0 inactivation whereas at least a portion of the late-acting synergizing TRF activity is

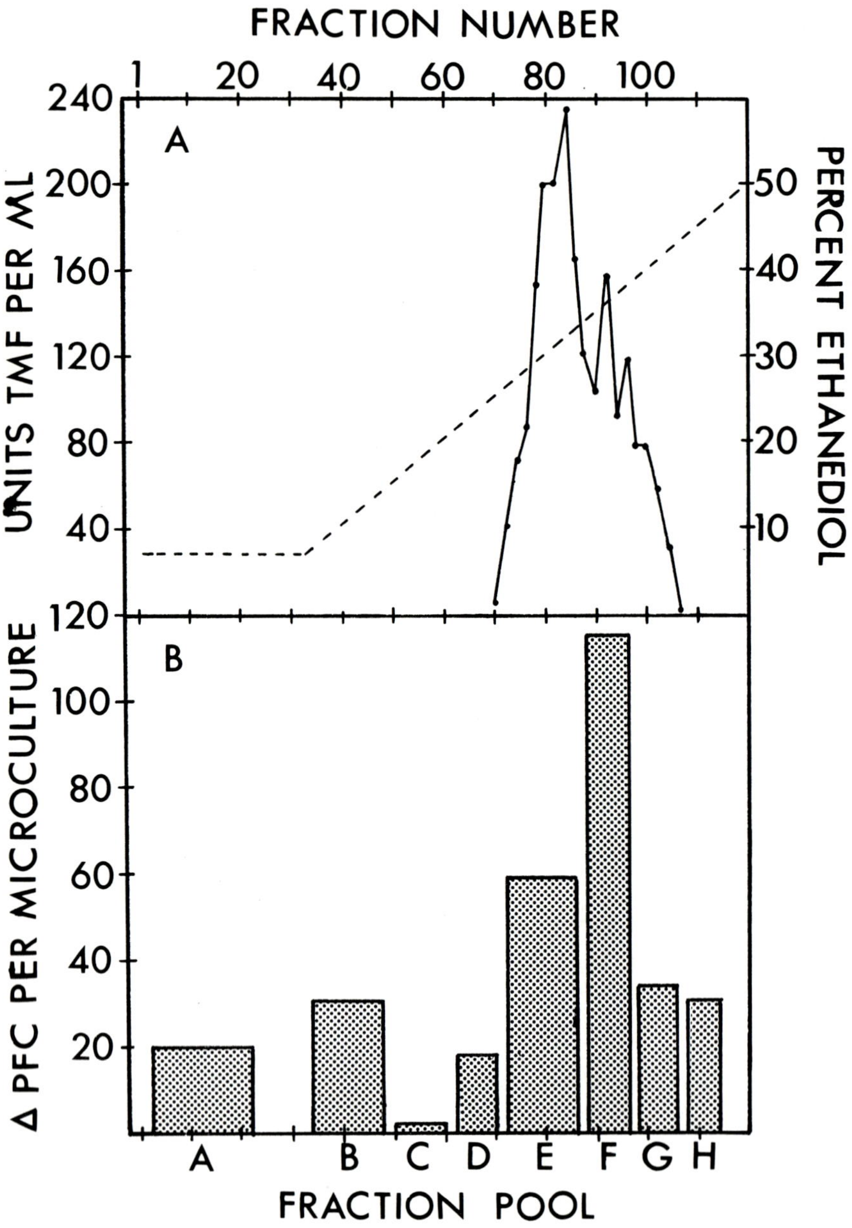

Fig. 1. Phenyl sepharose chromatography of a Con A-induced mouse spleen cell supernatant. TMF activity (Panel A) is expressed as units/ml. Late-acting TRF activity (Panel B) = PFC of LAF + Fraction Pool (added Hour 48) - PFC of Fraction Pool (added Hour 48). PFC of LAF = 6.

TABLE II. SYNERGISTIC HELPER EFFECTS OF LAF AND 25-45,000 M.W. FRACTION POOLS ON THE ANTIBODY RESPONSE OF B CELL ENRICHED MOUSE SPLEEN CELLS.[a]

Factor Additions		*PFC Per Culture at Hour 92*
LAF at Hour 0	*Fraction Pools at Hour 49*	
-	-	3 ± 3
+	-	21 ± 4
-	+	16 ± 7
+	+	522 ± 58

[a] *1.2 x 10^6 nude mouse spleen cells in 0.2 ml microcultures with 10^6 SRC.*

sensitive to pH 2.0. Thus, on the basis of functional and biochemical evidence, we have concluded that TMF and late-acting TRF are distinct molecular entities.

REFERENCES

1. Hunter, P., and Kettman, J.R. (1974). *Proc. Natl. Acad. Sci. 71,* 512.
2. Hubner, L., Muller, G., Schimpl, A., and Wecker, E. (1978) *Immunochemistry. 15,* 33.
3. Koopman, W.J., Farrar, J.J., Oppenheim, J.O., Fuller-Bonar J., and Dougherty, S. (1977). *J. Immunol. 119,* 55.
4. Koopman, W.J., Farrar, J.J., and Fuller-Bonar, J. (1978) *Cell. Immunol. 35,* 92.
5. Farrar, W.L., Mizel, S.B., and Farrar, J.J. (1979) *Fed. Proc. 38,* 1006.
6. Männel, D.N., Farrar, J.J., and Mergenhagen, S.E. (Submitted for publication).
7. Farrar, J.J., Simon, P.L., Koopman, W.J., and Fuller-Bonar J. (1978). *J. Immunol. 121,* 1353.
8. Simon, P.L., Farrar, J.J., and Kind. P.D. (1979). *J. Immunol. 122,* 127.

DISCUSSION

WECKER: I am glad that we all now agree on a late acting T-helper factor, the target cell of which is the B lymphocyte. Regarding the early-acting factors there seem to be two possibilities: (1) Generation of T-helper cells even in the nu/nu spleen cell system; (2) Shifting of the immature B cells into the compartment of mature antigen reactive B cells.

FARRAR: I believe that LAF activates a population of T or pre-T cells in the B enriched population. These T cells are then involved in a sequence of events which culminate in the initiation of the B cell response. Subsequent to this activation they become susceptible to the terminal signal provided by the late-acting TRF.

WAKSMAN: But Farrar's factor could be a proteolytic enzyme, and we know that many of these are directly mitogenic for B cells.

WEBB: With reference to the issue of sequential action of LAF and TRF. Has Farrar performed the following experiments?

(1) Reversing the order of addition of LAF and TRF - adding TRF followed by LAF.
(2) Adding LAF and TRF together, as late as 33 hours.

FARRAR: Unfortunately, the experiment proposed in the first part of Webb's question cannot be satisfactorily performed with mouse late-acting TRF, because the late-acting factor is contaminated with early-acting TMF which then elevates the PFC response to such an extent that synergism is difficult to observe. We have, however, done the experiment with human MLC-derived late-acting helper factor which is not contaminated with early-acting helper factor. In these experiments, if the factors were applied in the reverse order, no synergism was observed. In answer to the second part of Webb's question, the later one adds LAF to cultures receiving TRF at hour 48 the less synergism is obtained so that by the time LAF addition has been delayed to the point where both factors are being added at the same time (day two), the effect is only slightly above additive.

WOOD: We have data which are complementary to those of Hoffmann. In the plaque assay, purified BAF and purified TRF from Watson added at time zero synergize. This synergy is chromatic in BAF unresponsive cultures of nude splenocytes after passage over G10. It is difficult to rationalize these data with Farrar's hypothesis that LAF stimulates TRF release unless it is assumed that the early- and late-acting TRF differ. Would he tell us if there are any manipulations which allow one tc dissociate these two activities?

FARRAR: Yes, I believe we can differentiate the early and late-acting helper factors. In addition to partial separation achieved on phenyl sepharose, the early-acting helper factor (TMF) is insensitive to pH 2 whereas the late-acting factor (TRF) which synergizes with LAF is sensitive to pH 2. Therefore, with regard to the observed synergism between LAF and TRF, we would argue that LAF might be able to stimulate the endogenous production of sufficient early-acting helper factor (TMF) but that the response was still dependent on the exogenous addition of the biochemically and functionally distinct late-acting TRF.

MOLECULAR CHARACTERIZATION OF LYMPHOKINES THAT ENHANCE IMMUNE RESPONSES

James Watson*, Steven Gillis, and Kendall Smith

*Department of Microbiology
University of California, Irvine
Irvine, California 92717
and
The Hematology Research Laboratory
Dartmouth Hitchcock Medical Center
and
The Norris Cotton Cancer Center
Hanover, New Hampshire 03755

Lymphokines secreted by Concanavalin A-treated mouse spleen cells have been purified by salt precipitation, gel filtration, ion-exchange chromatography, and isoelectric focusing. Two classes of lymphokines have been distinguished. One class, termed T cell growth factor (TCGF), stimulates proliferation of antigen- or mitogen-activated T cells and may exert all regulatory activities by the clonal expansion of different subclasses of T cells. A second class, termed T cell-replacing factor (TRF) stimulates antibody synthesis in T cell-depleted spleen cultures, and may not require T cells to exert activity. The molecular and biological properties of these two classes of lymphokines are presented.

Introduction

A large number of lymphokine-like activities have been detected in the supernatants of cultured murine, rat, and human lymphocytes. Such lymphokines enhance a variety of B and T cell responses, but little attention has been directed toward the association of defined biological activity with purified material.

An excellent source of murine lymphokines is the supernatant from cultures of Concanavalin A (Con A)-stimulated mouse spleen cells (1-3), which enhance a variety of B and T cell responses (4-12). Such assays used appear to detect both proliferation and differentiation-inducing activities in these culture supernatants. The biological activity of lymphokines in Con A supernatants from murine, rat,

ISBN 0-12-213950-X

and human has been purified by successive gel filtration and isoelectric focusing, in an attempt to separate molecules with different activities from each other (1-3). In the course of these separative procedures, the biological activities measured in murine systems included: (i) T cell growth factor (TCGF) activity (8), (ii) the promotion of Con A-induced mitogenesis in thymocyte cultures (5), (iii) helper T cell-replacing factor (TRF) activity in athymic spleen cell cultures (4,5), and (iv) the induction of cytotoxic lymphocytes (CTL) in both thymocyte (9) and nude mouse spleen cell cultures (10). The results of these studies are summarized here.

Purification of Murine Lymphokines

Fractionation of murine Con A supernatants by gel filtration (Fig. 1) and isoelectric focusing (Fig. 2) revealed a class of molecules with an apparent molecular size of approximately 30,000 daltons, which was separable into two components which differ in charge having isoelectric points of 4.3 and 4.9 (Fig. 2). Both components support the continuous proliferation of cytotoxic and helper T cells (1), in culture (Fig. 2A), promote the proliferation of Con A-treated thymocytes (Fig. 2B), induce the generation of AFC in T depleted cultures (Fig. 2C), and cytotoxic cells in either thymocyte or nude spleen cell cultures (Fig. 2D).

In addition, within the factor(s) in the 30,000 dalton fraction, another subclass of molecules was detectable by their ability to induce antibody synthesis to heterologous erythrocyte antigens in cultures of spleen cells from nude mice. This material shows considerable heterogeneity in charge ranging from a pI of 3.0 to 4.2 (Fig. 2C). No activity was detected when these molecules were tested in the other assay systems (1).

Properties of Rat and Human Lymphokines

The data summarized in Table 1 compares the molecular properties of lymphokines isolated from Con A-activated rat (2) and human (3) lymphoid cell populations. Both rat and human lymphokine activities were tested in the four murine lymphocyte assay systems detailed above. These data are extensively discussed in references 1-3.

TABLE 1

COMPARATIVE PROPERTIES OF MURINE, RAT AND HUMAN LYMPHOKINES

	Murine	Rat	Human
Size (Gel filtration)	30,000 daltons	15,000 daltons	15,000 daltons
Elution (DEAE ion-exchange resin pH 7.6)	0.15-0.2 M	<0.05 M	<0.05 M
Isoelectric points	4.3, 4.9	5.5	6.0

Discussion

Lymphokines isolated from mitogen-activated murine, rat, and human cells were found to stimulate (i) the growth of established murine T cell lines in culture, (ii) the proliferation of murine thymocytes in the presence of Con A under culture conditions where Con A alone is nonmitogenic, (iii) the induction of antibody responses to heterologous erythrocyte antigens in athymic (nude) spleen cultures, and (iv) the generation of cytotoxic T lymphocytes (CTL) in murine thymocyte cultures and in nude spleen cultures (1-3). The finding that lymphokine activities from each of these different species were inseparable in four different murine lymphocyte proliferation and differentiation assays following successive gel filtration, ion-exchange chromatography and isoelectric focusing (1-3), provides strong evidence that all four biological activites are mediated by the same molecules. The molecular properties of this class of lymphokine differ from each species. From mouse, this class of lymphokine had an apparent size of 30,000 daltons, and was separable into two components (pI 4.3 and 4.9) (Figs. 1,2). Rat (2) and human (3) lymphokines appeared smaller in size (15,000 daltons) but differed in isoelectric points (Table 1).

There is strong evidence that this class of lymphokine acts to enhance lymphocyte activity by the clonal expansion of T cells (7-12), therefore this lymphokine activity is referred to as T cell growth factor (TCGF). The following considerations of each assay support this contention:

(i) For the growth of cloned effector T cells in culture, there is an absolute requirement for TCGF, thus it can be assumed TCGF acts directly on T cells. This conclusion is further supported by the observation that activated T cells absorb TCGF whereas non-activated cells or activated B cells do not. It furthermore seems plausible that activation of T cells by antigen or mitogen results in the appearance of receptors for TCGF (13).

(ii) Both antigen and TCGF are required to generate cytotoxic effector T cells from nude mouse splenocytes. By definition, pre-T cells are present in the spleens of nude mice. In that T cell antigen or mitogen alone cannot initiate the proliferation of nude mouse lymphocytes (nude mice being incapable of producing TCGF) (13), it follows that addition of TCGF to responder pre-T cell populations promotes proliferation to the point where meaningful cytotoxic reactivity can be witnessed.

(iii) There may be antigen reactive pre-T cells other than those able to become cytotoxic cells in nude spleens. In the presence of TCGF and antigen, therefore, specific T helper cells may be generated which are able to subsequently contribute to antibody responses. In consideration of such a scheme of events, it is interesting that both TCGF production and the stimulation of nude spleen cells to produce antibody, require macrophage (6,8).

(iv) Finally with regard to the generation of thymocyte reactivity, helper T cells (Lyl+) and adherent cells have been shown to be required for both the polyclonal sensitization of murine T cells by Con A or PHA and the generation of cytotoxic T cells from thymocyte cultures. The T cells stimulated to proliferate and mature to effector cells are, in fact, antigen sensitive T cells from killer, suppressor, and helper subclasses. Con A activation may have two roles; the first being to mimic the signal normally provided by an antigen (5), and the second being to stimulate the production of the proliferative factor which we have designated TCGF (7-13).

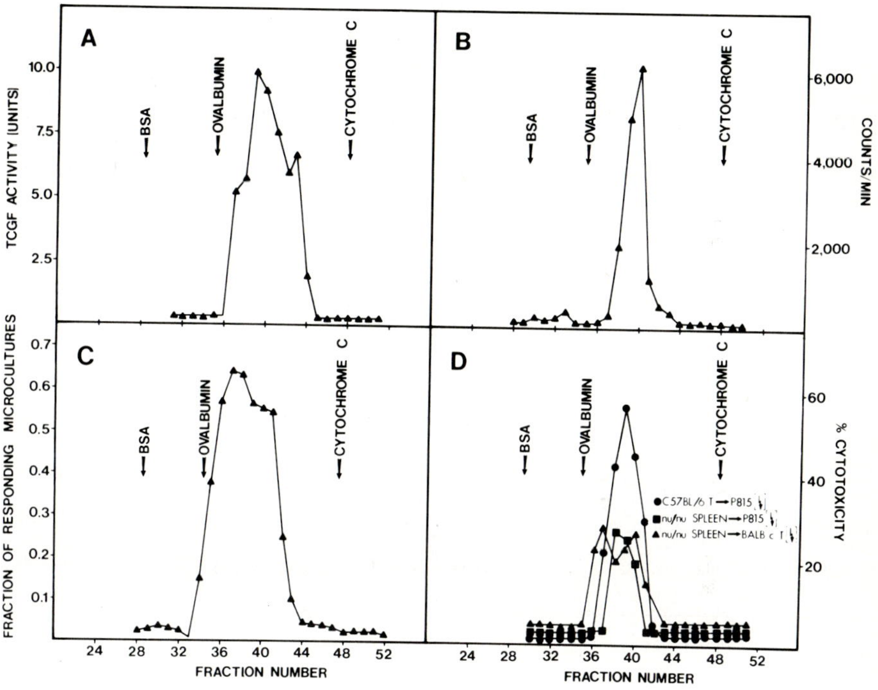

Figure 1: Lymphokine activities assayed following Sephadex G-100 gel exclusion chromatography of concentrated medium conditioned by Con A-stimulated mouse spleen cells. (A) TCGF activity. (B) Ability to promote thymocyte mitogenesis. (C) Ability to promote anti-erythrocyte antibody production in nude mouse spleen cell cultures. (D) Ability to induce CTL responses in C57BL/6 thymocyte P815 MTLC (●), NIH nude spleen by P815 MTLC (■) and NIH nude spleen by BALB/c thymocyte MLC (▲).

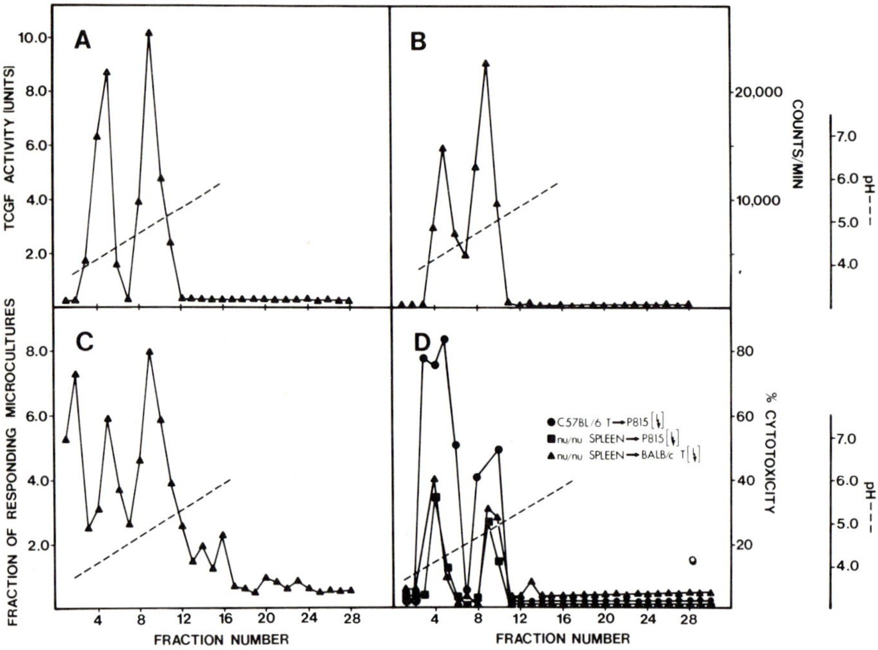

Figure 2: Lymphokine activities assayed following flat-bed IEF (pH 3-10) of active fractions pooled after Sephadex G-100 gel exclusion chromatography. (A) TCGF activity. (B) ability to promote thymocyte mitogenesis. (C) Ability to promote anti-erythrocyte antibody production in nude mouse spleen cell cultures. (D) Ability to induce CTL responses in C57BL/6 thymocyte P815 MTLC (■), NIH nude spleen P815 MTLC (●), and NIH nude spleen by BALB/c thymocyte MLC (▲).

The molecular properties of TCGF isolated from these three species are different, yet they possess identical biological activity when assayed on murine lymphocytes. It is possible that each of these TCGF may interact with common cellular receptors in murine cells, implying that murine, rat, and human TCGF share structural homologies. It is also possible that TCGF purified from these sources are an unrelated group of molecules that interact with common target cells at different receptor sites. It appears very likely from the biological assays that TCGF may be a class of T cell growth hormones. It may, therefore, be expected that there is some species conservation of a biologically active region in such a class of hormones.

Among the molecular entities present in the murine lymphokines with an apparent size of 30,000 daltons (Fig. 1C), there was an activity that may truly function to replace T cells in the induction of antibody synthesis, which was not observed in rat or human lymphokine preparations. After isoelectric focusing, within the pH range of 3.0 to 4.2, there was clearly an activity which was detectable in the TRF assay but which had no effect on either mature T cells (TCGF assay) or immature T cells. One explanation for this T cell-replacing activity, therefore, is that this factor may be acting directly on the B cell rather than indirectly causing the proliferative expansion of helper T cells. There may exist both species-specific and nonspecific TCGF and TRF molecules, and due to the use of murine assay systems, rat and human TRF activities may not be detected.

Further studies will be required to define the exact molecular characteristics of the murine TRF which has no apparent activity on T cells. One might predict that activated B cells would absorb TRF in much the same manner that activated T cells absorbed TCGF activity. Nonetheless, the results of the experimentation described herein suggests that at least two distinct molecular entities exist from murine sources that have similar molecular sizes yet differ in charge and biologic activity. Further studies of the nature of the target cells of these factors as well as their *in vitro* and *in vivo* immunobiological function should provide for an era of a hormonal approach to our understanding of the regulation of the immune response.

REFERENCES

1. Watson, J., Gillis, S., Marbrook, J., Mochizuki, D., and Smith, K. A. (1979) J. Expt. Med., submitted.
2. Gillis, S., Smith, K. A., and Watson, J. (1979) J. Expt. Med., submitted.
3. Gillis, S., Smith, K. A., Watson, J. (1979) J. Expt. Med., submitted.
4. Watson, J. D., Aarden, L., and Lefkovits, I. (1979) J. Immunol. 122:209.
5. Watson, J., Aarden, L., Shaw, J., and Paetkau, V. (1979) J. Immunol., in press.
6. Hoffman, M. K., and Watson, J. (1979) J. Immunol. 122:1371.
7. Gillis, S., and Smith, K. A. (1977) Nature 268:154.
8. Gillis, S., Ferm, M. M., Ou, W., and Smith, K. A. (1978) J. Immunol. 120:2027.
9. Baker, P. E., Gillis, S., Ferm, M. M., and Smith, K. A. (1978) J. Immunol. 121:2168
10. Gillis, S., Union, N. A., Baker, P. E., and Smith, K. A. (1978) J. Expt. Med., in press.
11. Gillis, S., and Smith, K. A. (1977) J. Expt. Med. 146:468.
12. Gillis, S., Baker, P. E., Ruscetti, F. W., and Smith, K. A. (1978) J. Expt. Med. 148:1093.
13. Smith, K. A., Gillis, S., Ruscetti, F. W., Baker, P. E., and McKenzie, D. Proc. N.Y. Acad. Sci., in press.

DISCUSSION

WAKSMAN: How does one get CTL from nude spleen? Does this mean that Watson's factor is also inducing differentiation (from T cell precursors to mature T cells) as well as proliferation?

WATSON: Since this part is the work of Gillis, and he deals with this issue in a separate report, I will ask him to answer.

GILLIS: We have found that stimulation of nude mouse spleen, lymph node and bone-marrow cells with either antigen or mitogen does not result in the production of T cell growth factor. Therefore we feel that antigen presentation to nude mouse spleen cells (incapable of TCGF production) results in acquisition of TCGF responsiveness (receptors) but only after addition of TCGF do these cells proliferate to the point where we are capable of detecting effector cell cytolytic reactivity.

OPPENHEIM: Has Gillis had the opportunity to test the effect of monocyte derived LAF on growth of CTLL cells or for its capacity to induce CTL in nu/nu mice?

GILLIS: Yes, both the high and low molecular weight LPS-induced LAF that Oppenheim provided, as well as purified material from Mizel, are incapable of stimulating the proliferation of CTLL cells in TCGF microassays. But we have tested neither material in nude mouse CTL-induction assays.

I would like to add that we have recently had some success in using different absorption to dissociate lymphokine activities. It appears that purified (i) TCGF activity, (ii) the ability to promote thymocyte mitogenesis, and (iii) the ability to induce CTL in thymocyte and nude splenocyte cultures, are all removed by absorption with antigen-specific, TCGF-dependent CTLL cells. However, the pI 3.0 - 3.0 pH material isolated by Watson et al., which has no activity in T cell assays and yet induces antibody production by nude spleen cells, is not absorbed. It is quite possible that this non-CTLL absorbable factor activity may be the true late-acting TRF described by Schimpl and Wecker and discussed previously by Farrar.

DOES LPS-INDUCED MONOKINE INITIATE B CELL DIFFERENTIATION AND THYMOCYTE PROLIFERATION THROUGH A COMMON PATHWAY?[1]

Michael K. Hoffmann
Kathleen Gilbert
Myung Chun

Department of Immunology
Memorial Sloan-Kettering Cancer Center
New York, NY

Macrophages respond to various endogenous and exogenous stimuli with the generation of factor which induce B cells to secrete antibody and thymocytes to proliferate. Macrophage factors with these functional properties received, depending on the laboratory and the functional aspects studied, different designations: lymphocyte activating factor (LAF, 1), B cell activating factor (BAF, 2), mitogenic protein (MP, 3), B cell differentiation factor (BDF, 4), and macrophage derived T cell replacing factor (TRF-M, 5). Biochemical studies indicate that those thymocyte and B cell responses are stimulated by the same macrophage-derived molecule (6, 12). It was, therefore, of interest to determine whether one biological mediator elicits different reactions on different targets or whether it initiates different biological responses through a common pathway. The experiments reported here favor the latter alternative.

Investigating the enhancement of antibody production in murine spleen cell cultures by an LPS-induced macrophage factor (TRF-M), we found that TRF-M induced phenotypic and functional differentiation of B cells (7). It increases the frequency of precursor B cells capable of interacting with helper T cells (8) (or T cell replacing factors released by them)

[1]*Supported in part by grants from the National Institutes of Health CA-08748 and CA-17673 and by a grant from the Cancer Research Institute.*

ISBN 0-12-213950-X

which is reflected in a marked synergism between macrophage derived (TRF-M) and T cell derived (TRF-T) helper factors (5).

The ability of TRF-M to stimulate proliferation of thymus cells is demonstrated in Fig. 1. TRF-M induces blast formation and ^{3}H-thymidine uptake (data shown) of C3H/HeJ thymus cells in concentrations ranging from 0.1 to 10%. In an attempt to verify that this response induced by a macrophage mediator was macrophage-independent (as in the activation of B cells), we passed thymocytes over Sephadex G-10 columns and found that thymocytes so treated no longer respond to TRF-M. The response was not reconstituted by peritoneal macrophages which were added in a concentration optimal in reconstituting antibody formation in macrophage depleted spleen cells (9). The Sephadex G-10 column is commonly used for the removal of macrophages from lymphoid cell suspensions (10); however, this

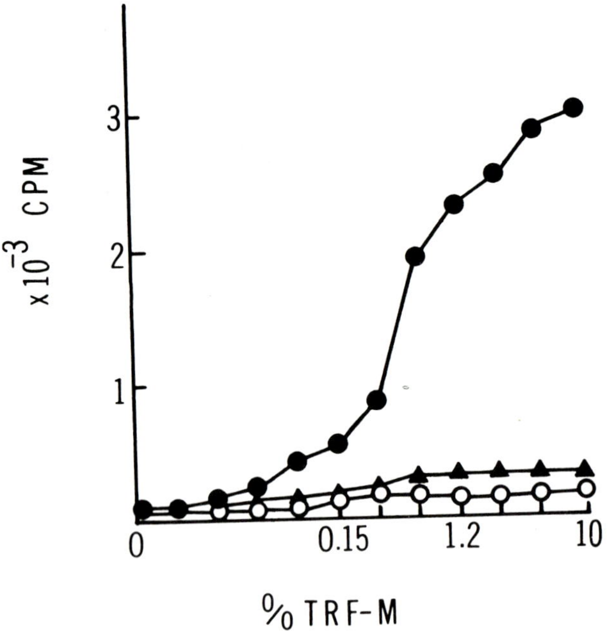

FIG. 1. 10^{6} C3H/HeJ thymocytes were cultured in 0.1 volumes of Mishell-Dutton medium (13) in the absence or presence of TRF-M (10%). After 3 days, triplicate cultures were pulsed for three hours with 0.1 μCi ^{5}H-thymidine. Incorporated tritium was counted in a Packard liquid scintillator spectrometer. Unseparated thymocytes: ●--●; Seph. 6-10 treated o--o; Seph. G-10 treated, reconstituted with 10^{4} peritoneal cells ▲--▲.

column has been shown to also retain certain fractions of B cells (PFC) (10) and T cells (suppressor cells) (11). The possibility that the effect of Sephadex G-10 filtration on thymocyte TRF-M responsiveness was due to the removal of cells other than macrophages was therefore considered. In order to test whether an accessory cell rather than TRF-M responding cell was removed from thymocyte suspensions by column filtration, we added graded numbers of mitomycin-c treated syngeneic spleen cells to the thymocyte cultures. It was found that 10^5 spleen cells (unresponsive themselves) reconstituted the TRF-M response of 10^6 Sephadex G-10 treated thymocytes to the level of the response of 10^6 unseparated thymocytes (Fig. 2). This finding indicated that it was not the thymus cell that proliferates in the TRF-M response, but rather an accessory cell which was retained on Sephadex G-10 column. The accessory

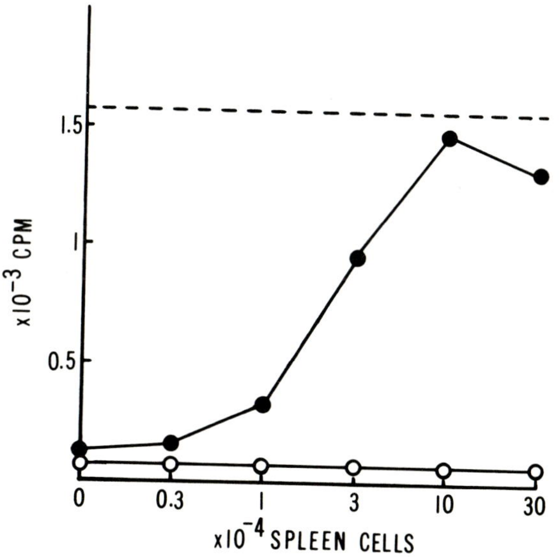

FIG. 2. 10^6 Sephadex G-10 filtered C3H/HeJ thymocytes were cultured and pulsed with ^{3}H-thymidine, as described under Fig. 1. C3H/HeJ spleen cells, treated with mitomycin-c (40 γ/ml, 30 min, 37°C) was added in concentrations ranging from 0.3 to 30 x 10^4 cells per culture. No addition: o--o; TRF-M (10%) ●--●. Dotted line indicates response in cultures of unseparated thymus cells.

cell occurs in the spleen and its nature could now be investigated. Initial experiments indicated that its activity does not depend on an intact thymic function; BALB/c·nu/nu spleen cells reconstituted the TRF-M response of heterozygous BALB/c·nu/+ thymocytes as efficient as BALB/c·nu/+ spleen cells (data not shown). Incubation of spleen cells in rabbit anti-mouse Ig coated plastic dishes (retaining > 80% B cells) did not reduce the ability of spleen cells to reconstitute the TRF-M response of thymocytes. In addition, the splenic accessory cell did not adhere to uncoated plastic surfaces. These observations suggest that the cell that mediates TRF-M dependent thymocyte proliferation is not typical of any of the major cell classes of the lymphoid system -- T cells, B cells or macrophages. It remains to be tested whether it is a pre-T cell (occuring in nu/nu spleen cells), a weakly Ig^+ or Ig^- end-differentiated B cell adherent to Sephadex G-10 columns but not to insolubilized anti-Ig reagents, or a weakly adherent macrophage subpopulation which occurs in the spleen but not in the peritoneal cavity.

Consideration must be given to an observation recently reported by D. Wood (12). He found that an LPS-induced human monocyte factor (BAF) which induces antibody production in culture of nu/nu mouse spleen cells (2) failed to do so when spleen cells were passed over a modified Sephadex G-10 column. In this modification cells are suspended prior to passage in medium containing Hepes buffer (12). He concluded that the modified Sephadex G-10 column (but not the original method) (10) retained an accessory cell which mediates the activity of BAF. This observation, when considered in conjunction with our finding in the thymocyte proliferation assay suggests that macrophage mediators may stimulate antibody production and thymocyte proliferation through a common pathway, namely through the activation of a Sephadex adherent cell. Given the fact that this accessory cell occurs in thymus in a lower frequency than in the spleen (10^5 spleen cells reconstitute 10^6 thymus cells), it is conceivable that the original Sephadex filtration method removes accessory cells from thymus cells, yet, a more efficient separation (D. Wood's modification) is required to deplete splenic accessory cells.

As cell separation procedures have so far failed in the classification of the accessory cell, attempts were made to replace this helper cell. It was found that a highly purified T cell-derived T cell replacing factor [TRF-T (14), obtained from Dr. James Watson, Irvine, California] circumvented the need of accessory cells for the TRF-M induced proliferation of thymocytes (Table 1). The possibility (suggested by this finding) that the accessory cell performs a T cell function and might in fact belong to the T cell lineage is currently under investigation. It should be noted that TRF-M and TRF-T act synergistically in this response much as both mediators were previously found to act synergistically in the generation of antibody forming B cells (PFC) (5).

THYMUS CELLS	*^{3}H-thymidine uptake (cpm)*			
	-	*TRF-M*	*TRF-T*	*TRF-M+TRF-T*
Unseparated	*30±14*	*1724±912*	*691±288*	*6754±1275*
Sephadex G-10	*65±27*	*266±156*	*543±230*	*6717±503*

TABLE 1. 10^6 C3H/HeJ thymus cells were cultured in Mishell-Dutton culture medium (13) in 0.1 ml volumes, unseparated or after passage over Sephadex G-10 columns (10). Additions: TRF-M (5,7), 10%; TRF-T (14), 4μl/ml. After three days triplicate cultures were pulsed for three hours with 0.1 μCi (6-^{3}H)-thymidine and incorporated Tritium was counted in a Packard liquid scintillation spectrometer.

REFERENCES

1. Gery, I., Gershon, R.K., and Waksman, B.H. (1972). *J. Exp. Med. 136*, 128.
2. Wood, D.D., and Gaul, S.L. (1974). *J. Immunol. 113*, 925.
3. Calderon, J., Kievy, J.M., Lefko, J.L., and Unanue, E.R. (1975). *J. Exp. Med. 142*, 151.
4. Finelt, M., and Hoffmann, M.K. (1979). *Clin. Immunol. and Tumor Pathol. 12*, 281.
5. Hoffmann, M.K., and Watson, J. (1979). *J. Immunol. 122*, 1371.
6. Mizel, S.B. (1979). In *"Molecular Mediators of Cellular Immunity"* (J.H. Hadden and W.E. Stewart, eds.), Humana Press, N.J.
7. Hoffmann, M.K., Koenig, S., Mittler, R.S., Oettgen, H.F., Ralph, P., Galanos, C., and Hammerling, U. (1979). *J. Immunol. 122*, 497.
8. Hoffmann, M.K. *Ann. N.Y. Acad. Sci.*, in press.
9. Hoffmann, M.K. (1970). *Immunology 18*, 791.
10. Ly, I.A. and Mishell, R.I.(1974). *Immunol. Methods 5*, 289.
11. Pickel, K., and Hoffmann, M.K.(1977).*J. Immunol. 118,* 653.
12. Wood, D.D. *Ann. N.Y. Acad. Sci.*, in press.
13. Mishell, R.I., and Dutton, R.W. (1967). *J. Exp. Med. 126*, 423.
14. Watson, J., Aarden, L.A., and Lefkovits, I. (1979). *J. Immunol. 122*, 209.

DISCUSSION

OPPENHEIM: How does Hoffmann know LAF is not a prerequisite for TRF production?

HOFFMANN: I cannot exclude that possibility. However, LAF cannot act through the generation of TRF. We have clearly shown that Watson's highly purified TRF induces antibody synthesis by B cells only in presence of either macrophages or their mediator TRF-M (LAF). TRF alone is inactive on B cells. I do think that LAF (or TRF-M, BAF etc.) acts directly on B cells inducing their differentiation. We have shown that LAF is a potent inducer of phenotypic differentiation of B cells in the Komuro-Boyse assay. However, LAF might not be capable of converting B cell precurser into antibody producing cells. In the latter reaction, LAF apparently synergizes with T cell derived signals (TRF) or with accessory cells (as shown by Wood and by us in an earlier report) which might perform T cell functions. We have shown recently that LAF increases the number of precursor B cells capable of responding to T cell dependent TRF.

A HUMAN T CELL FACTOR DRIVES DIFFERENTIATION OF PFC PRECURSORS[1]

Myron A. Leon
Tuan-Huey Kuo

Department of Immunology and Microbiology
Wayne State University, School of Medicine
Detroit, Michigan

Supernatants from the human T cell line HPB-ALL, contain a lymphocyte differentiation factor, LDF, which drives differentiation of antigen primed murine B lymphocytes to PFC. Effects of LDF are demonstrable in vivo and in vitro.

A. *In Vivo Activity Of LDF*

Mice were immunized on day 0. LDF was injected on various days and anti-dextran PFC measured on day 5. Maximal response

TABLE I. Effect of Time of Injection of LDF[a]

Day LDF Injected	*PFC/10⁷ Cells*
-	3480 ± 140
0	3970 ± 720
1	2850 ± 100
2	9870 ± 640
3	5870 ± 790
4	6080 ± 720

[a]*Mice were injected i.v. with 20 μg of dextran B1355S on day 0 and 0.75 ml LDF on day noted.*

[1]*Supported by NCI Grants CA-20812 and CA-18900.*

ISBN 0-12-213950-X

TABLE II. Dose-Responses For SRBC and Dextran

LDF	PFC/10^7 Cells Anti-SRBC	Anti-Dextran
-	2990 ± 290	3480 ± 90
0.1 ml	6530 ± 230	6930 ± 180
0.25 ml	3720 ± 250	7290 ± 460
0.75 ml	3270 ± 120	6080 ± 440

BALB/c Mice were primed i.v. with either 2.5 X 10^7 SRBC or 20 μg of dextran B1355S. Two days later LDF was injected i.v.

was observed when LDF was injected at day 2.

LDF also enhanced anti-SRBC responses. Table 2 shows dose-response data for mice immunized with either SRBC or B1355S. Response to LDF differs for the two immunogens, with the SRBC system more sensitive to inhibition by large doses of LDF.

B. *In Vitro Activity Of LDF*

Experiments in which human LDF has been added to in vitro cultures with or without antigen, have failed to demonstrate enhancement of PFC. In vitro activity of human LDF is demonstrable when cultured with spleen cells harvested from con-

TABLE III. Duration of Priming Influences Response

Days Primed	LDF	Anti-SRBC PFC/10^7 Cells
3	-	459 ± 67
3	+	1088 ± 37
4	-	1353 ± 50
4	+	9093 ± 621
5	-	349 ± 8
5	+	2473 ± 64

Mice were primed with 5X 10^7 SRBC. Spleen cells were cultured for 18 hrs before measuring PFC.

ventional or athymic animals primed with antigen. In vitro response to LDF as a function of length of in vivo priming is shown in Table 3. The data demonstrate a) that the size of the size of the cell population driven to differentiate to mature PFC by LDF is maximal in 4 day primed cells; b) the size of this pre-PFC population bears no obvious relationship to the number of mature PFC measured in the absence of LDF.

Hydroxyurea (1 mm) is useful for demonstrating whether LDF acts on dividing and/or non-dividing pre-PFC populations(2). Spleen cells from BALB/c mice primed for 3 or 10 days with dextran were cultured ± LDF and ± hydroxyurea. Table 4 shows that LDF drives differentiation to mature PFC of both dividing and non-dividing precursors.

TABLE IV. Effect of Hydroxyurea on in vitro enhancement

Days Primed	*LDF*	*Hydroxyurea*	*PFC*
3	-	-	159 ± 8
3	-	+	31 ± 3
3	+	-	916 ± 45
3	+	+	149 ± 3
10	-	-	63 ± 2
10		+	61 ± 2
10	+	-	676 ± 80
10	+	+	575 ± 60

Mice were primed with 20 μg of dextran. Spleen cells were cultured as described in Table 3.

REFERENCES

Leon, M. A. and Kuo, T.-H. (1979). *Ann. N.Y. Acad. Sci. in press.*
Sinclair, W.K. (1965). *Science. 150*, 1729.

HEMOLYTIC PLAQUE ASSAY FOR ACTIVATED T CELLS[1]

Daniele Primi[2]
George K. Lewis
Richard P. Triglia
Joel W. Goodman

Department of Microbiology and Immunology
University of California, San Francisco
San Francisco, California

I. HELPER AND SUPPRESSOR PRODUCTS RELEASED BY T CELLS ACTIVATED BY CONCANAVALIN A

Supernatants from unfractionated or B cell-depleted murine spleen cells cultured for 48 hours with 1.0 μg of Concanavalin A induced polyclonal antibody synthesis by B cells from normal and athymic mice in the absence of antigen (Primi et al., 1979). In contrast to antibody secretion, B cell proliferation induced by the supernatant was only discernible in low density cultures.

The Con A-induced supernatant also contained suppressive components, since the primary anti-sheep RBC response was markedly suppressed when the antigen added to cultures consisted of SRBC which had been used for absorbing the supernatant (Primi et al., 1979). Absorbed supernatants had enhanced helper activity, indicating that only the suppressor was removable by antigen. The absorbed suppressive component was eluted from SRBC with ammonium thiocyanate and was itself strongly suppressive when added to cultures with fresh SRBC. It proved to be highly antigen-specific, as the SRBC-absorbed factor did not affect the response to horse RBC.

[1] Supported by USPHS grant AI 05664.
[2] Recipient of a Dernham Postdoctoral Fellowship from the American Cancer Society.

ISBN 0-12-213950-X

Gel filtration of concentrated supernatant through Sephadex G-150 showed that the suppressor molecule eluted in a narrow peak reflecting a MW of 90-95,000 daltons whereas the helper activity eluted at a position of 20-30,000 daltons. The MW of the suppressive component was also determined by running ^{35}S-methionine-labelled supernatant on SDS-gel electrophoresis after absorption to and elution from SRBC. Again, a strongly enriched band of about 90K daltons was observed.

II. HEMOLYTIC PLAQUE ASSAY FOR CON-A-ACTIVATED T CELLS

A recently described modification of the Jerne plaque assay permits the detection of any cell secreting a product for which an antiserum is available (Gronowicz et al., 1976). The method employed SRBC coated with Staphylococcal protein A in a plaquing medium which also contained rabbit anti-mouse Ig, guinea pig complement and Ig-secreting mouse plasmacytoma cells. Plaques developed around a fraction of the cells, presumably as a consequence of Ig-anti-Ig complexes binding to the protein A-coated RBC and fixing complement.

Since Con A-activated T cells release a variety of products, including helper and suppressor substances, it seemed feasible that an antiserum could be generated against the Con A-induced culture supernatant containing the products, which might then be used to detect T cells secreting those products in a similar plaque assay. Accordingly, rabbits were immunized with concentrated culture supernatants and their sera tested for activity in a plaque assay of Con A-activated mouse spleen cells.

For the assay, cells were harvested, washed twice in cold BSS and adjusted to the desired concentration. Four tenths ml of 0.5% agar in BSS containing 0.5% DEAE-Dextran was added to 3 ml test tubes, which were kept at 46°C in a water bath. Thereafter, 0.025 ml of the indicator erythrocytes diluted 1:4 in BSS, 0.05 ml of the lymphocyte cell suspension, 0.025 ml of guinea pig serum diluted 1:5 in BSS and 0.025 ml of rabbit anti-supernatant serum (appropriately diluted) were added to each tube. The ingredients were mixed and evenly spread on 9 cm plastic petri dishes, which were then incubated for 1 h or 18 h (at which time fresh C was added at 37°C and scored for plaques.

Each of two rabbits injected four times subcutaneously with 1.0 ml of five-fold concentrated Con A supernatant produced antiserum which developed plaques by spleen cells cultured for 48 h in the presence of 10 μg/ml of Con A. The two sera differed in potency, and plaque formation by Con A-activated lymphocytes was dependent on the concentration of the developing serum. Omission of either the anti-supernatant serum or complement from the assay abrogated the appearance of plaques. Negative results were also obtained when serum from normal rabbits was substituted for the anti-supernatant serum, demonstrating the dependence of plaque formation on anti-supernatant antibody. Under the best conditions, 1-2% of cultured spleen cells (2-4% of T cells) formed plaques. In assessing the significance of this figure, it should be realized that the efficiency of the technique, as applied to the detection of Ig-secreting plasmacytoma cells, is not high (Gronowicz _et al._, 1976). In that study, only 10-70% of cells from various plasmacytomas formed plaques with anti-mouse Ig developing reagents.

III. NATURE OF THE PLAQUE-FORMING CELLS

The most immediate priority was to establish the identity of the PFC. For this purpose, the following experiments were carried out.

1. Cultured cells were assayed for the Thy-1 antigen by an indirect immunofluorescent technique and plaqued immediately after staining. One-tenth ml of the mixture was deposited as a drop on a microscope slide and a cover slip immediately put on the drop. This procedure gave a thin layer of agar which facilitated the scoring of stained lymphocytes in the plaques. About 50% of lymphocytes in the centers of plaques stained strongly for Thy-1. That this figure isn't higher can probably be ascribed to capping and internalization of Thy-1 during incubation at 37° in the plaque assay, as well as to the variable expression of Thy-1 by cultured T cells.

2. Cultured spleen cells were tested with anti-Thy-1 serum and complement, with a monoclonal anti-Ly-2.2 serum (from Dr. U. Hammerling) and complement or with complement alone. Dead cells were removed by Ficoll-Hypaque density gradient centrifugation prior to plaquing. Treatment with anti-Thy-1 or with anti-Ly-2.2 virtually eliminated PFC (>95% depletion) but had no effect on the polyclonal response to LPS.

3. Spleen cells were depleted of B cells by adherence to plastic surfaces coated with rabbit anti-mouse Ig antibody. The non-adherent population (less than 5% Ig-positive by fluorescence) was then cultured and assayed for PFC. Removal

of B cells doubled the number of PFC per culture, providing additional evidence that at least the majority of PFC detected by this procedure are T cells.

4. Absorption of the anti-supernatant serum with a polyvalent mouse Ig immunoadsorbent had no effect on the numbers of PFC, indicating that Ig-secreting cells were not being detected in the assay.

5. Selective T cell mitogens (Con A and PHA) induced vigorous PFC responses, whereas LPS, a B cell mitogen, did not. If B cells were being detected in the assay, it is very unlikely that LPS would have had no effect on the PFC response.

6. About 50% of spleen cells reacted with the anti-supernatant antibody in an indirect immunofluorescence assay, whereas 80% of spleen cells depleted of B cells were positive. These findings indicate that the antiserum detects products on cell surfaces and that at least the majority of reactive cells are T cells.

7. The lymphocytes which bound anti-supernatant antibody formed rosettes with SRBC coated with protein A. The rosetted cells were separated from the residual population, and the two fractions were cultured and plaqued. All the PFC were in the rosetted population. Since this population is almost exclusively T cells (from the fluorescent assay described above), the findings are consistent with the PFC being T cells.

8. Spleen cells from Balb/c mice sensitized to L929 cells were plated on monolayers of target cells. Adherent cells (putative T killers; >98% Thy-1+) plaqued at high efficiency (1.6×10^4 PFC/10^6 cells), whereas non-adherent cells yielded only 400 PFC/10^6 cells.

9. Enriched T cells were cultured for 8 days with Con A plus Con A-induced culture supernatant (which contains T cell growth factor). All surviving cells stained for Thy-1 and >2% produced plaques.

10. Rabbit antiserum against highly purified human lymphotoxin (LT) (Boulos _et al._, 1974) was used in a plaque assay of normal human PBL cultured for various times with different concentrations of Con A. A very rapid, dose-dependent increase in PFC was observed, reaching peak levels of about 1400 PFC/10^6 PBL, followed by a sharp decline to background

levels within hours. Since it has been shown that normal human B cells do not secrete LT (Rosenau et al., 1979), these results provide additional support for the T cell nature of PFC in this assay. They further illustrate the power of the technique for clonal and kinetic study of lymphokine production by T cells.

REFERENCES

Boulas, G.N., Rosenau, W., and Goldberg, M.L. (1974). J. Immunol. 112, 1347.

Gronowicz, E., Coutinho, A., and Melchers, F. (1976). Eur. J. Immunol. 6, 588.

Primi, D., Lewis, G.K., and Goodman, J.W. (1979). Eur. J. Immunol., in press.

Rosenau, W., Stites, D., and Jemtrud, S. (1979). Cell. Immunol. 43, 235.

DISCUSSION

PICK: I want to congratulate Goodman on being the first investigator to have developed a plaque technique for lymphokine producing T cells. Has Goodman tried to use this reverse passive haemolysis technique for detecting lymphokines in the supernatant itself? Judging from other systems, such as the titration of bacterial toxins, this appears to be a very sensitive technique which could provide an alternative to lymphokine radioimmunoassays.

GOODMAN: We have assayed antisera for reactivity with the supernatants by standard immunochemical procedures for purpose of determining that appropriate antibodies were present, but not by passive haemolysis. I can see no reason why it should not work, but it would be worth-while only with monospecific antisera; one antiserum obviously has multiple specificities. The comparative sensitivity of this technique and radioimmunoassay would have to be directly determined.

WAKSMAN: I would echo Pick in saying that this is a major technical advance. It is the first plaquing technique which will permit us to demonstrate (and enumerate) cells forming any particular LK.

PURIFICATION OF MURINE THYMOCYTE STIMULATING FACTOR[1]

Giovanni Di Sabato
Muzaffer Altin

Department of Molecular Biology
Vanderbilt University
Nashville, Tennessee

I. INTRODUCTION

TSF[2] is a factor produced in vitro by murine lymphocytes of spleen or lymph nodes stimulated in various ways (Di Sabato et al, 1975; Chen and Di Sabato, 1976; Chen and Di Sabato, 1977; Di Sabato et al., 1977; Di Sabato et al., 1978). TSF confers to murine thymocytes at least some of the characteristics of mature lymphocytes: the ability to respond to PHA or Con A with the dose-response profile characteristic of mature lymphocytes (Chen and Di Sabato, 1977; Di Sabato et al., 1977), the ability to participate in a MLR in vitro (Chen and Di Sabato, 1976) and to mount a graft vs. host reaction when injected into an appropriate hybrid (Chen and Di Sabato, 1977). Moreover, thymocytes incubated with TSF-containing supernatants show an increase in the expression of the H-2 antigens, while the expression of the TL antigen (in TL^+ strains) is decreased (Di Sabato et al, 1979). The experiments reported in this communication deal with the purification of the activity enhancing the PHA-responsiveness of thymocytes from the bulk of the proteins present in supernatants of MLC.

[1]*This work was supported by grant No. PCM 78-15987 from the National Science Foundation.*

[2]*Abbreviations: TSF, Thymocyte Stimulating Factor; PHA, Phytohemagglutinin; Con A, Concanavalin A; MLC, Mixed Lymphocyte Culture; MLR, Mixed Lymphocyte Reaction.*

ISBN 0-12-213950-X

II. RESULTS

In most experiments the amount of proteins was determined by the radioactivity of [^{35}S] methionine incorporated during the MLC. Lyophilized supernatants of MLC dissolved in 3 ml of water were applied to Sephadex G-100 columns eluted with 0.02 M Tris HCl buffer, pH 7.2. Most of the TSF activity (as measured by the enhancement of the PHA-responsiveness of murine thymocytes) eluted over a broad range of molecular weights with peaks at about 50,000-55,000 and 30,000-32,000 daltons (Chen and Di Sabato, 1977). Part (about 60%) of the proteins (measured as [^{35}S] methionine-containing material) was eluted in a sharp peak with a molecular weight of about 150,000, while the remaining 40% was eluted with the TSF activity.

The TSF activity-containing material obtained from Sephadex G-100 (fraction I) was concentrated in an Amicon ultrafiltration cell equipped with a PM 10 membrane. With this step more than 60% of the [^{35}S] methionine-containing material was removed, while only 25% of the TSF activity was lost. The concentrated material was applied to a Phenyl-Sepharose-CL-4B column and eluted with 25% saturated ammonium sulfate, followed by a linear gradient in which ammonium sulfate saturation was decreased from 25% to 0 and ethylene glycol concentration was increased from 0 to 50%. Finally, the column was eluted with a 50% solution of ethylene glycol to deabsorb most of the TSF activity.

The TSF activity-containing fractions from the Phenyl-Sepharose column (fraction II) were pooled and applied to a Con A-Sepharose column. The column was eluted first with 0.02M Tris HCl buffer, pH 7.2, and subsequently with 1M α-methyl-D-mannoside. Most of the [^{35}S] methionine-containing material was eluted with Tris buffer, while most of the TSF activity was eluted with α-methyl-D-mannoside (fraction III). The TSF activity, however, was eluted in several peaks. Occasionally, some TSF activity was eluted also with Tris buffer. This behavior indicates a certain degree of molecular heterogeneity in the amount of terminal mannose and/or glucose residues (for which Con A has specific affinity) in TSF.

In separate experiments, the proteins present in the supernatants of MLC were labeled with [^{125}I]. The recoveries of radioactivity were then measured at each purification step. As shown in Table I, the recoveries of [^{35}S] methionine-labeled material and of [^{125}I]-labeled material closely agree, thus indicating that the measurement of [^{35}S] radioactivity is an accurate determination of the amount of proteins present in the system.

TABLE I. SUMMARY OF PURIFICATION OF TSF ACTIVITY

	Total activity	*Total protein*		*Specific activity*
	([^{3}H] thymidine)	[^{35}S]	[^{125}I]	*(based on [^{35}S] material)*
Crude Supernatant	100	100	100	1
Sephadex G-100	97	40	38	2.5
Amicon (PM10)	75	15	9	5
Phenyl-Sepharose	24	2	3	12
Con A-Sepharose	18	0.05	0.06	360

Electrofocusing of [^{35}S]-labeled or [^{125}I]-labeled crude supernatants of MLC showed 5-6 major peaks. Electrofocusing of [^{35}S]-labeled fraction III of TSF showed that both TSF activity and [^{35}S]-labeled material focused in two peaks with pI about 5.1 and 4.7. Experiments carried out with [^{125}I]-labeled material also showed two peaks with pI 5.1 and 4.7.

In conclusion, the work presented in this communication shows that a considerable purification (about 360 fold) of TSF activity from the bulk of the proteins present in supernatants of MLC has been achieved. The recovery of TSF activity was about 18%. Any comparison of the degree of purification achieved in this work with that achieved by other workers, should take into consideration the fact that the starting preparations used in this work contain no added proteins.

REFERENCES

D.-M. Chen and G. Di Sabato, Cell. Immunol. 22, 211 (1976).
D.-M. Chen and G. Di Sabato, Cell. Immunol. 30, 195 (1977).
G. Di Sabato, D.-M. Chen and J. W. Erickson. Cell. Immunol. 17, 495 (1975).
G. Di Sabato, M. Altin and D.-M. Chen, Cell. Immunol. 30, 204 (1977).
G. Di Sabato, D.-M. Chen and M. Altin, Cell. Immunol. 35, 340 (1978).
G. Di Sabato, E. K. Moraes and M. Altin, Cell. Immunol., In press (1979).

GENERATION OF AN IMMUNOSUPPRESSIVE ACTIVITY BY ALTERATION OF A PURIFIED IMMUNOENHANCING FACTOR

Arnold S. Rubin, Henry L. Mulcahy and A. Bruce MacDonald

Departments of Microbiology, University of Texas,
Austin, Texas and Harvard University School
of Public Health, Boston, Massachusetts

Herpesvirus saimiri inoculated into owl monkeys (*Aotus trivirgatus*) causes leukemia and lymphoma. Cultured peripheral blood lymphocytes isolated from leukemic monkeys have the properties of T cells, but not B cells, as determined by a variety of techniques (1-3). The supernatant fluid from these cultures contains a factor which non-specifically augments the plaque-forming cell (PFC) response of DBA/2 mouse B cells to sheep erythrocytes (SRBC) *in vitro* (3). The mediator, owl monkey enhancing factor (OMEF), must be added to Mishell-Dutton cultures at nanogram concentrations on day 2 of a 5-day culture period for its activity to be manifest. Here we report the generation and partial characterization of an immunosuppressive activity produced by alteration of OMEF.

RESULTS AND DISCUSSION

OMEF was purified to homogeneity by a combination of ammonium sulfate precipitation, DEAE-cellulose chromatography, gel filtration over Sephadex G-150 and polyacrylamide disc-gel electrophoresis (PAGE)(3). Careful analysis of gels used to purify OMEF revealed the presence of a material which was capable of suppressing the anti-SRBC PFC response *in vitro*. This inhibitory activity, owl monkey suppressor factor (OMSF), was widely separated electrophoretically from the enhancing factor. By using ^{125}I-labelled preparations of OMEF, in addition to confirming the location of the enhancing mediator, we were able to detect a small peak of radioactivity in the exact location where suppressor activity had been found in the gel eluate. Early observations indicated that aged, or frozen and thawed preparations of OMEF were markedly reduced in enhancing activity and suggested a possible alteration in biological

ISBN 0-12-213950-X

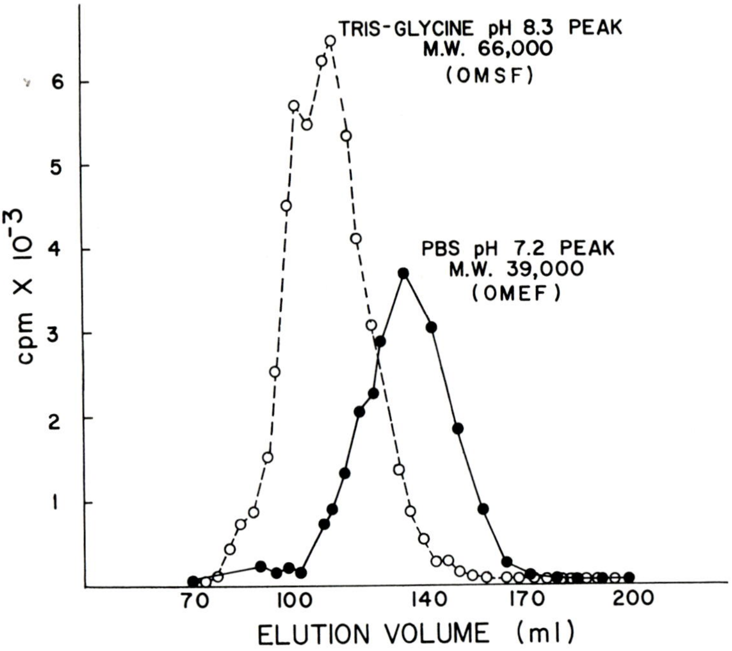

FIGURE 1. Generation of OMSF from OMEF by buffer dialysis.

properties. Indeed, the effect of repeated freeze-thaw cycles on OMEF was a ten-fold enrichment in radiolabelled OMSF in a region of the gel known to contain the inhibitor. More dramatic results were obtained by buffer dialysis of a purified preparation of radiolabelled OMEF. Figure 1 demonstrates that an aliquot of ^{125}I-OMEF, dialyzed *vs.* PBS, pH 7.2, and then subjected to gel filtration over a column of Sephadex G-150 equilibrated in the same buffer, eluted at a position consistent with its molecular weight of ∿39,000d (3). The radiolabel in the sample treated in an identical manner with Tris-glycine buffer, pH 8.3, eluted with molecules of ∿66,000d. There was no significant radiolabel present at the 39,000d position indicating that a complete shift in molecular weight had occurred. When the 66,000d (OMSF) peak was tested for suppressor activity, it was found to inhibit the anti-SRBC PFC response of DBA/2 spleen cells by 50-70% when added at a concentration of 0.3-0.6 ng/culture on day 0 of a 5-day culture period.

Our data suggested that OMEF was capable of associating into molecules of OMSF. To further demonstrate the interchange of molecules between these two species, ^{125}I-OMEF was mixed with an unlabelled pool (Sephadex G-150 eluate) known to contain both factors. Figure 2A shows that when labelled OMEF

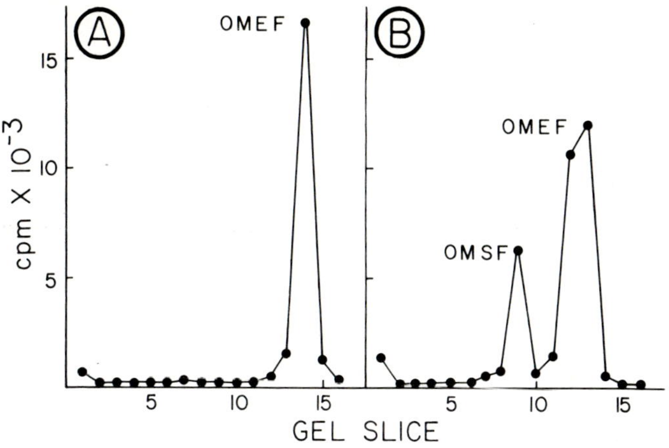

FIGURE 2. Association of ^{125}I-OMEF with unlabelled OMSF.

was subjected to PAGE, one rapidly migrating radiolabelled species was observed. In contrast, PAGE of the mixed preparation resulted in two peaks of radiolabel with electrophoretic mobilities characteristic of OMEF and OMSF (Figure 2B). The peak OMEF fractions contained ∿2X the radiolabel of the OMSF gel slice. But the concentration of proteins eluted from the OMEF and OMSF gel sections containing peak activity were quite comparable. Based on these data and the molecular weight of each mediator, we have determined that the specific activities (cpm/mM) of OMEF and OMSF in the gel were identical. These results suggest (a) ^{125}I-OMEF can spontaneously distribute itself equally between the two unlabelled species, and (b) OMSF is composed of two non-covalently bound OMEF molecules. Consistent with this hypothesis is the observation that OMSF binds to antiserum raised specifically against OMEF, and competitively inhibits the binding of OMEF to this antiserum. Moreover, each factor has been shown to be a glycoprotein with an isoelectric point of pH 6.5. We conclude from these data that a T cell-derived mediator can either augment or suppress antibody synthesis depending on its molecular configuration.

REFERENCES

1. Wallen, W.C., Neubauer, R.C., Rabin, H. and Cicmanec, J.L. *J. Nat. Cancer Inst. 51*:961, 1973.
2. Wallen, W.C., Russell, H., Neubauer, R.C. and Rabin, H. *J. Med. Prim. 3*:41, 1974.
3. MacDonald, A.B., Fraser, C.E.O. and Rubin, A.S. *Immunology 34*:137, 1978.

DISCUSSION

WAKSMAN: This finding by Rubin et al. is reminiscent of the increased "tolerogenicity" of larger or more aggregated B cell antigens, for B cells and Con A at higher concentrations or at higher states of aggregation for T cells.

MAURER: It seems appropriate to express a word of caution as to the use of ^{3}H-thymidine (^{3}H-Tdr) when one wants to measure cell proliferation. We ran into several problems when we tried to test endogenous inhibitors on bone-marrow cell suspensions incubated with ^{3}H-Tdr. A subsequent search through the literature revealed that one can collect at least 14 different ^{3}H-Tdr antifacts which can stimulate cell proliferation, e.g. enzymes are known which metabolize ^{3}H-Tdr. ^{3}H-Tdr can unspecifically bind to TCA precipitable proteins. Cold Tdr may dilute the Tdr pool size. ^{3}H-Tdr must be transported through the cell membrane and be phosphorylated to get incorporated into DNA; these processes can be inhibited or stimulated by added factors. ^{3}H-Tdr may be heavily incorporated into mycoplasma and not into cellular DNA. ^{3}H-Tdr may be reutilized from degraded ^{3}H-DNA of dead cells.

To me it seems, therefore, absolutely necessary to make sure that the cells under test are multiplying in fact. For that reason we have developed a T and B lymphocyte and a granulocyte-colony assay using glass capillary tubes. With these methods we have extracted from calf thymus a factor of < 1,400 d, probably a peptide, which inhibits T lymphocyte but not granulocyte colony growth, which is non-cytotoxic and reversible as to its inhibitor activity at the nanogram level.

WOOD: Rubin's figures did not show biological activity. How precisely do the biological activity and radioactivity coincide?

RUBIN: Biological activity, either enhancing or suppressor activity, was always found to co-chromatograph (on columns of Sephadex G-150 or DEAE-cellulose) or co-electrophorese (on polyacrylamide gels) with the corresponding radioiodinated factor.

SCHIMPL: Would Rubin please specify his assay system for enhancement and suppression? Would it be possible to interpret his results by assuming that denatured enhancing factor blocks the receptor for native enhancing factor? Or do enhancement and suppression act at different levels?

RUBIN: The soluble factors derived from supernatants of cultured leukemic owl monkey T cells were tested for biological activity in SRBC-stimulated Mishell-Dutton spleen cell cultures. OMEF augmented the PFC response by 3 - 5-fold when added at 15 - 30 ng/culture on day 2 of a 5-day culture period. OMSF, generated from OMEF, produced a 50 - 70 % inhibition of the anti-SRBC PFC response when added at 0.3 - 0.6 ng/culture on day 0 of 5-day culture period. While OMEF can replace T cell helper activity in nylon wool purified B cell cultures, we have not, as yet, tested the effects of OMSF on the PFC response of T cell-depleted cultures of lymphocytes.

We do not feel that OMSF is generated by denaturation of OMEF. Rather, our data indicate that OMSF is an aggregate, probably a dimer of OMEF. OMEF (39,000 daltons) can readily associate, under non-denaturing conditions, into OMSF molecules; OMSF (66,000 daltons), at least in SDS-polyacrylamide gels, can dissociate into molecules of 39,000 daltons mol. wt. with electrophoretic mobilities characteristic of OMEF activity. Moreover, OMEF and OMSF are serologically cross-reactive as determined by radioimmunoassay.

We have no data at present regarding the mechanism of action, target cell or receptors involved in binding of OMSF. We know that OMEF can directly affect B cell PFC responses. The fact that OMEF and OMSF have different optimal addition times may suggest that they have different target cells and/or bind to different cellular receptors since by day 2 of culture, the cells affected by OMSF or day 0 are probably in an altered state of reactivity of differentiation, i. e. by the time OMEF is most effective.

ACTIVATION OF MOUSE SPLENIC SUPPRESSOR CELLS BY ENDOGENOUS PROSTAGLANDIN

David R. Webb
Kenneth Wieder
Thomas J. Rogers
Irene Nowowiejski

Department of Cell Biology
Roche Institute of Molecular Biology
Nutley, New Jersey

I. PROSTAGLANDIN ACTIVATED SUPPRESSOR CELLS

We have recently demonstrated that the mouse spleen contains a population of glass-adherent T cells which, when stimulated by prostaglandin E_1 or E_2 suppress mitogen induced DNA synthesis in non-adherent T lymphocytes. The production of prostaglandin by mitogen activated non-adherent T lymphocytes is also capable of activating the glass-adherent T suppressor cell (1,2). This had led us to postulate the existence of a regulatory feedback loop in which activated lymphocytes release prostaglandin which, in turn stimulates the prostaglandin sensitive suppressor cell. This suppressor cell then releases a soluble lymphokine which can suppress DNA synthesis in the activated lymphocytes thus closing the loop (2,3). The present communication deals with the nature of the prostaglandin induced suppressor. A list of the biological and biochemical properties of the suppressor is presented in Table 1.

Original molecular weight estimates suggested the suppressor had two forms: M.W. 38,000 and $\leq$5000. Refractionation of the material under high ionic strength conditions (1 M acetic acid, 3 M pyridine) on Sephadex G-25 suggested the previous estimates were not correct. Figure 1 shows fractionation of the suppressor on BioGel P-2 in 0.5 M acetic acid 25% methanol. Under these conditions the M.W. appears to be 500.

ISBN 0-12-213950-X

Table 1

BIOCHEMICAL & BIOLOGICAL PROPERTIES
OF PGE_2 INDUCED GAT SUPPRESSOR

1. HEAT STABLE (100°C, 10 MIN)
2. SENSITIVE TO:
   A. TPCK TRYPSIN
   B. PRONASE
   C. PROTEASE K
   D. CARBOXY PEPTIDASE A (DFP)
   E. LEU-AMINOPEPTIDASE
   F. CLOSTRIPAIN (ARG-SPECIFIC)
   G. CHYMOTRYPSIN
3. NOT SENSITIVE TO:
   A. DNASE
   B. RNASE
4. MOLECULAR WEIGHT 500-1000 DALTONS (G-25 SEPHADEX, BIOGEL P-2)
5. MODERATELY HYDROPHOBIC (REVERSED PHASE LIQUID CHROMATOGRAPHY)
6. SENSITIVE TO BOROHYDRIDE
7. INHIBITS DNA SYNTHESIS IN PHA STIMULATED NON-GLASS ADHERENT SPLENIC T LYMPHOCYTES
   A. NO EFFECT ON EARLY RNA OR PROTEIN SYNTHESIS
8. INHIBITS LPS INDUCED DNA SYNTHESIS
9. INHIBITS MLR
10. INHIBITS ACROSS HISTOCOMPATIBILITY SPECIFICITIES
11. GENERATED IN THE PRESENCE OF CYCLOHEXIMIDE
12. APPEARS WITHIN HOURS FOLLOWING EXPOSURE OF GAT LYMPHOCYTES TO PGE_2.

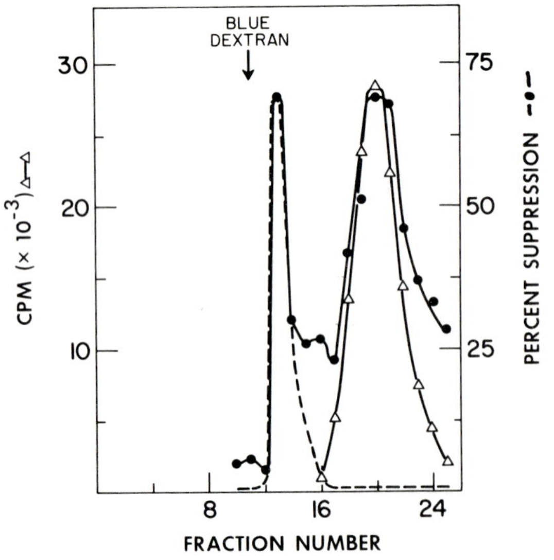

Fig. 1. Fractionation of suppressor on Sephadex G-25

This peptide has now been purified to apparent homogeneity by the use of fluorescence detection and reversed phase high performance chromatography (RPLC) on Lichrosorb RP-18 (acetic acid 0.5 M, pyridine 1.0 M) (4). Figure 2a and b shows the results of experiments in which supernatants from PGE_2-stimulated suppressor cells prepared as previously described (3), were fractionated by RPLC. Figure 2a shows the results of a single passage over the column. The peptide is eluted with 35% propanol. In Fig. 2b are shown the results of a chromatography run in which 500 mls of supernatant which had been purified previously by one passage over the RP-18 column, was rechromatographed on a RP-18 column. The biologically active material migrates as a single homogeneous peak. This peak appears to consist of a single molecular species as assessed by N-terminal labeling using ^{3}H-Dansyl chloride.

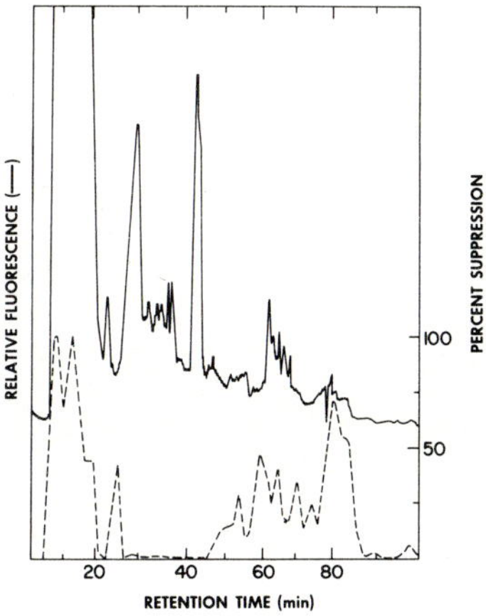

Figure 2a

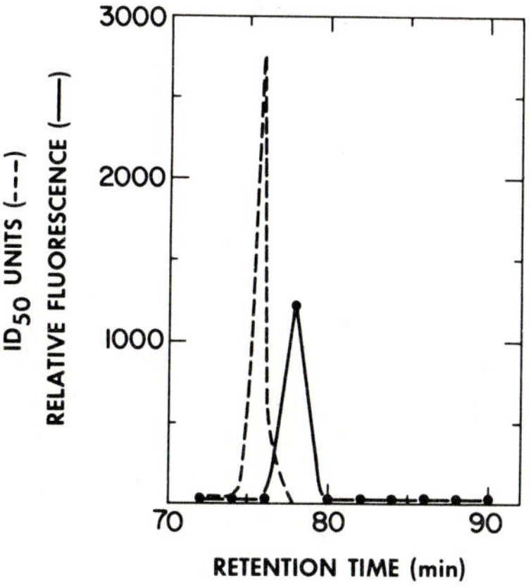

Figure 2b

In conclusion, we have shown that PGE_2 which is itself immunosuppressive, can induce a glass-adherent T cell to release a highly suppressive peptide. This peptide appears to be unlike any other previously reported lymphokine and has now been purified to near homogeneity using high performance liquid chromatographic techniques.

1. Webb, D.R. & Jamieson, A.T. Cell. Immunol. 24:45 (1976)
2. Webb, D.R. & Nowowiejski, I. Cell. Immunol. 41:72 (1978)
3. Webb, D.R., Rogers, T.J. & Nowowiejski, I. New York Academy of Sciences (in press)
4. Stein, S. The Peptides (E. Gross, ed.) (in press)

BIOCHEMICAL CHARACTERIZATION OF SUPPRESSIVE IMMUNOGLOBULIN BINDING FACTOR (IBF)

Wolf Herman Fridman
Mireille Joskowicz
Chantal Rabourdin-Combe
Catherine Neauport-Sautès

Laboratoire d'Immunologie cellulaire
Institut de Recherches Scientifiques sur le Cancer
Villejuif, France

Antibody production by B cells to T dependent antigens is regulated by antigen specific factors acting in the early phase of the response and by non specific factors acting in the late phase of the response (1). Among the non specific factors, Fridman and Golstein (2) have described a factor, named Immunoglobulin Binding Factor, which suppresses primary and secondary *in vitro* antibody response to T dependent and T independent antigens, by acting directly on already differentiated B cells (3-5). IBF has the property to bind specifically to the Fc portion of IgG and represents the soluble form of the Fcγ receptor expressed on activated T cells (6,7).

At the present time, the prerequisite for a better knowledge of the mode of action of these factors will probably be their biochemical characterization. Most of them are difficult to isolate since they are: (i) produced in small quantity by an heterogeneous population of T cells and (ii) very labile. In this context, the facts that IBF: (i) was shown to be produced by an Fcγ receptor positive thymoma line, L-5178-Y, and recently by hybridomas between T-lymphoma cells and activated T cells (8) and (ii) is rather stable and can be purified on IgG immunoadsorbents, allowed us to undertake its biochemical characterization.

Acknowledgements. This work was supported by grants from INSERM (ATP n° 59-78-91), DGRST (ATP n° 76-7-0965), and CNRS (ATP n° A-651-2890.

ISBN 0-12-213950-X

Using supernatants of L-5178-Y thymoma cells internally labelled by *in vitro* incorporation of radioactive amino acids and/or sugars, we could show that both the suppressive and IgG binding activities eluted at peaks of 140 000 d and 300 000 d (9). However, on SDS polyacrylamide gels, after precipitation with antigen antibody complexes, IBF was found in a single peak of 80 000 d which could be dissociated, in the presence of mercaptoethanol into units of 38-40 000 d and 18-20 000 d. These two bands were also found on SDS polyacrylamide gels of IBF prepared by passage of supernatants of alloantigen activated T cells on IgG immunoadsorbents and radiolabelled with ^{125}I (10). We therefore concluded that IBF is a glycoprotein, of 80 000 d which contains chains of 40 000 d and 20 000 d and which exists, in the supernatants under polymeric forms.

Using internally labelled IBF, we could show that IBF, as revealed by its ability to bind IgG, is sensitive to proteolytic enzymes (pronase, trypsin) and resistant to neuraminidase. Furthermore, the presence of the 38-40 000 d chain was necessary for the binding to IgG (10).

T cell factors have been shown to bear Ia determinants. In this context, we found that when purified IBF was applied on immunoadsorbents of antisera directed against the I region products, the acid eluates suppressed the *in vitro* antibody response to SRBC and contained the two chains characteristics of IBF (39 000 d and 18 000 d) (10). As a control no suppressive activity and no bands on SDS polyacrylamide gels were found when IBF was applied on immunoadsorbents of anti - H-2D antisera. These data indicate that IBF bears, or is associated to Ia determinants.

In an attempt to obtain clones of T cells producing continuously IBF, hybridomas were prepared between an Fcγ receptor negative T lymphoma line and alloantigen activated T cells. The hybridomas and their clone derivatives bear receptors specific for the Fc portion of IgG, as determined by rosette formation, and produce suppressive IBF which can be purified on immunoadsorbents of IgG (8). Such hybridomas may provide a useful homogeneous source to undertake characterization of IBF by other biochemical and immunochemical techniques.

REFERENCES

1. Rabourdin-Combe, C., and Fridman, W. H., *Annales d'Immunol. 129 C,* 591 (1978).
2. Fridman, W. H., and Golstein, P., *Cell Immunol. 11,* 442 (1974).
3. Gisler, R. H., and Fridman, W. H., *J. Exp. Med. 142,* 507 (1975).
4. Gisler, R. H., and Fridman, W. H., *Cell Immunol. 23,* 99 (1976).
5. Yagello, M., Rabourdin-Combe, C., and Fridman, W. H., *Transpl. Proc. 11,* 895 (1979).
6. Guimezanes, A., Fridman, W. H., Gisler, R. H., and Kourilsky, F. M., *Eur. J. Immunol. 6,* 69 (1976).
7. Fridman, W. H., Neauport-Sautès, C., and Gisler, R. H., *in* "Protides of the biological Fluids" (Peeters, ed.) *25,* 669 (1978).
8. Neauport-Sautès, C., Rabourdin-Combe, C., and Fridman, W. H., *Nature 277,* 656 (1979).
9. Neauport-Sautès, C., and Fridman, W. H., *J. Immunol. 119,* 1269 (1977).
10. Joskowicz, M., Rabourdin-Combe, C., Neauport-Sautès, C., and Fridman, W. H., *J. Immunol. 121,* 777 (1978).

DISCUSSION

PICK: Has Fridman tested whether IBF might be identical with a Cl fragment? Was this done by using an anti-Cl antiserum?

FRIDMAN: IBF interferes with Cl by inhibiting the binding of Cl_9 to the Fc fragment of IgG. Therefore, we investigated whether IBF could be an analog of Cl_q. By physiochemical comparisons, IBF was clearly different from Cl_q. In answer to Pick's second question, IBF does not react with anti-Cl serum.

THE ROLE OF SOLUBLE MEDIATOR IN THE DIFFERENTION OF CYTOTOXIC CELLS IN PRIMARY AND SECONDARY CULTURES

Christopher S. Henney
Masaji Okada

Program in Basic Immunology
Fred Hutchinson Cancer Research Center
Seattle, Washington

Within 10-12 hours of establishment of a murine mixed lymphocyte culture (MLC), a soluble mediator was produced which was capable of augmenting primary cytotoxic responses to alloantigen (1). The mediator produced was not H-2 restricted. Thus, supernatants harvested from cultures of C57BL/6 + CBA/J augmented the primary response of mice of all H-2 haplotypes (including C57BL/6; DBA/2; BALB/c and CBA/J) to all alloantigens tested. The MLC-induced factor did not induce cytotoxic T lymphocyte (CTL) responses in primary cultures in the absence of alloantigen, and the amplified response seen in the presence of antigen was specific. The factor did not therefore appear to function by polyclonal activation of cytotoxic precursor cells.

Primary cytotoxic responses to u.v. irradiated and to sonicated spleen cell populations could be induced in the presence of the MLC-induced soluble factor, but not in its absence (Fig 1). On the other hand, neither u.v. irradiated nor sonicated cells could induce mediator production when such cells were used as stimulators in an MLC (1). It thus seems likely that this deficiency is the basis of the well documented failure of u.v. irradiated and sonicated stimulator cells to induce primary cytotoxic responses (2, 3).

The amplifying effects of the MLC-induced factor were distinctive from, but synergistic with, those of 2-mercaptoethanol. Production of the amplifying mediator did not require cell division, but was dependent upon the presence of Lyt 1+ cells. On the other hand, Lyt 2+ cells were not needed for mediator production, but served as a target cell population on which the factor exerted its action (1).

It thus appears that the production of a soluble mediator during a primary MLC is needed in order to produce an optimal cytotoxic response to alloantigen. Thus, that Lyt 1+ cells are needed to elicit optimal responses from the Lyt 2+3+ compartment.

We were interested in asking whether such mediators were also produced on stimulation of alloantigen-primed ("memory") cell populations and, if so, whether they played a role in the differentiation of

ISBN 0-12-213950-X

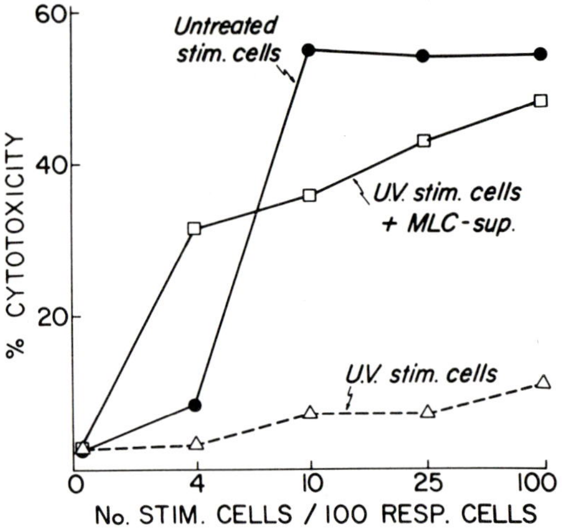

Fig. 1. Induction of primary cytotoxic response by MLC-induced soluble factor.

memory cells into CTL. The latter issue is an intriguing one, because of the observation that u.v. treated spleen cells can provide an adequate alloantigenic stimulus to memory cells but do not induce augmenting factors from normal spleen cells.

In studies on the appearance of augmenting factors following stimulation of alloantigen-primed (memory) cell populations we observed:

(i) that mediator production occurred earlier (peak 9 hrs) than during primary MLC (peak 24 hrs), and

(ii) that less alloantigen was needed to elicit mediator production from memory cell populations than from normal (unprimed) spleen cells.

Furthermore, in keeping with earlier reports (4, 5), supernatants from secondary MLC were capable of causing the direct differentiation of memory cells into CTL whereas supernatants from primary MLC did so with much less efficiency (Table I).

Thus, if augmenting factors are induced in secondary MLC cultures they can amplify CTL formation. Is mediator production then a prerequisite for CTL differentiation? In an attempt to address this issue we confronted an observation made earlier by Cerrottini et al. (6): that memory cell populations induced in vivo could respond to a wider range of alloantigenic stimuli than could memory cell populations induced in long-term mixed lymphocyte cultures. This is clearly shown in Table II, where memory cells harvested after in vivo priming with alloantigen form CTL in response to heated (45°, 60 min) and to sonicated spleen cell populations in addition to those subjected to u.v. irradiation. In contrast, memory cell populations harvested from long-term MLC responded only to untreated spleen cells and to those subjected to u.v. irradiation.

TABLE I

Response of "memory" cells to 1° and 2° MLC supernatants

BL/6 Responder Cells	Augmenting Factor	% Specific Cytolysis 12:1
Normal	None	1
	from 1° MLC	0
	from 2° MLC	-1
In vitro memory	None	8.0
(BL/6 + BALB/c_{mit} 14 days)	from 1° MLC	21.2
	from 2° MLC	41.0
In vivo memory	None	3.3
(BL/6 2 months after P815)	from 1° MLC	12.5
	from 2° MLC	38.5

Augmenting factors:

1° BL/6 + CBA/J_{mit}

2° BL/6 + CBA/J in vivo 4 wks → ( ) + CBA/J_{mit}

A satisfying rationale for this phenomenon was reached when the same memory cell populations and alloantigenic stimuli that had been used to follow CTL formation were used to generate augmenting factors (Table III). Although normal spleen cells failed to make mediator in response to u.v. irradiated spleen cells, memory cell populations did so readily. Furthermore, memory cell populations harvested following in vivo priming formed mediator in response to heated and sonicated spleen cell preparations whereas the memory cell populations harvested from long-term MLC did not. There was then complete concordance between CTL formation and mediator production.

TABLE II

RESPONSE OF MEMORY CELLS AFTER IN VITRO OR IN VIVO PRIMING

BL/6 Responder Cells	Stimulating Antigen 5×10^6 Cells	Cytolysis of H-2[d] Targets 12:1
In vitro memory	BALB/c spleen$_{mit}$	64
	u.v. treated	59
(BL/6 + BALB/c 14 days)	heated (45°, 60')	5
	sonicated	2
	none	9
In vivo memory	BALB/c spleen$_{mit}$	81
	u.v. treated	67
(BL/6 3 months after P815 I.P.)	heated	69
	sonicated	24
	none	4
Normal	BALB/c spleen$_{mit}$	22
	u.v. treated	3
	heated	5
	sonicated	-1
	none	0

These findings raise the interesting possibility that the failure of memory cell populations induced *in vitro* to respond to either heated or sonicated spleen cells, lies not in the failure to trigger CTL precursor cells but in a failure to generate soluble mediators within these populations. It remains to be established whether, in memory cell cultures as in primary MLC, mediator production is dependent on cells of the Lyt 1+ phenotype.

These findings do not refute the autonomy of Lyt 2, 3 cells in producing CTL from memory cell populations, but they do suggest that soluble mediators might play a more crucial role in CTL differentiation than has hitherto been suspected.

TABLE III

Effect of form of alloantigen on augmenting factor generation

Supernatant from BL/6 cultures stimulated with:	% Specific Cytolysis in cultures containing normal BL/6 T cells u.v. irradiated BALB/c spleen and supernatants from:		
	Normal	*in vitro* memory	*in vivo* memory
CBA_{spl}	92	83	75
u.v. CBA_{spl}	13	55	63
heated CBA_{spl}	-2	16	64
sonicated CBA_{spl}	1	17	40
BL/6 alone	-2	16	15

In vitro memory $BL/6_{spl}$ + CBA/J 14 days

In vivo memory $BL/6_{spl} \xrightarrow{CBA/J}$ 4 wks

REFERENCES

1. Okada, M., Klimpel, G.R., Kuppers, R.C. and Henney, C.S. J. Immunol. 1979, in press.
2. Bach, F.H., Grillot-Courvalin, C., Kuperman, O.J., Sollinger, H.W., Hayes, C., Sondel, P.M., Atler, B.J. and Bach, M.L. Immunol. Rev. 35:76, 1977.
3. Engers, H.D., Thomas, K., Cerottini, J-C. and Brunner, K.T. J. Immunol. 117:2213, 1975.
4. Ryser, J-E., Cerottini, J-C. and Brunner, K.T. J. Immunol. 120:370, 1978.
5. Wagner, H. and Rollinghoff, M. J. Exp. Med. 148:1523, 1978.
6. Cerottini, J-C., Ryser, J-E., Engers, H.D. and Brunner, K.T. Prog. in Immunol. 3:217, 1977.

ACKNOWLEDGEMENT: This work was supported by Grant AI 15383 from the NIH.

DISCUSSION

GERMAIN: One cannot explain all data on stimulation of memory CTL by liposome-associated viral antigens, since primed memory cells from F_1 mice can be stimulated by viral protein in liposomes containing only *one* set of parental H-2 molecules to yield CTL specific for only the virus plus that parental H-2 haplotype. If triggering of helper cells by liposomes plus virus was causing "non-specific" activation of memory CTL, then cytotoxicity against *both* parental haplotypes plus virus would have been expected. Therefore, such studies do look at CTL, and not helper cell, specificity.

HENNEY: For experiments showing such one way stimulation of primed F_1 cells, I would agree with Germain that helper effects cannot explain the data, and it is CTL specificity that is apparently being studied.

ALTMAN: Is it possible that the differential requirements for stimulation between *in vivo*-primed and *in vitro*-primed CTL-memory cells are due to an accessory cell? I am thinking of a cell such as the macrophage that is present in an *in vivo*-primed spleen cell population but will not be present, or only to a much lesser extent, in a long-term *in vitro*-primed memory cell population.

HENNEY: Yes, I think that is possible. Alternatively, there could be differences in the Ly 1.1 compartment in those two populations.

WAKSMAN: In a previous report Smith mentioned 4 types of T cells, but matters are really much more complex. At last count there were at least 8 types of T cells, including amplifier cells, feedback-inducer cells etc. These have had virtually no attention so far in LK research. They could account, in part, for the difference between in vitro and in vivo memory.

SECONDARY MIXED LEUKOCYTE CULTURE-INDUCED FACTORS ACTIVE IN CYTOLYTIC AND/OR PROLIFERATIVE T CELL RESPONSES IN VITRO

Jean-Charles Cerottini

Unit of Human Cancer Immunology
Ludwig Institute for Cancer Research
Epalinges s/ Lausanne, Switzerland

K. Theodor Brunner
Jean-Etienne Ryser[1]

Department of Immunology
Swiss Institute for Experimental
Cancer Research
Epalinges s/ Lausanne, Switzerland

I. QUANTITATIVE DETERMINATION OF ACTIVITIES

Although it is well established that the formation of cytolytic T lymphocytes (CTL) depends on proliferation and differentiation of non-lytic precursor cells, our understanding of the molecular and cellular events involved in CTL responses is still very limited. In this respect, studies of long-term unidirectional mixed leukocyte cultures (MLC) have provided useful information as to the differentiation pathway of memory CTL upon specific secondary (2°) antigenic stimulation (1). Thus, our earlier studies showed that memory CTL, which are operationally defined as the non-lytic progeny of CTL generated during a primary (1°) response, differentiated rapidly into highly active effector cells upon specific secondary stimulation and then

[1] *Present address: Dept. of Pathology, Uni. of Geneva, Geneva*

ISBN 0-12-213950-X

underwent extensive proliferation (2-4). In addition, we reported that similar 2° CTL responses could be induced in the absence of antigenic stimulation by exposure of long-term MLC cells to culture supernatants (SN) obtained from 2° MLC (5). Comparative analysis of the early phase of 2° CTL responses induced either by specific antigenic stimulation or 2° MLC SN showed that in both instances CTL formation was independent of DNA synthesis and accompanied by the enlargment of the small-sized memory cells (6). In more resent studies, Wagner and Röllinghoff (7) found that 2° MLC SN induced a 2° CTL response in long-term MLC cell populations which had been depleted of T cells expressing the Ly 1^+ phenotype. Moreover, recent experiments from our laboratory showed that, like SN from cultures of concanavalin A-stimulated lymphocytes, 2° MLC SN supported the continuous growth of CTL clones (8). It is thus likely that the soluble factors present in 2° MLC SN are able to trigger directly the differentiation and proliferation of memory CTL.

In our earlier studies, it became apparent that stringent culture conditions had to be used for the production of active 2° MLC SN (5). In order to further document these findings on a quantitative basis, we have recently developed two microassays which allow the quantitative determination of SN activities on either the cytolytic or the proliferative response of long-term MLC cells. Based on the microassay described by Gillis et al. (9) for measuring T cell growth factors in supernatants of mitogen-stimulated lymphocytes, these two assay techniques have been used to assess in quantitative terms the activities of 2° MLC SN produced under various culture conditions.

The microassays are based on (a) the short-term induction of CTL activity in long-term MLC cells as measured with a 3 hr ^{51}Cr release assay 24 hr after incubation with serial dilutions of SN, and (b) the proliferative response of the same population as measured by ^{3}H-TdR incorporation (4 hr pulse) 72 hr after incubation with serial dilutions of SN. In the present report, we will illustrate the use of such microassays for comparing the activities of two SN samples obtained from the same set of MLC restimulated at two different time intervals.

Unidirectional 1° MLC were set up using C57Bl/6 responding spleen cells and irradiated DBA/2 stimulating spleen cells as previously described (10). Long-term MLC cells recovered either at 7 or 14 days of 1° culture were used as the source of responding cells for SN production. The detailed conditions used for the production of 2° MLC SN have been described previously (5). Briefly, cultures were set up using 10 x 10^6 long-term MLC cells and 40 x 10^6 irradiated DBA/2 spleen cells in 10 ml culture medium in 25 cm^2 horizontal flasks. The supernatants were collected after 24 hours of culture at 37°C.

The activities of 2° MLC SN were tested on long-term MLC C57Bl/6 anti-DBA/2 cells which had not been re-exposed to allogeneic cells using two techniques (a) 50 x 10^3 cells (100 µl) were placed in round-bottomed microwells together with serial dilutions of SN (100 µl). After 24 hr of culture at 37°C, the lytic activity generated in each well was assayed using a short-term ^{51}Cr release assay. To this end, 100 µl of the culture medium were removed from each well and 10 x 10^3 ^{51}Cr labeled P-815 (DBA/2) target cells (100 µl) were added. After incubation at 37°C for an additional 3 hr, ^{51}Cr release in the supernatant was determined as previously described (10). (b) 10 x 10^3 cells (100 µl) were placed in round-bottomed microwells together with serial dilutions of SN (100 µl). After 72 hr of culture at 37°C, 1 µCi of ^3H-TdR was added to each well. After an additional 4hr culture at 37°C, the cells were collected on glass fiber filters for the determination of thymidine incorporation. The results of a representative experiment in which the activities of two 2° MLC SN samples have been compared are shown in Figure 1. The two samples were derived from the same set of C57Bl/6 anti-DBA/2 MLC cells which had been restimulated for 24 hr with irradiated DBA/2 spleen cells either on day 7 or on day 14 after the onset of the primary cultures.

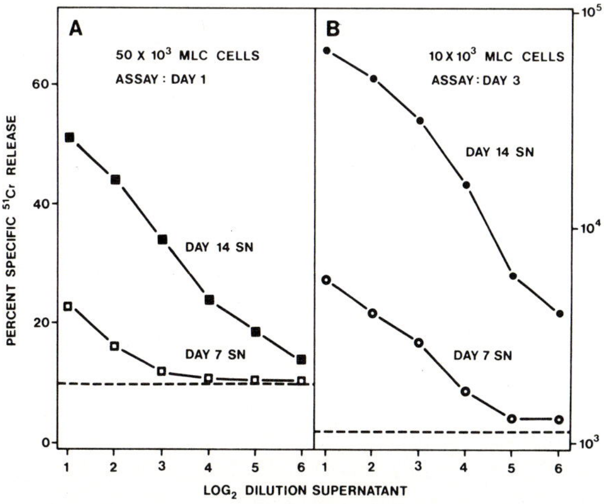

FIGURE 1. Cytolytic (A) and proliferative (B) responses of long-term C57Bl/6 anti-DBA/2 MLC cells to 2° MLC SN.

It can be seen that dose-response effects were observed with both assays, thus allowing for a quantitative comparison between the activities displayed by the two samples. In both instances, the SN derived from restimulated 14-day long-term MLC cells was 4-8 fold more active than the corresponding SN produced in 7 day cultures. As previously reported (5), SN from 24 hr cultures of normal C57Bl/6 spleen cells and irradiated DBA/2 spleen cells had no detectable activity (data not shown).

Additional experiments confirmed that the concentration of long-term MLC cells and of the stimulating cells was of critical importance to obtain 2° MLC SN with high activities (5). For example, the activities of 2^oMLC SN were reduced 4-fold when 10 x 10^6 long-term C57Bl/6 anti-DBA/2 cells were restimulated with 10 x 10^6 (instead of 40 x 10^6) irradiated DBA/2 spleen cells. It is thus evident that minor modifications of the conditions used for the production of SN can greatly influence the level of activities displayed by such SN. As described here, the use of quantitative microassays should be very helpful for defining the conditions necessary for optimal production of active SN.

II. EFFECT OF 2^oMLC SN ON NORMAL CTL PRECURSORS

We previously reported that 2° MLC SN induced a CTL response not only in long-term MLC cells but also in spleen cells from alloimmune mice (5). It was therefore of interest to determine whether CTL precursors in unprimed, normal population could be activated by 2° MLC SN. To this end, normal C57Bl/6 spleen cells which had been cultured for 5 days in the presence of 2° MLC SN were assayed for lytic activity on ^{51}Cr labeled P-815 target cells in the presence or absence of PHA. In the absence of PHA, significant, although low, lytic activity (4 lytic units/ 10^6 cells) was observed, whereas much higher activity (60 lytic units/10^6 cells) was detected in the presence of the lectin (6). In contradistinction to these findings, no lytic activity was found by Wagner and Röllinghoff (7) in cultures of normal CBA spleen cells incubated with similar SN. In this study, however, lytic activity was assayed on day 3 of culture and in the absence of PHA, i.e. under conditions which do not allow for the detection of polyclonal CTL responses.

As pointed out previously (6), our results showing that CTL precursors in normal spleen were susceptible to activation by 2° MLC SN did not rule out the existence of qualitative differences between normal and memory CTL precursors as to the requirement for alloantigen for optimal responses. In order to approach this question at the level of individual CTL precursors, we used a recently developed micro MLC system which allows for the generation of CTL under limiting dilution conditions (11). It was found that CTL were generated in microcultures containing either 500 normal C57Bl/6 spleen cells or 20 long-term MLC cells (11-12). The response of normal cells required the presence of both DBA/2 irradiated spleen cells <u>and</u> 2° MLC SN. No positive microcultures were found when the same number of responding cells were incubated with syngeneic irradiated spleen cells and 2° MLC SN (or allogeneic cells without 2° MLC SN). In contrast to normal cells, however, long-term MLC cells responded to the same extent to 2° MLC SN in the presence of either allogeneic or syngeneic irradiated spleen cells. It is thus evident that, under these conditions, there exists a fundamental difference between unprimed and primed CTL precursors. In view of these results, further work is needed to ascertain whether the factors in 2° MLC SN provide any activation signal or simply promote the proliferation of antigen-activated CTL.

1. Engers, H.D., and MacDonald, H.R., *Contemp. Top. Immunobiol.* *5*, 145 (1976).
2. MacDonald, H.R., Engers, H.D., Cerottini, J.-D., and Brunner, K.T., *J. Exp. Med.* *140*, 718 (1974).
3. MacDonald, H.R., Cerottini, J.-C., and Brunner, K.T., *J. Exp. Med.* *140*, 1511 (1974).
4. MacDonald, H.R., Sordat, B., Cerottini, J.-C., and Brunner, K.T., *J. Exp. Med.* *142*, 622 (1975).
5. Ryser, J.-E., Cerottini, J.-C., and Brunner, K.T., *J. Immunol.* *120*, 370 (1978).
6. Ryser, J.-E., MacDonald, H.R., Engers, H.D., Cerottini, J.-C., and Brunner, K.T., in "Immunology 1978" (J. Gergely, G.A. Medgyesi, and S.R. Hollan, eds.), p. 157.
7. Wagner, H., and Röllinghoff, M., *J. Exp. Med.* *148*, 1523 (1978).
8. Nabholz, M., Engers, H.D., Collavo, D., and North, M., *Contemp. Top. Microbiol. Immunol.* *81*, 176 (1978).
9. Gillis, S., Ferm, M.M., Ou, W., and Smith, K.A., *J. Immunol.* *120*, 2027 (1978).
10. Cerottini, J.-C., Engers, H.D., MacDonald, H.R., and Brunner, K.T., *J. Exp. Med.* *140*, 703 (1974).
11. Ryser, J.-E., and MacDonald, H.R., *J. Immunol.* *122*, 1691 (1979).
12. Ryser, J.-E., and MacDonald, H.R., *J. Immunol.* *123*, in press (1979).

THE SPONTANEOUS INDUCTION OF PRIMARY CYTOTOXIC T LYMPHOCYTE RESPONSES *IN VITRO* BY ALLOGENEIC EFFECT FACTOR[1]

Amnon Altman[2]
Jose M. Cardenas
Thomas E. Bechtold
David H. Katz

The Department of Cellular
and Developmental Immunology
Scripps Clinic and Research Foundation
La Jolla, CA 92037

Allogeneic effect factor (AEF), a soluble mediator derived from allogeneic cell interactions, was studied for its effects on T lymphocyte functions in vitro. *AEF could facilitate the induction of a primary cytotoxic T lymphocyte (CTL) response against syngeneic tumor cells. Furthermore, unprimed T lymphocytes cultured with AEF for 5 days in the* absence *of exogenous stimulating cells differentiated autonomously into CTL capable of lysing target cells in a short term ^{51}Cr release assay (CRA). These CTL lysed preferentially, but not exclusively,* H-2-*compatible target cells. A short exposure of spleen cells to AEF before culture was enough for triggering the induction of CTL, and this induction did not require heterologous serum determinants. "Cold" target inhibition experiments indicated the polyclonal nature of the AEF-induced CTL. In addition to its ability to induce primary CTL, AEF was also found to be a potent T cell mitogen. However, the mitogenic and the CTL-inducing activities of AEF could be experimentally dissociated. These studies suggest that AEF triggers a polyclonal CTL response, consisting predominantly of self-*H-2-*reactive CTL.*

[1]*This is publication number 116 from the Department of Cellular and Developmental Immunology and publication number 1809 from the Immunology Departments, Scripps Clinic and Research Foundation, La Jolla, CA. This work was supported by NIH grants CA-24911, AI-13781, Biomedical Research Support Grant RRO-5514, and by grants from the Pardee Foundation and the National Leukemia Association, Inc.*

[2]*Supported in part by NIH Institutional Research Service Award T32-AI-07065.*

ISBN 0-12-213950-X

INTRODUCTION

AEF, a soluble mediator derived from short-term mixed lymphocyte cultures (MLC) of *in vivo* alloantigen-activated T cells (ATC) was extensively studied by this laboratory for its effects on B lymphocyte responses *in vitro* (reviewed in 1). It was capable of replacing helper T cells in the antibody response to sheep erythrocytes. Similar MLC-derived soluble mediators were also found to contain helper factor(s) capable of enhancing weak CTL responses (2-10). Consequently, we decided to study the effects of AEF on T lymphocyte functions *in vitro*. Early during these studies we discovered that AEF, in contrast to other helper factors (2-10), was capable of triggering *autonomously* the differentiation of primary CTL in the absence of exposure to exogenous stimulating cells. It should be pointed out at the outset that by the term AEF we are referring to biological activity(ies) contained in short term MLC supernatants prepared under well-defined conditions (1,11); as yet, we do not know whether the effects of AEF on T cell responses, as presented below, are mediated by the same or distinct molecules as those shown previously to act on B cells (1,11).

MATERIALS AND METHODS

AEF was prepared by injecting mice intravenously with a mixture of syngeneic thymocytes and irradiated semiallogeneic or allogeneic spleen cells, and culturing the resulting ATC, recovered one week later, for 24 hours with appropriate target cells under serum-free conditions (11). Normal spleen cells were cultured with various concentrations of AEF for 5 days, and then tested for their ability to lyse target cells in a 4-hour CRA, or for their level of proliferation by the uptake of tritiated thymidine (12,13).

RESULTS AND DISCUSSION

Induction of Primary CTL in Vitro *by AEF*

The first clue that AEF was able to autonomously trigger the differentiation of cytotoxic lymphocytes *in vitro* was obtained in experiments in which we were trying to facilitate the primary sensitization of T lymphocytes against syngeneic tumor cells by adding the AEF to the cultures. While AEF enabled the development of such responses against syngeneic lymphoma cells, it also induced a significant level of cytotoxic activity in cultures that did not contain stimulating tumor cells (12). In subsequent experiments, it was found that unprimed spleen cells of various mouse strains, when cultured with concentrations of AEF ranging from 0.1-20% (depending on the particular AEF preparation), acquired within 4-5 days a substantial cytotoxic activity. The presence of AEF during the initial 24 hours of culture was critical for the induction of the response and, in fact, pretreatment of fresh spleen cells with AEF for only one hour was sufficient to trigger an efficient cytotoxic response (13).

Several lines of evidence documented that the cells involved in this process are T lymphocytes. First, treatment of spleen cells with anti-Thy 1.2 antibodies plus C before culture abolished their ability to develop cytolytic activity when cultured with AEF. Second, hydrocortisone-resistant thymocytes could be stimulated by AEF to develop into cytotoxic lymphocytes. Finally, depletion of T cells from AEF-activated spleen cell populations completely abolished the resulting cytotoxic activity (12,13).

The induction of CTL by AEF is not a fetal calf serum (FCS)-related artifact since a significant CTL response can be induced by AEF (prepared under serum-free conditions) in medium containing fresh syngeneic or allogeneic mouse serum. However, the CTL response induced in mouse serum is less efficient than that induced in FCS and, furthermore, mouse serum was found to inhibit the high level of CTL response induced in FCS (14), indicating the existence of potentially suppressive factor(s) for this process in mouse serum.

The Mitogenic Effects of AEF

Our observation that the AEF-stimulated spleen cell cultures contained a significantly higher proportion of lymphoblasts than the control cultures prompted us to test the mitogenic potential of AEF. Indeed, AEF was found to be a potent mitogen for thymocytes, spleen and lymph node cells. Mitogenic responses induced by AEF were quite often of the same order of magnitude as those induced by known T cell mitogens, such as concanavalin A and phytohemagglutinin. AEF was markedly mitogenic for whole, and hydrocortisone-resistant, thymocytes as well as for nylon wool-purified, T cell-enriched, spleen cells, indicating that the mitogenic effect of AEF was exerted on T lymphocytes. However, in agreement with the initial reports from this laboratory, which clearly demonstrated the ability of AEF to serve as a differentiative signal for B cells in the antibody response (1,11), we found that AEF was also mitogenic for T cell-depleted, anti-Thy 1.2 + C-treated whole, or nylon wool-adherent, spleen cells (13).

Dissociation between the Mitogenic and CTL-Inducing Activities of AEF.

In view of the above findings documenting the ability of AEF to a) induce CTL, and b) exert a mitogenic effect on T lymphocytes, we were interested in determining whether these two activities could be dissociated. Previous studies on the T cell response to alloantigens determined by the major histocompatibility complex (MHC) have indicated that two separate subpopulations of T cells are involved in the proliferative response to *I*-region determinants and in the differentiation of CTL directed against the *K* and *D* regions of the MHC (15). Our experiments demonstrate that the mitogenic and the CTL-inducing activities of AEF can be experimentally distinguished by at least two different approaches (13). First, nylon wool-purified spleen cells respond to the mitogenic stimulus of AEF as well as, or better than, whole spleen cells. However, AEF induces no, or only a minimal, CTL response in this population. Induction of CTL in nylon wool-purified spleen cell populations by AEF can be fully restored by adding small numbers of glass-adherent spleen cells. Secondly, whole thymocytes do not differentiate into CTL under the influence of AEF but are fully susceptible to its mitogenic effect. It remains to be determined whether the mitogenic and the CTL-inducing activities of AEF are mediated by the same or by a different molecular entity(ies).

The Specificity of AEF-Induced CTL

Our experiments indicate no MHC restriction in the induction of CTL by AEF. Thus, AEF derived from allogeneic interactions between T cells of two given *H-2* haplotypes retained full mitogenic and CTL-inducing activities for lymphocytes of a third-party strain (14). In our initial experiments, the AEF-induced CTL were routinely tested against *H-2*-compatible, or even fully syngeneic, tumor target cells. We analyzed in detail the specificity of the AEF-induced CTL to determine whether a) the antigenic determinants recognized by these CTL are unique to tumor cells; and b) such CTL could also lyse *H-2*-incompatible target cells.

Such experiments clearly indicate that mitogen-stimulated normal T or B lymphoblasts are fully susceptible to the cytolytic effects of the AEF-induced CTL (14). We then compared the lysis of target cells of different *H-2* haplotypes by *H-2*-compatible *vs.* incompatible AEF-stimulated spleen cells. Representative results from one of these experiments are presented in Table I. These results clearly indicate that there is a marked preference for *H-2*-compatible target cells in the lytic activity mediated by the AEF-induced CTL. Thus, target cells of a given *H-2* haplotype were most efficiently lysed by CTL of the same *H-2* haplotype. However, the lysis was not restricted and there was some killing of target cells by *H-2*-incompatible CTL. In fact, in certain effector-target cell combinations, the preference in lysis for *H-2*-compatible targets was not clear. The specificity of the AEF-induced CTL was further analyzed by applying the competitive "cold" target inhibition assay. The results of these experiments established a specific pattern of inhibition, i.e., the lysis of a given target cell was most efficiently inhibited by the homologous "cold" target cells or by other target cells of the same *H-2*-haplotype (14). An additional indication for the involvement of *H-2* antigens in the lysis was provided by our finding that the lysis of target cells by AEF-induced CTL could be specifically inhibited by anti-*H-2* alloantisera added to the CRA (14). These results strongly suggest that AEF induces a polyclonal CTL response which consists predominantly of self *H-2*-reactive CTL.

Several mechanisms could be involved in the autonomous primary induction of CTL by AEF. One interesting possibility, which is currently being tested, is that, in the absence of exogenous stimulating antigens in the cultures, AEF facilitates and helps the induction of autoreactive CTL clones. Additional studies in our laboratory focus on the characterization of the molecular entity(ies) responsible for the various biological effects of AEF.

Finally, our findings about the ability of AEF to induce autonomously, *i.e.*, in the absence of an exogenous antigen source, primary CTL capable of efficiently lysing MHC-compatible tumor target cells raise the possibility that AEF, or similar mediators, may serve as a useful tool in the management of malignant diseases.

TABLE I. *The Specificity of Lysis by AEF-Induced CTL*[a]

AEF-Induced CTL	% Specific lysis ± S.E. of target cells (E:T=72:1)		
	Thy-56 ($H-2^d$)	CBA-D1 ($H-2^k$)	EL4 ($H-2^b$)
B10.D2 ($H-2^d$)	35 ± 8	-4 ± 1	0 ± 1
B10.BR ($H-2^k$)	-3 ± 1	20 ± 1	3 ± 2
B10 ($H-2^b$)	15 ± 2	12 ± 1	17 ± 1

[a] Cultured for 5 days with 1% AEF (DBA/2 → $C3D2F_1$).

REFERENCES

1. Katz, D.H. (1977). In "Lymphocyte Differentiation, Recognition and Regulation", pp. 598-630, Academic Press, New York.
2. Altman, A. and Cohen, I.R. (1975). *Eur. J. Immunol. 5,* 437.
3. Plate, J. M.D. (1976). *Nature (London) 260,* 329.
4. Finke, J.H., Orosz, C.G. and Battisto, J.R. (1977). *Nature London 267,* 353.
5. Sopori, M.L., Alter, B.J., Bach, F.H. and Bach, M.L. (1977). *Eur. J. Immunol. 7,* 823.
6. Simon, P.L., Farrar, J.J. and Kind, P.D. (1977). *J. Immunol. 118,* 1129.
7. Ryser, J.-E., Cerottini, J.-C. and Brunner, K.T. (1978). *J. Immunol. 120,* 370.
8. Wagner, H. and Röllinghoff, M. (1978). *J. Exp. Med. 148,* 1523.
9. Fyfe, D.A. and Finke, J.H. (1979). *J. Immunol. 122,* 1156.
10. Friedman, S.M., Kuhns, J., Irigoyen, O. and Chess, L. (1979). *J. Immunol. 122,* 1302.
11. Armerding, D., and Katz, D.H. (1974). *J. Exp. Med. 140,* 19.
12. Altman, A., Bechtold, T.E., Cardenas, J.M. and Katz, D.H. (1979). *Proc. Natl. Acad. Sci. U.S.A.,* in press.
13. Altman, A., Cardenas, J.M., Bechtold, T.E. and Katz, D.H. (1979). *Submitted for publication.*
14. Altman, A., Cardenas, J.M., Bechtold, T.E. and Katz, D.H. (1979). *Submitted for publication.*
15. Cantor, H. and Boyse, E.A. (1975). *J. Exp. Med. 141,* 1390.

DISCUSSION

WECKER: This is neither a question nor a comment but a statement in order not to further confuse an already complex situation. AEF as originally described by Armerding and Katz has never been defined as a late, only as an early-acting factor in T cell-reduced normal spleen cultures. It contains Ia antigen and McDevitt suggested that this factor is the product of either B cells or macrophages. It is true, however, that AEF which we received from Katz also contains true TRF as defined in our assay system.

ALTMAN: I fully agree with Wecker's comment.

DI SABATO: In the interpretation of Altman's data, did he consider the possibility of the production of inhibitor(s) for some of the activities of AEF?

ALTMAN: In mixing experiments we clearly found that an "inactive" AEF prepared according to the method of Delovitch does not suppress at all the activation of T lymphocytes by the AEF prepared according to our conventional method.

WOOD: Do anti-Ia columns absorb the mitogenic or cytotoxicity inducing activity of "conventional" AEF?

ALTMAN: We are now in the process of doing such experiments, but I do not yet have the relevant information.

CHARACTERIZATION OF LYT^{+} T CELL DERIVED LYMPHOKINE (S) AS SECOND SIGNAL IN PRIMARY IN VITRO CYTOTOXIC T LYMPHOCYTE (CTL) RESPONSES AND AS AN AUTONOMOUS TRIGGER SIGNAL IN SECONDARY RESPONSES

Martin Röllinghoff
Klaus Pfizenmaier
Hermann Wagner

Institute of Medical Microbiology
University of Mainz
Mainz, West-Germany

It is widely accepted that two separate events occur during the induction of murine cytotoxic T lymphocytes (CTL) (1-3). Two distinct T cell subsets are triggered by two distinct antigenic determinants. In the allograft response Lyt 23^{+} CTL-precursors react preferentially to K/D region-dependent determinants of the MHC (Signal 1), whereas Lyt 1^{+} helper cells respond primarily to I region coded determinants, thereby providing an amplification signal (Signal 2) for the differentiation of alloantigen-triggered Lyt 23^{+} cells. It was postulated that signal 2 is mediated by a soluble product secreted by Lyt 1^{+} helper T cells.

Evidence has been obtained by others (4-11) and by ourselves (12,13), that upon polyclonal (ConA) or antigen-specific (MLC) stimulation murine T cells release in the supernatant a soluble factor, which, after transfer, allows thymocytes in the presence of antigen (alloantigen, TNP and virus) to differentiate into antigen-specific CTL; similarly it allows antigen-primed non-lytic secondary T cells to regain their lytic activity in the absence of newly added antigen.

Recently we have reported that it is the Lyt 1^{+} T cell subset, which upon stimulation produces within 18-24 hours the factor which induces the differentiation of CTL (12). The production requires an intact protein metabolism of the producing cells, but no DNA metabolism. Once induced the functional activity is not antigen-specific, nor is it H-2 restricted (12). As far as primary cytolytic thymocyte responses are concerned, the factor has to be present during the initial 24-48 hours of the culture period in order to allow CTL responses comparable in magnitude to mature peripheral T cells. In regard to secondary CTL responses , the factor allows experimental growth and within certain limits

ISBN 0-12-213950-X

long term cultivation of CTL (12). Even cloning of CTL and propagation of cloned CTL has been achieved (Wagner et al., to be published).

Although attempts have been made to purify and to characterize the helper factor for the induction of CTL our present knowledge is still rather limited (11,12,14). We know that the factor precipitates between 50-80% ammonium sulfate saturation, it can be concentrated by ultrafiltration on An.icon Diaflo UM 30 membranes, it is stable at 4°C, it elutes from sephadex G100 with an approximate molecular weight of 35 - 40 000 D, it can be further purified by hydroxyl apatite chromatography, by isoelectric focussing it exhibits a pI value in the range of 4.6 - 5.2. Work is in progress to purify the factor in quantities sufficient to induce heterologous antibodies. It is hoped that a specific antibody will allow a further characterization of the active principle itself and will facilitate the analysis of its relation to other factors, produced under rather similar condition, such as the classical T-cell replacing factor (TRF) (15), immune interferon (IF) (16), thymocyte mitogenic factor (TMF) (17), and the lymphocyte-activating factor (LAF) (17).

Nothing is known about the mode of action of the helper factor. We know it has to be present during the initial phase of the T cell activation, we also know that only antigen-activated T cells but not virgin T cells absorb the factor, indicating that upon antigen exposure responder T cells express a receptor for the factor. Since there exists some evidence that the factor is identical to TRF, it may be that one and the same T helper cell is able to produce the helper signal for T and B cells.

ACKNOWLEDGMENTS

This work is supported by the Deutsche Forschungsgemeinschaft SFB 107 (Mainz) and a grant of the Stiftung Volkswagenwerk.

REFERENCES

1. Wagner, H., Röllinghoff, M., and Nossal, G.J.V. (1973). Transplant. Rev. 17,3.
2. Bach, F.H., Bach, M.L., Alter, B.J., Lindahl, K.F., Schendel, D. J., and Sondel, P.M. (1975). In "Immune Recognition" (A.S. Rosenthal, ed) p. 175, Academic Press, New York.
3. Cantor, H., and Boyse, E.A. (1975). J. Exp. Med. 141, 1390.

4. Altman, A., and Cohen, I.R. (1975). Eur.J.Immunol.5, 437.
5. Plate, J.M.D.(1976).Nature (Lond.) 260,329
6. Finke, J.H., Orosz, C.G., and Battisto, J.R.(1977).Nature (Lond.) 267, 353.
7. Bonavida, B. (1977).J.Exp.Med.145, 293.
8. Tartof, D., and Fitch, F.W.(1977).J.Immunol.118, 43.
9. Gillis, S., and Smith, K.A.(1977).Nature(Lond.) 268, 154.
10. Ryser, J.E.Cerottini, J.-C., and Brunner,K.T.(1978).Eur.J. Immunol. 120,370.
11. Farrar, J.J., Simon, P.L., Knoopman,W.J., and Fuller-Bonar,J. (1978). J.Immunol. 121, 1353.
12. Wagner, H., and Röllinghoff, M.(1978).J.Exp.Med.148,1523.
13. Wagner,H., Röllinghoff,M., Schawaller,R., Hardt,C.,and Pfizenmaier,K. (1979). Nature(Lond.) in press.
14. Watson,J., Aarden, L.A., and Lefkovits, I.(1979).J.Immunol. 122, 209.
15. Schimpl, A., and Wecker, E.(1972). Nature(London) 237,15.
16. Neumann, C., and Sorg, C.(1977).Eur.J.Immunol. 7, 719.
17. Gery, I., and Waksman, B.H.(1972). J.Exp.Med.136,143.

DISCUSSION

SMITH: Does the cell which elaborates the mitogenic factor proliferate?

RÖLLINGHOFF: We know that the cell does not necessarily have to proliferate in order to produce the helper activity for killer-cell differentiation. Whether it actually does proliferate we do not yet know.

SMITH: When PNA^+ Ly $1,2,3^+$ cells respond to the mitogenic factor, do they change their surface markers?

RÖLLINGHOFF: We do not have specific data to answer Smith's question. I would however assume that the PNA^+ thymocytes change their surface markers to become Ly^+ $2,3^+$ since it is known from other experiments that alloreactive cytotoxic T cells are of the Ly^+ $2,3^+$ type.

MIZEL: Röllinghoff stated that the target of his factor is a PNA^+ cell. Oppenheim has found that LAF-containing column fractions activate PNA^- thymocytes. Smith has some data to suggest that LAF-containing macrophage supernatants activate TCGF production. The thinking has been that PNA^+ cells are more immature than PNA^- cells. Are we to conclude that more mature thymocytes can activate immature thymocytes to become cytotoxic?

RöLLINGHOFF: Yes, that would be logical reasoning.

TUMOR SECRETED MEDIATORS[1] - ROLE IN INDUCTION OF THE TUMOR MICROENVIRONMENT

Harold F. Dvorak
Neil S. Orenstein
Angela C.Carvalho
Winston H. Churchill
Ann M. Dvorak
Stephen J. Galli

Departments of Pathology & Medicine
Harvard Medical School
Boston, Massachusetts USA

Joseph Feder

Monsanto Company
St. Louis, Missouri USA

Recent morphologic studies have demonstrated that two well-characterized, diethylnitrosamine-induced hepatomas, line 1 and line 10, induce a fibrin gel about themselves within hrs of transplant into the subcutaneous space of syngeneic strain 2 guinea pigs (H.Dvorak et al. 1979a,b). This fibrin gel forms a variably-thick, cocoon-like investment that separates tumor from the host and its defense mechanisms. It was reasonable to hypothesize that this gel might result from an interaction between mediators secreted locally by the tumor cells and host plasma proteins.

[1]This work was supported by USPHS grants CA-16881, CA-19403, and HL-21460. Dr. Churchill is National Institutes of Health Career Development Awardee KO4-CA-00116. Dr. Galli is a Research Fellow of The Medical Foundation, Inc., Boston, Mass., and is supported in part by NIH Fellowship 1 F32 CA-06145.

ISBN 0-12-213950-X

MEDIATOR SECRETION BY LINE 1 AND LINE 10 TUMORS

Line 1 and line 10 tumor cells do in fact secrete at least four mediators in short term tissue culture, at least three of which may be linked to the induction and modulation of the tumors' fibrin gel investment: a vascular permeability factor (VPF), a procoagulant (PC), a plasminogen activator (PA), and an MIF-like activity.

Purification and characterization of these molecules is presently at an early stage but certain properties are known. VPF secretion was dramatically inhibited by culture at 4°C and by puromycin, an inhibitor of protein synthesis. It is a heat labile molecule (70°C, 30 min) unaffected by diisopropylfluorophosphate (DFP) and quantitatively retained on dialysis. VPF does not cause basophils to release histamine nor is it inhibited by H-1 antihistamines.

PC may be separated from the other mediators by ultracentrifugation at 100,000x g for 90 min. Total PC secretion was little affected by culture with puromycin. The bulk of the procoagulant activity is probably lipid and it is therefore not surprising that PC affects multiple steps in the clotting cascade.

Secretion of PA activity was substantially reduced by cold or puromycin and was significantly enhanced by cytochalasin B and by EDTA. The line 10 PA, like others that have been described, is a serine esterase inhibited by DFP.

Finally, line 10 tumor cells, like SV-40 transformed fibroblasts (Hammond et al., 1974; Bigazzi et al., 1975), secrete an MIF-like activitity. This activity is heat stable and dialyzeable and its relationship to that of other anti-inflammatory, macrophage-subverting mediators awaits further experimentation (Fauve et al.,1974; North et al., 1976; Snyderman & Pike, 1976).

POSSIBLE ROLE OF TUMOR MEDIATORS IN INDUCTION OF A FIBRIN GEL, ANGIOGENESIS, AND PROTECTION FROM HOST DEFENSE MECHANISMS

Line 1 and 10 tumors growing in vivo create a microenvironment characterized by leaky blood vessels, by a cocoon-like investment of fibrin gel, and by angiogenesis. The in vitro studies summarized here suggest a mechanism by which this microenvironment may be established and maintained; namely, by tumor cells secreting mediators that act in concert and trigger various pathways of the host's inflammatory system. VPF is thought to initiate the sequence by enhancing local microvascular permeability. Heightened vascular permeability, in turn, leads to the extravasation of plasma proteins, particularly fibrinogen and plasminogen. PC then clots extravasated fibrinogen to form the fibrin gel which envelops tumor cells. Finally, tumors are able to regulate the fibrin gel by secreting PA that converts extravasated plasminogen to the active fibrinolytic protease, plasmin. Plasmin digests fibrin, allowing local tumor expansion, and at the same time generates fibrin degradation products known to possess a variety of biologic activities.

What is the importance of the fibrin gel to tumor growth and survival? Precise answers to this question are presently unavailable but several possibilities come to mind: The fibrin gel may create a mechanical diffusion barrier affecting both affarent and efferent limbs of the immune response. With regard to the latter, host inflammatory cells require a mechanism for triggering fibrinolysis in order to penetrate the gel and reach tumor; neutrophils, macrophages and basophils have cell-associated plasminogen activators but lymphocytes, the principal effector cells of the immune response, do not. Also, an association between fibrin deposition and new vessel formation was established in older studies of wound healing and we have confirmed these data in guinea pigs; i.e., fibrinogen clotted in the subcutaneous space induced neovascularization closely resembling in quantity and kinetics that induced by tumors. Thus, fibrin deposition may initiate the angiogenesis required for tumor growth. Finally, the MIF-like activity may act to prevent the accumulation of macrophages important for immune tumor killing. Taken together, our data suggest that tumors, like microorganisms, are sophisticated parasites capable of eluding host defense systems by subverting these very systems to their own advantage.

REFERENCES

Dvorak, H.F., Orenstein, N.S., Carvalho, A.C., Churchill, W.H., Dvorak, A.M., Galli, S.J., Feder, J., Bitzer, A.M., Rypysc, J., and Giovinco, P. (1979a). J. Immunol. 122, 166.

Dvorak, H.F., Dvorak, A.M., Manseau, E.J., Wiberg, L., and Churchill, W.H. (1979b). J. Natl. Cancer Inst., in press.

Hammond, M.E., Roblin, R.O., Dvorak, A.M., Selvaggio, S.S., Black, P.H., and Dvorak, H.F. (1974). Science 185, 955.

Bigazzi, P.E., Yoshida, T., Ward, P.A., and Cohen, S. (1975). Am. J. Pathol. 80, 69.

Fauve, R.M., Hevin, B., Jacob, H., Gaillard, J.A., and Jacob, F. (1974). Proc. Natl. Acad. Sci. (USA) 71, 4052.

North, R.J., Kirstein, D.P., and Tuttle, R.L. (1976). J. Exp. Med. 143, 559.

Snyderman, R. and Pike, M. (1976). Science 192, 370.

INTERACTION OF SPECIFIC HELPER T-CELLS AND ANTIGEN: CONVERSION OF SPECIFIC INTO NON-SPECIFIC SIGNALS

Max H. Schreier

Basel Institute for Immunology
Basel, Switzerland

The analysis of possible mechanisms by which T-cells and macrophages interact with B-cell precursors in the induction of an antibody response requires a system of defined and individually variable components. This amounts to an exact definition and quantitation both of the cell populations involved in these cooperative processes and an exact definition of the medium, components of which may affect these cell populations in a positive or negative way.

I have recently described an *in vitro* culture system which meets most of these requirements (1). Its essential features are lower cell density and replacement of fetal bovine serum by highly purified serum components. In this system no non-specific T-cell help is induced (2) and the induction of PFC directed against sheep red blood cells (SRC) or horse red blood cells (HRC) depends absolutely on specific helper T-cells, antigen and B-cells. The system is suited for the evaluation of antigen-dependent induction of B-cells, ennumeration of B-cell precursors, the quantitation of T-cell help, and studies on H2-restriction; it is also applicable to the study of mediators induced upon specific interaction of helper T-cells and antigen.

As seen in Table I, low number of B-cells (5×10^4 in a volume of 0.2 ml) cannot be induced to form PFC against the antigens SRC or HRC in the presence of low numbers of unprimed T-cells (up to $1\text{-}2 \times 10^5$). This is both due to the low total cell density and the nonstimulatory culture medium, in which FBS is replaced by the purified serum components albumin, transferrin and a mixture of lipids (3,4,1). With T-cells primed *in vivo* to SRC or HRC, as previously described (1), a significant specific response can be induced with the homologous antigen: T'_S will promote an antibody response to SRC but not HRC, while T'_H support a response against HRC but not against SRC.

ISBN 0-12-213950-X

This specific in vitro helper assay has been used to ennumerate B-cell precursors in various organs of syngeneic mice. One in about 3000 splenic B-cells can recognize antigenic determinants on SRC, a figure to be considered in assessing the efficiency of T-cell help. Priming of B-cells in vivo is not required.

As shown in the lower panel of Table I, T'_S which do not support a response against HRC in this specific helper assay, promote equally well the induction of an antibody response against SRC and HRC in the presence of both antigens. Similarly, in the crossover experiments T'_H support an antibody response to both antigens, if both are simultaneously present.

This phenomenon, the "bystander effect", has been observed by several investigators (5-9). However, in my experience, it has often been marginal and poorly reproducible under Mishell-Dutton type culture conditions (10) and no significant "T-cell replacing" activity could be revealed in supernatants of such cultures. The phenomenon could be readily explained by an adjuvant effect of the ongoing specific immune response, providing a stimulus for residual specific T-cells to mature to functional helper T-cells and/or produce sufficient specific T-cell factor for the induction of a response to the second antigen (11).

TABLE I. The Specificity of Helper T-Cells and the "Bystander-Effect"

T-cells (5×10^4/culture)	Antigen		PFC directed against	
	SRC	HRC	SRC	HRC
T	+	+	0	0
T'_{SRC}	+	-	2080 ± 556	0
T'_{SRC}	-	+	0	0
T'_{HRC}	+	-	0	0
T'_{HRC}	-	+	0	1010 ± 430
T'_{SRC}	+	+	3760 + 811	1840 ± 601
T'_{HRC}	+	+	2193 ± 705	1450 ± 577

All cultures contained 5×10^4 B-cells + 5×10^5 RBC

This phenomenon raises three questions.
1) Are stable products generated during a specific antibody response capable of promoting a response to unrelated antigens? Supernatants, removed at various times after onset of an *in vitro* helper assay, and added to anti-theta- and complement -treated spleen cells, have a potent T-cell replacing activity. The activity peaks after a 48 hour culture period and is absent by 96 hours. Irrespective of its origin, the supernatant promotes about equally well an anti SRC or an anti HRC response (Table II).

Table II. Effect of Supernatant* of T'_S and SRC or HRC on the the Induction of PFC in nude spleen cells (2×10^5 cells/culture)

Antigen added to T'_S	Antigen added to nude spleen cells	PFC directed against SRC	PFC directed against HRC
	SRC	30020 ± 3966	0
SRC	HRC	0	24400 ± 3290
	SRC	0	0
HRC	HRC	0	0

* 10^6 *in vivo* generated T'_S (containing adherent cells) were incubated for 48 hrs with 2.5×10^6 SRC or HRC in 1 ml medium. The supernatant was filtered through a 0.2 μ filter.

2) What are the requirements for the induction of supernatant activity?
Single omissions of components of the *in vitro* helper assay revealed that B-cells are not required for the induction of supernatant activity: It depends only on antigen, specific helper T-cells and adherent cells. Using longterm cultured or cloned helper T-cells (see below), the adherent cells were derived from nude mice and irradiated prior to use (3300 R), and the number of PFC induced by these supernatants was about as high as the number induced by helper T-cells. Supernatant activity and helper T-cells dilute out similarly.

3) Is the supernatant activity specific or nonspecific? Since the frequency of specific *in vivo* generated helper T-cells in T'_S or T'_H preparations is at best about 10^{-3} (1), the possibility of T-cell-T-cell interactions triggering release of specific helper factors from committed T-cells cannot be entertained and can be formally excluded by using longterm-cultured, highly enriched specific T-cell populations or clones of T'_S or T'_H (Table III) (M.H. Schreier and R. Tees, to be published). Longterm cultured T'_S (and clones of these cells) can still induce an anti HRC response in the simultaneous presence of both antigens.

These helper T-cells retain their biological function and specificity after up to one year of *in vitro* culture: nude mice are specifically reconstituted by an injection of cloned helper T-cells (R. Tees and M.H. Schreier, to be published). However, no bystander effect is observed *in vivo*. This difference may rest on strict compartmentalization within the lymphoid tissues and/or on the lack of dilution and degradation allowing accumulation of biological mediators *in vitro*.

Table III. Induction of an α HRC-Response by SRC-Specific Helper T-Cells*

Number of T'_S / culture	Antigen added to cultures: SRC		HRC		SRC + HRC	
	PFC Directed against					
	SRC	HRC	SRC	HRC	SRC	HRC
$10^{3.5}$	4760±1452	0	0	0	22827±7716	3613±298
10^{3}	16370±2114	0	0	0	22890±7963	7453±1730
$10^{2.5}$	883±205	0	0	0	1440±510	175±5
10^{2}	35±8	0	0	0	45±15	0
$10^{1.5}$	4±2	0	0	0	0	0

* after 4 months in culture

Taken together, these results suggest that the specificity of helper T-cells is not more than the interaction of a specific T-cell-receptor and antigen. This specific interaction leads to the release of nonspecific, biologically active mediators which promote T-cell proliferation, antigen-dependent induction of B-cell precursors, B-cell proliferation and growth of nonlymphoid cells. Whether these factors are exclusively T-cell products, remains to be established.

ACKNOWLEDGEMENT

The author is indebted to Ms. R. Tees for excellent technical assistance.

REFERENCES

1. Schreier, M.H., J. Exp. Med. 148, 1612 (1978)
2. Schreier, M.H., and Lefkovits, I., Immunology 36, 743 (1979)
3. Guilbert, L.J., and Iscove, N.N., Nature (Lond.) 263, 594 (1976)
4. Iscove, N.N., and Melchers, F., J. Exp. Med. 147, 923 (1978)
5. Hartmann, K.U., J. Exp. Med. 132, 1267 (1971)
6. Vann, D.C., and Kettmann, J.R., J. Immunol. 108, 73 (1972)
7. Hunter, P.C., Munro, A.J., and McConnell, I., Nature (New Biol.) 236, 52 (1972)
8. Waldmann, H., and Munro, A.J., Nature (Lond.) 243, 356 (1973)
9. Rubin, A.S., and Coons, A.H., J. Immunol. 108, 1597 (1972)
10. Mishell, R.I., and Dutton, R.W., J. Exp. Med. 126, 423, (1967)
11. Miller, J.F.A.P., Int. Rev. Cytol. 33, 77 (1972)

DISCUSSION

WATSON: Would Schreier tell us whether the B cell growth factor allows B cells to grow permanently in culture just as the T cell growth factor does for T cells?

SCHREIER: We have worked on this issue and I can say that the B cells grow longer than we have ever observed previously. However, before we do more work on this aspect we want to purify this factor to exclude the possibility that our supernatants are contaminated with other activities, already described, which drive B cells to maturation. At present, the implication of our findings is that we will be able to get continuous growth of B cell blasts.

SMITH: How long after the injection of the helper T cells into the nude mouse were the spleen cells removed for the plaque assay?

SCHREIER: The data I have presented were obtained on day 5 after simultaneous injection of helper T cells and antigen.

TAUSSIG:

(1) Did Schreier titrate the supernatant of helper T cells? I ask this because specificity might become apparent only on dilution.

(2) Did he attempt to absorb the supernatant with antigen? I was surprised that when Schreier found that the T-helper cells acted strictly specifically *in vivo*, he suggested that this was due to lymphoid architecture. It would rather imply, perhaps, that non-specific factors are not relevant *in vivo*, and that if factors are involved *in vivo* they are antigen-specific.

SCHREIER: The supernatant activity titrates out quite rapidly. As Taussig may have noticed in Table 3, at marginal input of helper activity (this holds both for cells or supernatant) one may favor one or the other activity. Since the presented results did not indicate a specific factor, I had no rationale for attempting absorption with antigen.

ROLE OF GRF IN T HELPER CELL INDUCTION IN VITRO[1]

Peter Erb

Institute for Microbiology
University of Basel
Basel, Switzerland

Marc Feldmann

ICRF Tumour Immunology Unit
Dept. of Zoology, University College
London, England

INTRODUCTION

The induction of T helper cells (HC) in vitro requires either antigen and macrophage-like accessory cells (MØ) or genetically related MØ factor which is obtained from antigen-incubated MØ (1,2). GRF is a complex of Ia antigen and immunogenic fragment-(s) with a MW of about 55,000 daltons (3). Like the MØ-T cell interaction (4) GRF-T cell interaction is genetically restricted in that only GRF obtained from MØ similar at the I-A subregion of the H-2 complex is capable of generating HC (2). As only Ia positive MØ induce HC (5) and one site of Ir gene expression is at the level of MØ (6) the question arises whether GRF is a mediator of Ir gene function.

In this communication we provide additional information about the site of action of GRF and suggest that GRF is an Ir gene product.

RESULTS AND DISCUSSION

Previously we demonstrated that GRF adsorbed short lived T_1 cells (phenotyped as Ly $1^+2^+3^+$ amplifier cells obtained from ALS treated mice) incubated with normal recirculating T_2 cells (typed as Ly $1^+2^-3^-$ helper cell precursors obtained from adult

[1]supported by the JDF (grant no 78R085), the NIAID (grant no. 1 R01 AI14513-01A1) and The Imperial Cancer Research Fund

ISBN 0-12-213950-X

thymectomized mice) generated HC, but not if GRF adsorbed T_2 cells were added to normal T_1 cells (7). From that we concluded that GRF activates T_1 cells which stimulate T_2 cells to become HC (7). Genetic restriction was found in the GRF-T_1 interaction but not in the T_1-T_2 interaction (7,8).

However the possibility was not excluded that GRF binds to T_1 as well as to T_2 cells, but that T_2 cells require an additional signal from stimulated T_1 cells in order to be activated. To test this hypothesis T_1 cells were adsorbed with GRF-KLH (=S/N of MØ incubated with KLH for 4d) for 1h, washed twice and incubated in Marbrook flasks. As a control unadsorbed T_1 cells were cultured. After 3d supernatants (S/N) of each culture were collected and incubated with T_2 cells and GRF-KLH, with GRF-KLH adsorbed T_2 cells or with T_2 cells alone. 4d later the T_2 cells were tested for helper activity with B cells and TNP-KLH. A typical result is shown in Table I. Only T_2 cells either preadsorbed or incubated with GRF-KLH and S/N obtained from GRF incubated T_1 cells became KLH-specific HC. The interpretation of this result is that GRF simultaneously binds to both T1 and T_2 cells, and thus both T subpopulations must have the same capacity to recognize GRF. The function of binding of GRF to T_1 cells would be to generate a mediator which provides a 'signal' to T_2 cells, necessary for their differentiation into HC. This amplifier-mediator is nonspecific and works across the histocompatibility barrier (data not shown). The physical and chemical nature of the T_1 mediator is not yet known.

TABLE I. GRF binds to both T_1 and T_2 cells.

Helper cell induction [a]	AFC $\pm$ SD / 10^6 [b]
T_1 + T_2 + KLH	95 $\pm$ 5
T_1 + T_2 + KLH + MØ	435 $\pm$ 75
T_1 + T_2 + GRF-KLH	475 $\pm$ 95
T_1 + T_2 ads GRF-KLH	70 $\pm$ 10
T_2 + GRF-KLH + S/N(T_1 ads GRF-KLH)	390 $\pm$ 40
T_2 ads GRF-KLH + S/N (T_1 ads GRF-KLH)	360 $\pm$ 60
T_2 + GRF-KLH + S/N(T_1)	125 $\pm$ 5
T_2 + S/N(T_1 ads GRF-KLH)	170 $\pm$ 70
T_2 + KLH + S/N(T_1 ads GRF-KLH)	25 $\pm$ 5
T_2 + KLH + MØ	95 $\pm$ 20
NIL	70 $\pm$ 30

[a]HC were induced in the Mini-Marbrook system ($3x10^6$ cell per culture). Doses used per culture were: 0.1μg KLH, $5x10^4$ MØ, 10μl GRF-KLH, 20μl S/N (T_1 ads GRF-KLH) or S/N (T_1); for adsorption $3x10^6$ T_2 cells were incubated with 20μl GRF for 1h, then washed twice.

[b]HC induction as well as helper activity was measured by the anti-TNP-response of B cells after incubation with 'HC' and TNP-KLH for 4d. The Mini-Mishell-Dutton system was used for cooperation (10^6 spleen cells as source of B cells and $5x10^4$ 'HC')

The activity of GRF closely parallels that of MØ and antigen (1,3,7,9). For example, GRF obtained from nonresponder (NR) MØ does not induce responder (R) T cells to become HC. This is also shown in Table II. H-2^b mice are NR to pork insulin, while H-2^d or F_1 (bxd) are R to pork insulin (10). H-2^b (b) MØ or GRF obtained from b-type MØ do not induce pork insulin specific HC if incubated with F_1 (bxd) T cells, while H-2^d (d) MØ or GRF do. The simplest interpretation of that result is that GRF is an Ir gene product and may mediate Ir gene function. Alternatively, F_1 (bxd) T cells might lack an appropriate receptor for NR GRF. Thus nonresponsivness would then be a property of the T cell receptor and not of the MØ. Which of these possibilities is correct is not yet known.

TABLE II. Is GRF an Ir gene product?

HC induced F_1 (bxd) T cells +	NIL	MØ or GRF from F_1 (bxd)	b	d
		(AFC±SD/10^6 cells)		
pork insulin + MØ	43 ± 17	167 ± 7	43 ± 7	165 ± 33
GRF-pork insulin		208 ± 55	43 ± 20	170 ± 15

REFERENCES

1 Erb, P., and Feldmann, M. (1975). Nature 254, 352
2 Erb, P., and Feldmann, M. (1975). Eur. J. Immunol. 5, 759
3 Erb, P., Feldmann, M., and Hogg, N. (1976). Eur. J. Immunol. 6, 365.
4 Erb, P., and Feldmann, M. (1975).J. Exp. Med. 142,460.
5 Stern, A.C., Erb, P., and Gisler, R.H. (1979). J. Immunol. in press.

6 Rosenthal, A.S., Barcinski, M.A., and Blake, J.T. (1979). Nature 267, 156.
7 Erb, P., Vogt, P., Meier, B., and Feldmann, M. (1977). J. Immunol. 119, 206.
8 Feldmann, M., and Erb, P., (1977). Z. Immun.-Forsch. 153,217.
9 Erb, P., Meier, B., and Feldmann, M., (1979). J. Immunol. in press.
10 Keck, K., (1975). Nature 254, 78.

DISCUSSION

WATSON: Work with the T cell growth factor implies that in the nude spleen there is some kind of precursor T cell which can be stimulated to become an effector cell. Can Erb take GRF and generate within nude spleen populations any type of helper activity?

ERB: I have not tried that.

WATSON: It would be interesting to test in such populations whether helper activity can be generated in the absence of the thymus and whether in that situation the genetic restriction of GRF would still hold.

FARRAR: Erb has shown that GRF containing supernatants are active at apparently two distinct sites; on the T_1 and T_2. Is there any evidence which points toward only one factor being active at both sites or could two biochemically distinct macrophage products be operative, only one of which is genetically restricted.

ERB: The evidence so far available is more in favor of one factor being active at both sites. Thus T_1 cells after adsorbing GRF provide a differentiation signal which activates T_2 cells in the presence of GRF. For the latter step T_2 cells can be used which have been preabsorbed with GRF. The restriction acts at both sites, GRF-T_1 as well as GRF-T_2. T-helper cells once generated in that way are also genetically restricted. Very preliminary evidence suggests that GRF can be used for stimulation of helper cells.

CROSS REACTIVE IDIOTYPIC DETERMINANTS ON ANTIBODIES AND T CELL HELPER FACTOR SPECIFIC TO (T,G)-A--L

Edna Mozes

Department of Chemical Immunology
The Weizmann Institute of Science
Rehovot, Israel

Antigen specific T cell helper or suppressor factors have been utilized as tools in the efforts aimed at the elucidation of the T cell recognition system. Since these factors replace T cell activity and are specific for the antigen in the presence of which they are produced, it is very likely that they represent the molecular recognition component of T cells - namely the T-cell receptor.

A factor produced by T cells "educated" either *in vivo* or *in vitro* to the synthetic polypeptide (T,G)-A--L, has been shown to replace T cell helper activity when mixed with B cells and antigen and transferred into irradiated recipients (1). Mice of the $H\text{-}2^k$ haplotype, which are low responders to (T,G)-A--L are capable of producing an active cooperative factor to this antigen (1), whereas T cells of mice of the $H\text{-}2^s$ haplotype cannot be activated to (T,G)-A--L and do not produce helper factors (2). The (T,G)-A--L specific factor possesses determinants coded by genes mapped in the I region of the mouse major histocompatibility complex (H-2) and more specifically in the I-A subregion (3,4). Although the (T,G)-A--L specific factor lacks conventional immunoglobulin determinants (4), one of its important features is its antigen specificity which was demonstrated by the removal of its activity on specific antigen-Sepharose columns (5) and also by demonstrating that its helper effect was specific to the antigen used in the T cell education (6). In view of the suggestions that B and T cells share idiotypic determinants (7,8) it was of interest to find out whether the (T,G)-A--L specific factor will share idiotypes with antibodies of the same specificity. For this purpose, anti-idiotypic sera to C3H.SW ($H\text{-}2^b$, $Ig\text{-}1^a$) anti-(T,G)-A--L antibodies

ISBN 0-12-213950-X

have been produced in guinea-pigs (9). The anti-idiotypes were shown to bind specifically 30% of the iodinated antibodies of C3H.SW against (T,G)-A--L and to inhibit antigen binding of these antibodies (9). The (T,G)-A--L specific idiotypes were found to be linked to heavy chain constant region allotypes (9). These anti-idiotypic sera were used to look for the presence of idiotypic determinants on the (T,G)-A--L specific T-cell factor. Table I demonstrates the ability of (T,G)-A--L specific T cell factors to cooperate with B.M. cells and antigen for eliciting antibody response to (T,G)-A--L in irradiated recipients after passage through different immunoadsorbents. As can be seen, the activity of a factor produced by C3H.SW educated T cells was removed after passage through an

TABLE I. Removal of the activity of a (T,G)-A--L specific T cell factor by anti-idiotypic serum

C3H.SW bone marrow cells and (T,G)-A--L transferred with:[a]	*No. of animals*	*Log_2 H.A. titers Means ± S.E.*
No addition	*20*	*0.55 ± 0.20*
C3H.SW factor	*30*	*4.37 ± 0.03*
C3H.SW factor passed on an anti-idiotype Sepharose column	*30*	*1.03 ± 0.21*
C3H.SW factor passed on a guinea pig anti-mouse IgG-Sepharose column	*6*	*3.07 ± 0.34*
C3H/DiSn factor	*11*	*4.0 ± 0.22*
C3H/DiSn factor passed on an anti-idiotype Sepharose column	*11*	*1.09 ± 0.39*
C3H/DiSn factor passed on a guinea pig anti-mouse IgG-Sepharose column	*6*	*3.75 ± 0.18*

a) Each recipient group was injected with 2 x 10^7 B.M. cells and 10 μg (T,G)-A--L together with factor at an amount produced by 5 x 10^6 "educated" T cells. Mice were bled 12 days after transfer and their sera assayed by passive H.A. (hemagglutination) with (T,G)-A--L coated sheep red blood cells.

anti-idiotype-Sepharose immunoadsorbent, whereas no effect on the activity of the factor was observed when guinea pig anti-mouse IgG was used as an immunoadsorbent. A factor from C3H/DiSn ($H-2^k$,$Ig-1^a$) low responder mice to (T,G)-A--L, also lost its helper activity following passage through the anti-idiotype Sepharose column. The activity of this factor was completely retained after passage through guinea pig anti-mouse IgG immunoadsorbent as observed with the C3H.SW derived factor. Thus, the similarity between the factors of high ($H-2^b$) and low ($H-2^k$) responder origin has been confirmed (10).

CWB ($H-2^b$,$Ig-1^b$) mice are high responders to (T,G)-A--L. They are congenic with C3H.SW ($H-2^b$,$Ig-1^a$) mice and differ only in their heavy chain allotypic markers. However, (T,G)-A--L specific antibodies of CWB do not share idiotypic determinants with antibodies of C3H.SW mice. Similarly, a (T,G)-A--L specific factor produced by CWB "educated" T cells, did not react with the anti-idiotypic antibodies against C3H.SW anti-(T,G)-A--L (10). The above described results suggest the presence of similar variable regions on B cell products (antibodies) and T cell products (factors), which are probably coded by the same variable region genes.

The cross reactivity between B and T cells on the level of idiotypic determinants has been recently confirmed using a different approach: C3H.SW and C3H/DiSn mice were immunized with syngeneic (T,G)-A--L "educated" T cells. The antibodies produced in both mouse strains against the (T,G)-A--L activated cells, reacted with (T,G)-A--L specific antibodies of C3H.SW mice (idiotypes). Thus, T cells of low responder mice possess antigen specific receptors to (T,G)-A--L and antibodies to high and low responder T cell receptor cross-react with specific antibodies to (T,G)-A--L (R. Lifshitz and E. Mozes).

The antigen specific T cell helper factors have been shown to possess Ia determinants. Thus, these factors are coded by two unlinked genes. The molecular basis of the combination between I region gene products and immunoglobulin variable region gene products is not yet understood. Table II represents experiments in which effluents of factors passed separately on anti-Ia and anti-idiotype immunoadsorbents were mixed and injected with B.M. cells and antigen into irradiated recipients. As can be seen the combination of the two effluents did not result in an active helper factor suggesting that the two determinants are part of one entity.

It appears that only a biochemical analysis of the antigen specific factors will shed light on the molecular properties of these T cell products. The minute amounts of antigen specific factors obtained from normal "educated" cells, were the drawback towards the elucidation of this problem. To this end, we were able recently to obtain T-cell hybridomas between

TABLE II. *Activity of (T,G)-A--L specific T cell factor after passage on anti-Ia and anti-idiotype immunoadsorbents*

C3H.SW bone marrow cells and (T,G)-A--L transferred with[a]:	No. of animals	Log_2 H.A. titers Means ± S.E.
No addition	8	0.6 ± 0.12
C3H/DiSn factor	15	4.1 ± 0.23
C3H/DiSn factor passed on an anti-idiotype-Sepharose column	9	0.6 ± 0.21
C3H/DiSn factor passed on an anti-Ia immunoadsorbent	7	1.8 ± 0.18
C3H/DiSn factor - mixture of effluents of anti-idiotype and anti-Ia immunoadsorbents	6	1.7 ± 0.20

a) Each recipient group was injected with 2 x 10^7 B.M. cells and 10 μg (T,G)-A--L together with factor at an amount produced by 5 x 10^6 "educated" T cells. Mice were bled 12 days after transfer and their sera assayed by passive H.A. (hemagglutination) with (T,G)-A--L coated sheep red blood cells.

the BW 5147 line and "educated" T-cells which were enriched on (T,G)-A--L bearing adherent cells. Preliminary results indicated that supernatants of one hybridoma cooperate specifically with (T,G)-A--L primed B cells and antigen for the production of anti-(T,G)-A--L antibodies in irradiated recipients, whereas an additional hybridoma and its supernatant suppress the production of (T,G)-A--L specific antibodies of antigen primed spleen cells in adoptive transfer experiments (Z. Eshhar, R.N.Apte and E. Mozes). The characterization of these functional T cell products is under investigation.

REFERENCES

1. Taussig, M.J., Mozes, E., and Isac, R., *J. Exp. Med. 140*, 301 (1974).
2. Mozes, E., Isac, R., and Taussig, M.J., *J. Exp. Med. 141*, 703 (1975).
3. Taussig, M.J., Munro, A.J., Campbell, R., David, C.S., and Staines, N.A., *J. Exp. Med. 142*, 694 (1975).
4. Isac, R., Dorf, M.E., and Mozes, E., *Immunogenetics 5*, 467 (1977).

5. Mozes, E., in "The role of products of the histocompatibility gene complex in immune responses" (Katz, D.H. and Benacerraf, B., eds.), p. 485. Academic Press, New York, (1976).
6. Isac, R., and Mozes, E., *J. Immunol. 118,* 584 (1977).
7. Binz, H., and Wigzell, H., *J. Exp. Med. 142,* 197 (1975).
8. Eichmann, K., and Rajewsky, K., *Eur. J. Immunol. 5,* 661 (1975).
9. Schwartz, M., Lifshitz, R., Givol, D., Mozes, E., and Haimovich, J., *J. Immunol. 121,* 421 (1978).
10. Mozes, E., and Haimovich, J., *Nature 278,* 56 (1979).

PROPERTIES OF T-SUPPRESSOR FACTOR SPECIFIC FOR L-GLUTAMIC ACID^{60}-L-ALANINE^{30}-L-TYROSINE^{10} (GAT)[1]

Ronald N. Germain
Michel Pierres[2]
Shyr-Te Ju
Martin E. Dorf
Baruj Benacerraf

Department of Pathology
Harvard Medical School
Boston, Massachusetts

I. INTRODUCTION

L-glutamic acid^{60}-L-alanine^{30}-L-tyrosine^{10} (GAT) is a synthetic polypeptide antigen, the immune response to which is under dominant H-2 linked Ir gene control. Kapp *et al.* (1) first demonstrated that nonresponder strains of mice primed with GAT develop potent suppressor T cell (T_s) responses able to prevent plaque forming cell (PFC) responses to the immunogen GAT-methylated bovine serum albumin (GAT-MBSA). Cell free extracts from such T_s (T_sE), prepared by sonication and centrifugation, also mediate specific suppression (2). The suppressive component of this T_sE has been shown to be a protein of 40-60,000 m.w., lacking C_H or C_L determinants, but with specific antigen binding capacity, and bearing determinants coded for by H-2 (I-J subregion) genes (3). GAT-T_sE has been found to mediate its effect at least in part by inducing new suppressor T cells (T_{s_2}) in both nonresponder (4) and responder mice (5).

[1] *Supported in part by NIH grants AI-14732, NSF grant PCM-22422 and PHS fellowship FO5TW2381-02.*
[2] *Present address: Centre D'Immunologie, INSERM-CRNS, Marseille, France.*

ISBN 0-12-213950-X

II. PRODUCTION OF GAT-T_sF USING RESPONDER SPLEEN CELLS

Attempts to elicit a predominant GAT-T_s response *in vivo* in responder mice have been unsuccessful. However, following the demonstration of an important role for macrophages (MØ) in regulating GAT responsiveness (6), an *in vitro* method for generating responder GAT-T_s was developed. Responder spleen cells were depleted of adherent cells (MØ), cultured with 10-50 μg/ml GAT for 2 days, and tested for suppressor activity in fresh cultures (7). This technique leads to excellent GAT specific suppressor T cell generation.

To obtain a specific suppressor factor from responder T_s cells, the responder GAT-T_s induced using MØ depleted spleen cells were washed and recultured without antigen for 24 hr. The supernatant of these T_s cells, or control cells educated without antigen, was then tested for suppressive activity *in vitro* (8). Such supernatants were found to contain a soluble factor which also can specifically suppress GAT PFC responses. This responder derived GAT-T_sF possesses antigen binding capacity and I-J determinants as illustrated in Table 1. Further studies showed that responder GAT-T_sF, like nonresponder derived T_sE, can also induce T_{s_2}.

III. IDIOTYPIC CROSS-REACTIVITY BETWEEN GAT-T_sE AND ANTI-GAT ANTIBODIES

To characterize more precisely the material responsible for the biological effects detailed above, experiments were carried out to determine if GAT-T_sE shared idiotypic determinants with anti-GAT antibodies. Ju *et al.* previously characterized a common cross-reactive idiotype (CGAT) on anti-GAT antibodies of both responder and nonresponder mice. However, the CGAT idiotype was not detected in anti-GA antibodies (9-11). This anti-idiotype antiserum (anti-CGAT) was coupled to Sepharose. Nonresponder GAT-T_sE from DBA/1 or SJL mice was then passed over the immunoadsorbent, and retained material eluted with acid. The filtrate and eluate of the anti-CGAT column, or a control column, were then tested for either direct suppression of nonresponder PFC responses or induction of T_{s_2} (Table 2) (12). All T_sE activity was removed by and recovered from the anti-CGAT adsorbents. Furthermore, it was shown that GA-T_sE, as predicted from the antibody data, failed to bind to the anti-CGAT immunoadsorbents. By passing the $CGAT^+$ GAT-T_sE over an anti-I-J antiserum immunoadsorbent, it could be shown that GAT-T_sE bears *both* I-J and idiotypic determinants in a single molecular complex.

TABLE 1. *Characterization of Responder GAT-T_sF*

Responding cells[a]	*Factor source*[b]	*Treatment of factor*[c]	*Specific IgG anti-GAT PFC/culture*	
			Response	*% suppression*
BALB/c	—	—	925	—
	BALB/c	None	<20	98
		Filtrate from GAT-Sepharose	1060	0
		Eluate from GAT-Sepharose	<20	98
		Filtrate from BSA-Sepharose	<20	98
		Eluate from BSA-Sepharose	960	0
$(B6D2)F_1$	—	—	300	—
	B10.BR	None	10	97
		Filtrate from anti-I-J^k-Sepharose	620	0
		Eluate from anti-I-J^k-Sepharose	10	97
		Filtrate from anti-I-J^s-Sepharose	20	94
		Eluate from anti-I-J^s-Sepharose	300	0

[a]*Responding cells in Mishell-Dutton assay culture.*

[b]*Factor from indicated strain, tested at a final dilution of 1/100.*

[c]*Anti-I-J^k = B10.A(3R) anti-B10.A(5R), anti-I-J^s = [B10.A(3R) × B10.S(9R)]anti-B10.HTT.*

TABLE 2. Idiotypic (CGAT) Determinants on GAT-T_sE

A. Direct Suppression Assay

Treatment of GAT-T_sE	Responding cells	Antigen	% of control response[a]
Filtrate of control adsorbent	SJL	GAT-MBSA	6.8 ± 1.8
Eluate of control adsorbent	SJL	GAT-MBSA	121 ± 12
Filtrate of anti-CGAT adsorbent	SJL	GAT-MBSA	148 ± 18
Eluate of anti-CGAT adsorbent	SJL	GAT-MBSA	14.5 ± 3.3

B. T_{s_2} Induction

Treatment of GAT-T_sE	T_{s_2}[b]	Responding cells[c]	Antigen	PFC/culture[d]
Filtrate of control adsorbent	BALB/c	BALB/c	GAT	80
Eluate of control adsorbent	BALB/c	BALB/c	GAT	675
Filtrate of anti-CGAT adsorbent	BALB/c	BALB/c	GAT	565
Eluate of anti-CGAT adsorbent	BALB/c	BALB/c	GAT	<10

[a] Pooled, normalized data from several experiments; control response = PFC in the absence of T_sE.

[b] Cells used for T_{s_2} induction.

[c] Cells used for assaying T_{s_2} activity.

[d] Specific GAT IgG PFC/culture.

IV. CONCLUSION

These studies indicate that both responder and nonresponder mice can produce a GAT-specific T cell derived suppressor factor, with antigen binding activity, and I-J subregion coded determinants. These factors act at least in part by inducing a new set of suppressor T cells, a process that requires both the H-2 coded product and GAT. Certain constraints on molecular models of GAT suppressor factor derive from the demonstration that the same molecular complex bears I-J coded and V_H related determinants, as assessed by binding to anti-alloantiserum or anti-idiotype immunoadsorbents. The simplest model consists of a two chain structure, in which the V_H product provides antigen-specificity and the H-2 product biological effector function.

REFERENCES

1. Kapp, J.A., Pierce, C.W., Schlossman, S., and Benacerraf, B. (1974). *J. Exp. Med. 140*, 648.
2. Kapp, J.A., Pierce, C.W., de la Croix, F., and Benacerraf, B. (1976). *J. Immunol. 116*, 305.
3. Germain, R.N. (1979). *In* "The Role of the Major Histocompatibility Complex in Immunobiology" (M.E. Dorf, ed.), Garland Press, New York, in press.
4. Germain, R.N., Theze, J., Kapp, J.A., and Benacerraf, B. (1978). *J. Exp. Med. 147*, 123.
5. Germain, R.N., and Benacerraf, B. (1978). *J. Immunol. 121*, 608.
6. Germain, R.N., and Benacerraf, B. (1978). *J. Exp. Med. 148*, 1324.
7. Pierres, M., and Germain, R.N. (1978). *J. Immunol. 121*, 1306.
8. Pierres, M., Benacerraf, B., and Germain, R.N. (1979). Manuscript in preparation.
9. Ju, S.-T., Kipps, T.J., Theze, J., Benacerraf, B., and Dorf, M.E. (1978). *J. Immunol. 121*, 1034.
10. Ju, S.-T., Benacerraf, B., and Dorf, M.E. (1978). *Proc. Natl. Acad. Sci. 75*, 6192.
11. Ju, S.-T., Dorf, M.E., and Benacerraf, B. (1979). *J. Immunol. 122*, 1054.
12. Germain, R.N., Ju, S.-T., Kipps, T.J., Benacerraf, B., and Dorf, M.E. (1979). *J. Exp. Med. 149*, 613.

ANTIGEN SPECIFIC T-CELL DERIVED HELPER FACTOR

C. Shiozawa, S. Sonik, B. Singh and E. Diener

Department of Immunology and MRC Group on Immunoregulation, University of Alberta, Edmonton, Alberta, Canada.

We have shown earlier that carrier specific helper factor (Hf) extracted from carrier primed thymus derived (T) cells specifically triggers unprimed bone marrow derived (B) cells to produce anti-hapten antibodies *in vitro* in the presence of haptenated carrier. Such helper factor-B cell interaction was found to be allogeneically restricted (1). In this communication, we shall extend the validity of our experimental model from the use of soluble, polymeric to monomeric protein carriers as well as to the histocompatibility antigens of chicken red blood cells (CRBC). We shall furthermore discuss parameters bearing on the biochemical and serological properties of Hf.

1. *Conditions for Hf Mediated Hapten Specific Priming of B Cells in vitro in the Presence of Monomeric Haptenated Carrier*

As previously demonstrated, the conditions for optimal Hf mediated B cell triggering to hapten derivatives of various proteins such as RGG, HGG, BSA, or OVA depends on the focusing of Hf molecules by multiple carrier determinants so as to have them interact in a sufficiently large number with the B cell surface membrane. This was brought about by having the antigen present during the entire culture period in the form of a sequence of hapten carrier conjugates attached to a linear carbohydrate backbone (1). We have since extended these studies to the use of monomeric hapten-carrier conjugates. In contrast to the polymeric antigen, however, its monomeric form failed to cooperate in B cell triggering when admixed to the cultures together with Hf. Instead, optimal *in vitro*

ISBN 0-12-213950-X

immune induction was obtained only when the recognition step of antigen by the B cell was separated from the events of factor mediated help. Thus TNP specific primary plaque forming cell (PFC) responses were obtained when normal or T cell depleted spleen cells were first incubated with TNP-RGG for 30 minutes at 37°, washed free of antigen and cultured for three days in the presence of RGG specific Hf derived from RGG primed T cells. The requirements in these experiments for the temporal separation of the antigen recognition event by the B cell from the Hf mediated effect is reminiscent of the physiological sequence of cooperative mechanisms known to occur in immune induction *in situ*; here the interaction of antigen with B cells also preceeds the availability of effector T cell mediated help. Current experiments are designed to arrive at a conceptual understanding of the above described observations (2).

2. *Triggering of B Cells in vitro against Histo-compatability Antigens of Chicken Red Blood Cells by Antigen Specific T Cell Derived Helper Factor*

It has recently been found by colleagues in this department that mouse spleen cells are capable of generating specific humoral antibodies against allelically determined antigens of the major histocompatability locus of the chicken (3). We have exploited this finding to initiate helper factor-dependent triggering of unprimed B cells (anti-Thy-1 and C' treated spleen cells) *in vitro* to the products of either the B2 or the B13 allele present on chicken red blood cells (CRBC). It was found that helper factor induced by B2/2 CRBCs is effective in helping an immune response in the presence of B2/2 but not B13/13 CRBCs in culture. The degree of specificity of these responses compared favorably with that of *in vitro* responses to CRBCs by normal spleen cells (Table I).

Helper factor induced by B2/2 CRBCs was successfully absorbed by B2/2 but not by B13/13 CRBCs. Experiments were also carried out to test for the presence of mouse histocompatability antigens on helper factor. It was found that the biological activity of helper factor derived from CBA/J (H-2^k) T cells could effectively be removed by anti-IA^k but not by anti-H-2^d antibodies. No Ig determinants on helper factor could be recognized by means of anti-IgG antibodies (Table I).

TABLE I.

Hf Mediated Response to B^2/B^2 and B^{13}/B^{13} Chicken Erythrocytes (CRBC)
Antigen Specific Hf Replaces Specific T Cells

CRBC in Culture	CRBC in Assay	AFC/Culture (±SEM)				
		Hf to B^2/B^2 (x10-6 cell eq/culture)				
		0	0.1	0.2	1	2
B^2/B^2	B^2/B^2	8 ± 6	268 ± 30	476 ± 11	469 ± 39	400 ± 53
B^{13}/B^{13}	B^{13}/B^{13}	8 ± 11	32 ± 23	8 ± 20	32 ± 18	48 ± 2

Control Immune Response of Normal Spleen Cells to CRBC

Antigen in Culture	AFC/Culture (±SEM)	
	Assayed on B^2/B^2	Assayed on B^{13}/B^{13}
not added	44 ± 4	48 ± 6
B^2/B^2	360 ± 23	88 ± 27
B^{13}/B^{13}	48 ± 4	168 ± 46

Hf is Absorbed by B^2/B^2 CRBC and Anti-IA^k but not by Anti-H-2^d or Anti-IgG Antiserum

Hf Absorbed by	AFC/Culture (±SEM)
Sepharose 4B	248 ± 20
CRBC B^2/B^2	60 ± 23
CRBC B^{13}/B^{13}	244 ± 30
Anti-IA^k-Sepharose 4B	12 ± 18
Anti-H-2^d-Sepharose 4B	156 ± 32
Anti-IgG-Sepharose 4B	260 ± 25

3. *Radioresistant Cells are Necessary for Hf-B Cell Interaction*

B cells were separated from normal spleen cells by virtue of their capacity to form rosettes with CRBCs of either B2/2 or B13/13 histocompatability phenotype. The purified cells were then tested for immunocompetence *in vitro* in the presence of Hf specific for B2/2 in the presence of either B2/2 or B13/13 CRBC. It was found that rosette forming cells (RFC) when separated from non RFCs failed to generate a Hf dependent immune response in the presence of CRBC. Immunocompetence was restored, however, when RFCs were reconstituted with irradiated (1200 rad) non RFCs. It is noteworthy that such reconstitution was not possible with irradiated nylon purified cells, suggesting that the reconstituting elements in the above experiments represent radioresistant cells of the RES (Table II).

TABLE 2. Radioresistant Cells Necessary for Hf-B Cell Interaction

		AFC/culture ± S.E.			
Cells	*Hf specificity*	*0*[a]	*0.1*[a]	*0.5*[a]	*1.0*[a]
RFC(2/2)	Hf(2/2)	12±2	20±1	16±4	24±4
RFC(2/2) + nonRFC[b]	+ Hf(2/2)	52±13	88±11	180±35	404±1
RFC(13/13)	+ Hf(2/2)	12±2	20±2	16±2	20±2
RFC(13/13) +nonRFC[b]	+ Hf(2/2)	32±6	12±2	72±4	80±20

[a] *Hf($\times 10^{-6}$ cell eq/culture)*

[b] *irradiated (2/2, 13/13) histocompatability antigens*

This conclusion is in agreement with earlier findings by others (4) and with our predictions based on a hypothesis to explain the mechanisms underlying allogenic restrictions with respect to Hf-B cell cooperation (2).

4. *Physicochemical Characterization of Helper Factor*

We have reported elsewhere that purification of crude helper factor from RGG-primed T cells on a Sephadex G-100 column revealed three peaks (A,B,C) containing biological activity. However, carrier specific helper function was restricted to fractions B and C while the stimulatory activity of fraction A was mainly non-specific. As determined by isoelectric focusing, the specific component in fraction A had an isoelectric point (Ip) of 4.0 while the Ip's of the specifically active component in fractions B and C were 4.6 and 2.5 respectively. All non-specific components in fractions A, B and C were focused within a pH range of 5.5 to 7. It is interesting to note that purification of crude factor from CRBC primed T cells by G-100 Sephadex column chromatography yielded the same three fractions whose helper activity was entirely antigen specific. We are currently investigating the possibility that the non-specific contaminant of Hf extracted from RGG primed helper T cells may have derived from cells of the RES that had been stimulated by complete Freunds Adjuvant used for immunization. The most effective method of Hf purification was that of affinity chromatography. Crude factor from RGG primed T cells was applied at room temperature to a saline equilibrated column containing RGG coupled to Sepharose. Hf was best eluted with 2M NaCl at pH 6.5 and less effectively with 0.15 M Soerensen buffer at pH 2.5. It was furthermore found that the stability of Hf after purification was critically dependent on the presence of Ca^{++}.

REFERENCES

1. Shiozawa, C., Singh, B., Rubinstein, S., and Diener, E., *J. Immunol. 118,* 2199 (1977).
2. Shiozawa, C., Sonik, S., Singh, B., and Diener, E., *in* "T and B Lymphocytes: Recognition and Function", *Proc. ICN-UCLA Symposia on Molecular and Cellular Biology, 16,* Academic Press, N.Y. (1979), (in press).
3. Longenecker, B. M., Mosmann, T. R., and Shiozawa, C., (1979), (submitted for publication).
4. Feldmann, M., *J. Exp. Med. 135,* 1049 (1972).

PRODUCTION AND TESTING OF ANTIGEN SPECIFIC HUMAN HELPER AND SUPPRESSOR CELL FACTORS

James N. Woody[1]

Department of Pediatrics
and The Lombardi Cancer Center
Georgetown University School of Medicine
Washington, D.C.

Sirrka Kontianen

Department of Microbiology
University of Helsinki
Helsinki, Finland

Nathan J. Zvaifler

Department of Internal Medicine
University of California, San Diego
San Diego, California

Ann Rees
Marc Feldmann

Department of Zoology
University College
London, England

[1]This work was supported by the Naval Medical Research and Development Command Work Unit No. M0095.PN.001.1028 and Office of Naval Research Contract N000-14-77-C-0748.

ISBN 0-12-213950-X

I. INTRODUCTION

Because there are many human diseases with significant derangements of lymphoid function, there has been an interest in more efficient techniques for measuring human lymphocyte function.

We have investigated the responses of human T cells chiefly in the generation of antigen specific helper and suppressor T cells which release antigen specific factors. This communication will review our results in this area.

II. MATERIALS AND METHODS

Essentially these have been described elsewhere (Woody et al., 1979. In brief, human helper cells were produced by culturing human Ficoll-Hypaque purified blood lymphoid cells with low doses of antigen for four days, and suppressor cells were produced using similar culture techniques with a high dose of antigen, as described for the mouse (Kontianen et al., 1976). The helper or suppressor cells were recultured for 24 hours with a low dose of antigen and the supernatants collected, these were the factors described in our subsequent assay systems.

Factors were assayed on mouse spleen cells, helper factor by culturing on primed or unprimed spleen cells, with antigen, however without a source of mouse helper cells. Suppressor factor, was also tested on primed or unprimed spleen cells with antigen and a source of normal mouse helper cells (Kontianen et al., 1976, Feldmann et al., 1979).

III. RESULTS AND DISCUSSION

A. *Helper Factors*

Human helper factors have been produced with a variety of antigens, so far we have used proteins such as keyhole limpet haemocyanin (KLH), and synthetic antigens like (T,G)A--L or GAT. Depending on the type of antigen used, the frequency of responding individual varied with all healthy individuals responding to KLH, but only about a third to the synthetic polypeptides. This is analogous to the situation in rodents where these antigens are under MHC linked Ir gene control. We have consistently found, over a three year period, that the level of responses induced by human factors is not significantly less than that induced by mouse factors, although the concentration of helper factor necessary to give a response is somewhat higher. This lack of species specificity has been noticed previously with both specific and non-specific factors (Feldmann et al., 1977). A representative experiment demonstrating the antigen specificity of human helper factor is shown in Table 1.

TABLE I. Assay of Human Antigen Specific Helper Factor

Helper Factor	*Antigen*	*IgM Anti DNP AFC Per Culture ± SE*[a]
--	*DNP-BEADS*	*1020 ± 99*
--	*TNP-KLH*	*103 ± 11*
HuHF-KLH	*TNP-KLH*	*679 ± 18*
--	*DNP-TGAL*	*68 ± 14*
HuHF-KLH	*DNP-TGAL*	*275 ± 17*
--	*DNP-GAT*	*171 ± 48*
HuHF-KLH	*DNP-GAT*	*252 ± 26*

[a]*Assays were performed using spleen cells from mice primed monthly for three months with the antigen DNP-CgG.*

The cell interactions during the induction of human helper factor have been analyzed (Rees et al., 1979). Just as in the mouse there is a requirement for adherent cells, which can be replaced by monocytes. There is also a genetic restriction with preliminary data indicating a requirement for compatibility at the HLA-D region (Rees et al., 1979).

The structure of helper factor is still not fully understood. Immunoabsorbent analysis indicates that helper factor binds to antigen and rabbit anti-IA (human equivalent) antisera also absorbs helper factor, indicating that the basic structure is akin to that of the mouse helper factor (Feldmann et al., 1979).

B. *Suppressor Factors*

Human lymphoid cells, cultured with high concentrations of antigen release factors which inhibit mouse antibody responses of both primary and secondary nature. This suppression is antigen specific, inhibiting both IgM and IgG responses. A representative experiment is shown in Table 2, using KLH as antigen and testing primed spleen cells.

TABLE II. Assay of Human Antigen Specific Suppressor Factor

Helper[a] Cells	Suppressor Factor	Antigen	anti DNP AFC per culture ± SE[b] IgM	IgG
-	-	TNP-KLH	56± 29	267± 57
$3x10^5$	-	TNP-KLH	2433± 285	7000± 306
$3x10^5$	(A) Human SF_{KLH} 3%	TNP-KLH	983± 120	3933±1091
$3x10^5$	0.3%	TNP-KLH	1250±1247	6667±2008
$3x10^5$	(B) Human SF_{KLH} 3%	TNP-KLH	1000± 153	2933± 371
$3x10^5$	0.3%	TNP-KLH	1483± 292	5933±1267

[a]*Mouse helper cells were nylon wool passed spleen cells from mice primed three times (monthly) with KLH on bentonite*

[b]*Assays were performed using spleen cells from mice primed monthly for three months with the antigen DNP-CgG*

Characterization of this material and analysis of the mode of action is still preliminary but one observation of interest was that some antisera to mouse suppressor factor also react with human suppressor factors.

We have made rabbit and mouse antisera to mouse suppressor factor (Kontianen et al., 1979, Rees et al., 1979). These antisera react in distinct patterns and have helped formulate our ideas of factor structure. Thus mouse anti factor antisera are idiotype like and react only with factors with the appropriate strain and antigen specificity, thus defining a variable like region. Rabbit antisera react with factors of all strains and antigen specificity, thus defining a "constant region". Such antisera also react with human factors (unpublished observations) indicating that there is a conserved region of the factor with similar serologic determinants in man and mouse. This observation also explains the lack of species specificity of suppressor factor action, and presumably of helper factor activity as well.

IV. CONCLUSIONS

In the absence of appropriate human B cell assays we have chosen to assay human T cells with mouse B cells. Human T cell factors are not species specific (Woody et al., 1979). Thus these assays have provided evidence for the existence of the same regulatory pathways in man as established in rodents, and have provided a potential means of analyzing human Ir gene function. These techniques have a potential for investigating the increasingly obvious association between HLA and disease.

ACKNOWLEDGMENTS

The authors wish to thank Ms. Betsy Ketterer who helped with portions of the experiments and Bonita Minor who assisted in the preparation of the manuscript.

REFERENCES

Feldmann, M., Beverley, P., Erb, P., et al. (1977). Cold Spring Harbor Symp. Quant. Biol. 41, 113.
Feldmann, M., Cecka, J., Cosenza, H., et al. (1979). J. of Supramolecular Structure (Proc. 1979 ICN-UCLA Symposia) (C. Fox, ed.) (In Press).
Kontianen, S., and Feldmann, M. (1976). European J. of Immun. 6, 296.
Kontianen, S., and Feldmann, M. (1979). Thymus (In Press).
Rees, A., Erb, P., Woody, J. et al. (1979). Proc. New York Acad. Sci. (In Press).
Woody, J., Zvaifler, N., Rees, A. et al. (1979). Trans. Proc. 11, 382.

GENERAL DISCUSSION ON ANTIGEN-SPECIFIC HELPER FACTORS

GOODMAN: Does anyone who has worked with antigen-helper factors have any information about whether the I region coded determinants and the H_V markers are on a single polypeptide chain?

FELDMANN: No one knows conclusively how many polypeptide chains there are on these factors.

OPPENHEIM: It is not clear to me why Diener indicates that macrophages are not needed for the response to soluble hapten-carrier antigens. Since macrophage factors only augment the T cell response to antigens, how does he account for the response to soluble antigen in the absence of the macrophage presentation function?

DIENER: We have shown that when macrophages are removed from B cells, cooperation of these B cells with crude helper factor is unimpaired. As I pointed out in my report, crude extract from in vivo carrier-primed T cells contains both a specific helper factor and a non-specific, antigen-independent B cell stimulating factor; these factors are separable by affinity chromatography. Since in the experiment I have shown, macrophages have not been removed from the educated T cells prior to factor extraction, the aforementioned non-specific contaminant could have been of macrophage origin. If this is the case the apparent lack of a macrophage requirement in helper factor-B cell cooperation to soluble antigens could, in our experiments, have been due to macrophage-replacing factor derived from the contaminating macrophages at the time of helper-factor extraction.

FELDMANN: The lack of strain specificity of the GAT idiotype system suggests that the antibodies recognize the combining site for antigen. This may be the same for both T and B cells without these necessarily being controlled by the same gene cluster. Does Germain have any evidence for the combining site of SF being controlled by the Ig gene cluster?

GERMAIN: Without allotype linkage of CGAT expression, it is difficult to prove that GAT-TsF actually uses the *same* gene(s) as anti-GAT immunoglobulins for construction of its combining site. However, azobenzenearsenate (ABA) specific TsF of A/J mice has been shown to possess the characteristic cross-reactive idiotype of anti-ABA antibodies, and the presence of this

ISBN 0-12-213950-X

idiotype on the TsF is regulated by allotype-limited genes. Since ABA-TsF and GAT-TsF are extremely similar in functional properties, one might draw the analogy that a similar envolvement of allotype-linked genes occurs in the GAT model which cannot be shown directly due to the lack of polymorphism in the system.

FELDMANN: Before we continue to suppressor cells and suppressor factors, it may be useful to summarize what most workers in this field believe. Every other worker has reported that these helper factors carry Ia determinants of a type that has not yet been characterized; all these molecules have antigen-combining sites. There is evidence for some relationship between the antigen-combining sites of these factors and immunoglobulin-combining sites and Ig markers. But there are also a number of things which are still puzzling: It is not clear why some factors have strain restrictions, yet other factors do not even have species restrictions. It is not clear exactly how these factors stimulate B cells and least clear of all is the molecular weight of these factors. We hear a range of 50,000 - 70,000 MW but nobody has presented any extensive analysis and this is probably indicative that there is no great confidence in these figures.

CHARACTERISATION OF AN ANTIGEN-SPECIFIC SUPPRESSOR FACTOR FROM A HYBRID T-CELL LINE.

Michael J. Taussig
Andrew Holliman

Department of Immunology
ARC Institute of Animal Physiology
Babraham, Cambridge, England

Jose R.F. Corvalan

Lilly Research Center
Erl Wood Manor, Windlesham
Surrey, England

We describe here some of the properties of a factor present in the supernatant of a hybrid T-cell line, designated A1. The line arose as a result of fusion between a thymoma, BW5147, and mouse (C57Bl/10) spleen cells primed against sheep red blood cells (SRBC), (Holliman and Taussig, 1978; Taussig et al., 1979a,b). 48 hour supernatants of the growing line were added to cultures of either unprimed mouse thoracic duct lymphocytes (TDL) or of SRBC-primed mouse spleen cells, whereupon it was found that both the primary (IgM) and secondary (IgM and IgG) PFC responses to SRBC were totally suppressed by A1 supernatant, but not by supernatants of BW5147 or 38 other T-hybrid lines produced in the same fusion. The suppressive activity of fresh supernatants could be titrated out to a 50% end-point at a final dilution in the cultures of about 1:270. Specificity was demonstrated (a) in the lack of suppression

Supported in part by USPHS grant AI-13162 and MRC grant G 975/871/C

ISBN 0-12-213950-X

of the responses to other red cells or hapten-protein conjugates and (b) in the specific removal of activity following absorption of the supernatant with SRBC. Moreover, suppression by A1 factor was carrier-specific and extended to haptens coupled to SRBC.

The nature of the A1 factor was explored by passage over anti-Ig and anti-H2 immunoadsorbents (Figure 1). A variety of anti-Ig's failed to remove the suppressor activity including anti-IgM, anti-IgG_{2a}, anti-IgG_{2b} and anti-IgA. On the other hand, anti-H2 sera removed the activity, provided they were directed against the haplotype of the spleen cells used in the fusion (H2^b) rather than that of BW5147 (H2^k). In further experiments, anti-H2^b serum was absorbed with spleen cells of recombinant mice to produce reagents capable of reacting with restricted regions of H2 only, (Figure 2). The reagents were used as immunoabsorbents to remove A1 activity and, as shown in Fig. 2, the A1 factor was

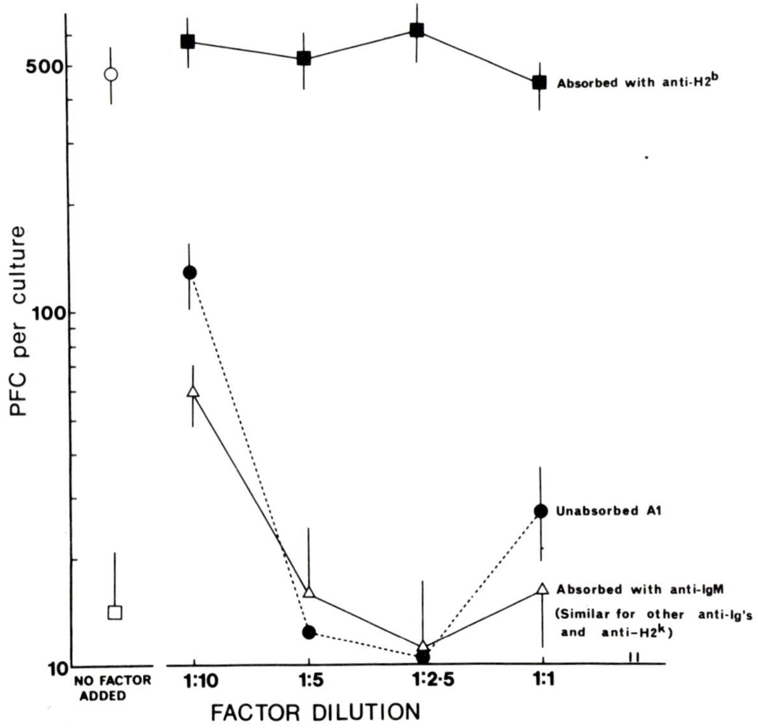

Fig. 1. Titration of A1 supernatant, before and after absorption with anti-Ig or anti-H-2 absorbents, in the primary response of mouse (CBA) TDL to SRBC in vitro. Open square and circle are negative and positive control responses.

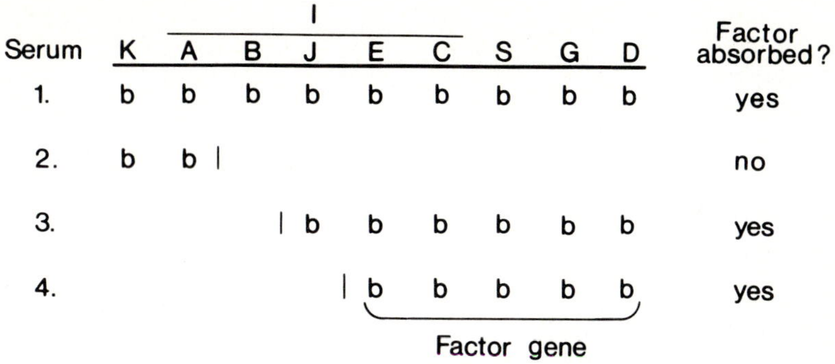

Fig. 2. Mapping a gene coding for A1 suppressor factor. A1 supernatant was absorbed with the following anti-H-2 reagents as sepharose absorbents. 1: B10.A anti-B10, 2: B10.A anti-B10 absorbed B10.A(4R), 3: B10.A anti-B10 absorbed B10.A(5R), 4: B10.A anti-B10 absorbed B10.A(3R). Residual factor activity was then tested in vitro. The chart indicates the H-2 regions against which each reagent could in principle react.

removed by antibodies reacting with determinants coded by genes to the right of the I-J subregions. If the factor is an I-region product (and this has yet to be established), the result implies that it may map to the I-E/C subregion. This mapping distinguishes the A1 suppressor factor from the molecules described by Tada and coworkers produced from T cells or T hybrid lines, which have been shown to carry I-J determinants (Taniguchi et al. 1979).

In order to study the structure of the factor, A1 cells were cultured in the presence of ^{3}H-leucine for 20 hours; at the end of this time labelled molecules binding specifically to SRBC were detectable in the supernatant (Taussig and Holliman, 1979). Aliquots of the labelled supernatant were absorbed on to SRBC and, after washing, the latter were run on 10% and 15% polyacrylamide gels in sodium dodecyl sulphate (SDS-PAGE). As shown in Figure 3a and 3b, this revealed a two chain structure, with a large chain of apparent m.w. about 85,000 and a smaller chain of m.w. about 25,000. The chains were not disulphide bridged, similar profiles being obtained with and without 2-ME. If the supernatant was first precipitated with anti-H2^b serum and anti-mouse Ig, both chains were removed, suggesting that one or both carried H2 determinants (Fig. 6c). In subsequent experiments, A1 cells labelled with ^{3}H-leucine were lysed with the non-ionic

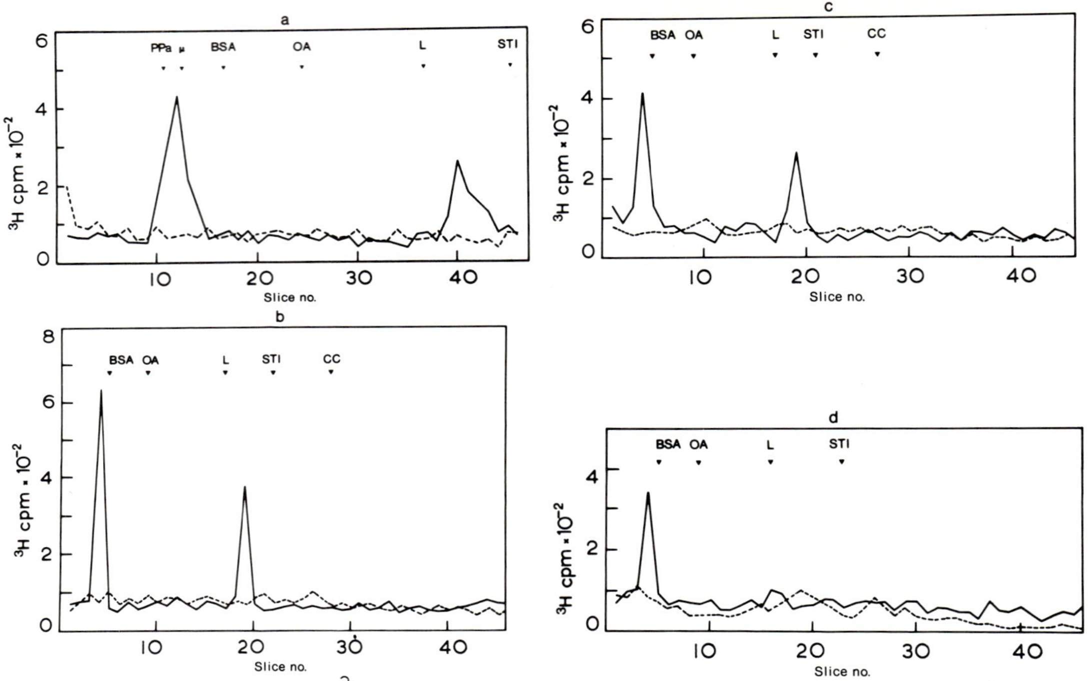

Fig. 3. SDS-PAGE profiles of ^{3}H-labelled SRBC-binding molecules of the A1 line. (a) 10% and (b) 15% SDS-PAGE of labelled supernatant of A1 (solid line) or BW5147 (dashed) absorbed onto SRBC. (c) 15% SDS-PAGE of labelled A1 supernatant absorbed onto SRBC after precipitation with anti-H-2^k serum (solid line) or anti-H-2^b serum (dashed) and anti-mIg serum. (d) 15% SDS-PAGE of NP-40 lysate of labelled A1 cells (solid line) or BW5147 cells (dashed) absorbed onto fixed SRBC. Markers: phosphorylase a (PPa); μ and L chains of MOPC 104E; bovine serum albumin (BSA); ovalbumin (OA); soyabean trypsin inhibitor (STI); cytochrome c (CC).

detergent NP-40; the extracts were absorbed onto SRBC which had been fixed by treatment with glutaraldehyde (to prevent their lysis in NP-40) and the latter again run, after washing, on SDS-PAGE. In contrast with the profiles obtained with labelled supernatant, the SRBC-binding molecules in NP-40 lysates appeared to consist only of a single chain of molecular weight about 85,000. Moreover, this large chain was unaffected by precipitation with anti-H2 serum. Thus, if this chain corresponds to the large chain of the supernatant molecule, we conclude that the H2 specificities of the latter are probably carried by its smaller (25,000) chain. Finally, the m.w. of the native factor molecule was determined by passage of (unlabelled) supernatants through an ultrogel AcA-34 gel filtration column. Suppressor activity emerged in the m.w. range of 7S IgM (about 200,000 daltons).

In conclusion, the A1 suppressor factor appears to be a larger molecule than antigen-specific factors described hitherto. It seems to consist of two types of polypeptide chain, of which the larger (85,000) combines specifically with SRBC but lacks H-2 specificities; the smaller (25,000) probably carries H-2 coded determinants, but there is no evidence that it contributes to SRBC binding. Elsewhere we have shown that the target of action of the factor is a B cell carrying an H-2 controlled acceptor site with which the factor combines (Taussig et al. 1979b). We speculate that the small factor chain is responsible for interacting with this acceptor and for suppressing the development of the antibody-forming cell, while the role of the large chain is to focus the factor to the surface of SRBC-binding B lymphocytes.

Acknowledgments We thank Dr. Peter Demant (Amsterdam) and Mr. J. Herbert (Babraham) for kindly providing anti-H-2 and anti-Ig sera respectively.

References

Holliman, A. and Taussig, M.J. (1978). J. Physiol. 284, 5P.

Taniguchi, M., Saito, T, Takei, I. and Tada, T. (1979). This volume.

Taussig, M.J. and Holliman, A. (1979) Nature 277, 308.

Taussig, M.J., Corvalan, J.R.F., Binns, R.M. and Holliman, A. (1979a). Nature 277, 305.

Taussig, M.J., Corvalan, J.R.F. and Holliman, A. (1979b). Anns. N.Y. Acad. Sci. in press

FUNCTIONAL ORGANIZATION OF I-J SUBREGION GENE PRODUCTS ON T CELL HYBRIDOMAS

Masaru Taniguchi [1)]
Izumi Takei
Takashi Saito
Keiichi Hiramatsu

Laboratories for Immunology
School of Medicine
Chiba University
Chiba, Japan

Tomio Tada

Department of Immunology
Faculty of Medicine
Tokyo University
Tokyo, Japan

A series of our previous studies have been centering around the mechanisms of suppression of antibody response by T cells and T cell-derived factors(1-4). In the antigen-specific suppression, it has been shown that the effect of an antigen-specific suppressor T cell is mediated by a soluble product from the suppressor T cells and that the active factor has antigen-binding site and products of genes mapped in *I-J* subregion of the mouse *H-2* complex(1-3). Similar findings were reported by several investigators(5-7). Much less is known about the chemistry and mode of action of the suppressor T cell factor, because of the limitation in collecting sufficient quantities of antigen-specific suppressor T cells and their factor. Application of the cell hybridization technique to establish I-J bearing T cell hybridoma with suppressive

1) *This work was partly supported by the International Cancer Research Data Bank Programme of NCI/NIH, No.NO1-CO-65341.*

ISBN 0-12-213950-X

function would provide great advantages for characterizing the suppressor factor at the molecular level. We have obtained several hybridoma cell lines producing I-J positive molecules which suppress the antibody response either in an antigen-specific or nonspecific fashion. The present communication deals with a characterization of suppressor factor derived from several I-J bearing T cell hybridoma lines. These studies indicated the heterogeneity of the I-J subregion gene products.

I. I-J SUBREGION GENE PRODUCTS EXPRESSED ON THE HYBRIDOMAS WITH SUPPRESSIVE FUNCTION

High frequency of I-J bearing fused cells with suppressive function was reproducibly attained by the combination of three procedures: 1) the use of the enriched population of the antigen-specific suppressor T cells for fusion with a T lymphoma cell line. 2) the selection of fused cells in HAT medium. 3) the separation of I-J positive hybrid cells by fluorescence activated cell sorter after the selection process with HAT medium(8).

The hybrids were made by fusion of an AKR thymoma cell line, BW5147(*H-2*^{k}) with the enriched suppressor T cells of C57BL/6(*H-2*^{b}) specific for keyhole limpet hemocyanin(KLH) by adsorption and elution on the antigen coated Petri dishes(9). After selection by HAT medium, fused cells grown in HAT medium were stained with anti-I-J^b(B10A(5R)anti-B10A(3R)) and fluorescence labelled rabbit anti-mouse immunoglobulins. I-J$^+$ hybrids were obtained by sorting out with fluorescence activated cell sorter(FACS) followed by the cloning with limiting dilution or single cell manipulation. The cell lines cloned

Table I. Selective Expression of I-J Subregion Gene Products on T Cell Hybridomas

Anti-I-J^b absorbed with	I-J haplotype	% Cytotoxicity on 34S-18	34S-15	34S-281
none	—	90	89	100
C57BL/6	b	2	N.D.	20
C3H	k	79	N.D.	74
B10.A(3R)	b	0	13	15
B10.A(5R)	k	75	76	80

at least twice were further investigated for surface markers by conventional dye exclusion cytotoxic assay using various alloantisera. The hybrid cell lines so far tested expressed $H\text{-}2^k$, $H\text{-}2^b$, $I\text{-}J^b$, Thyl.1 and Thyl.2 antigens, whereas no Immunoglobulins were detectable on their surface.

It is known that mouse alloantisera often contain anti-murine leukemia virus activity. Lymphoid cell lines are quite likely to bear viral determinants on their surface. Hence, in order to know whether *I-J* subregion gene products would selectively be expressed on the T cell hybridomas, anti-$I\text{-}J^b$ extensively preabsorbed with BW5147 was absorbed 4 times with 100 x 10^6 spleen cells of various strains of mice. The residual cytotoxic activity was then tested on the established T cell hybridomas. As shown in Table I, all cell lines tested were killed by anti-$I\text{-}J^b$ preabsorbed with BW5147 cells. Absorption with C57BL/6($H\text{-}2^b$) spleen cells however removed their cytotoxic activity, whereas that with C3H($H\text{-}2^k$) did not. Moreover, absorption with B10A(3R) but not B10A(5R) spleen cells also removed cytotoxic activity. In all cases, the absorption with $I\text{-}J^b$ haplotype cell populations always removed the antibody activity against T cell hybridomas.

We now have several T cell hybridoma lines expressing I-J determinants, some of which display suppressive activity in the in vitro secondary antibody response, either in an antigen-specific or nonspecific fashion. Some other hybridomas have no suppressive activity even though they express *I-J* subregion gene products on their cell surface. It is evident that these hybridomas have different functional properties, despite that they all express *I-J* subregion gene products.

Table II. Absorption of Hybridoma-Derived Antigen-Specific (34S-704) or Nonspecific(34S-44) Suppressor Factor with Various Immunoadsorbents Composed of Antigens or Antibodies

Factors Absorbed with	*Anti-DNP IgG PFC/culture*	
	34S-704 factor	*34S-44 factor*
——	2437 ± 205	2160 ± 243
Unabsorbed	725 ± 240	115 ± 92
KLH	2180 ± 134	273 ± 56
Asc	860 ± 289	201 ± 106
Anti-mouse Igs	634 ± 185	301 ± 37
Anti-$I\text{-}J^b$	2094 ± 83	1577 ± 373
Anti-$I\text{-}J^k$	363 ± 191	72 ± 42

II. HYBRIDOMA-DERIVED I-J BEARING SUPPRESSIVE FACTORS

Previous studies have shown that at least two subsets of T cells having *I-J* determined molecules are involved in the suppression of antibody response(10). T cells having I-J determinants and $Ly2^+3^+$ phenotype produce antigen-specific, I-J bearing suppressor factor. They induce new suppressor T cells which have accepted antigen-specific factor. The induced suppressor T cells act across *H-2* barrier and suppress the antibody response in antigen-nonspecific fashion in the final effector phase of the suppression. It is therefore of interest to examine immunochemical characteristics of hybridoma-derived antigen-specific and nonspecific suppressor factors. The factors derived from antigen-specific suppressor hybridoma 34S-704 or nonspecific suppressor hybridoma 34S-44 were absorbed with immunoadsorbents composed of specific antigen(KLH), irrelevant antigen(Ascaris extract), anti-I-J and polyvarent anti-mouse immunoglobulins(MIgs). Table II shows the results. The antigen-specific suppressor molecule from the hybridoma 34S-704 has an antigen-binding structure and *I-J* coded determinants, whereas antigen-nonspecific suppressor molecule from the hybridoma 34S-44 has only I-J determinants.

Another important observation with hybridoma derived suppressor factors is that there exsists a strict genetic restriction in an antigen-specific suppression. On the other hand, antigen-nonspecific suppressor factor acts across H-2 barrier. Since hybrids were made between BW5147 and $H\text{-}2^b$ suppressor T cells, suppressive effect of the hybridoma-derived factor was examined on the response of C3H, C57BL/6 or their F_1 mice. Table III summarizes the results. The antigen-specific factor from 34S-18 suppressed only the responses of $H\text{-}2^b$ and $H\text{-}2^{b/k}F_1$ mice, while antigen-nonspecific factor from 34S-44

Table III. Effects of Hybridoma-Derived Suppressor Factors on the Response of Syngeneic or Allogeneic Spleen Cells

Factor from	Suppressive activity	Anti-DNP IgG PFC/culture		
		C57BL/6	C3B F_1	C3H
not added	——	3035	9186	1450
BW5147	no	3368	8568	1183
34S-18	antigen-specific	469	1933	2014
34S-44	non-specific	224	1940	203

suppressed the responses of $H\text{-}2^k$ as well as those of $H\text{-}2^b$ and $H\text{-}2^{b/k}F_1$ spleen cells.

III. HETEROGENEITY OF I-J SUBREGION GENE PRODUCTS

The findings shown above indicate that functional differences of I-J bearing suppressor factors probably reflect the heterogeneity of *I-J* subregion gene products which are expressed on different subsets of T cells. In order to examine this possibility, anti-I-J^b antisera were absorbed with each I-J bearing hybridoma cell line having different activity. The residual cytotoxic activities of the absorbed anti-I-J^b antisera were tested on the panel of hybridoma lines. Table IV surmmarizes the results of this experiments. All cell lines tested were killed by anti-I-J^b antiserum. Absorption with hybridoma cells with antigen-specific suppressive function, (34S-704) removed the activity against themseleves, whereas the absorbed anti-I-J antisera still have cytotoxic activity against other functionally different hybridoma cell lines (eg. 34S-281, 34S-44). Similar result was obtained in the case of absorption with hybridoma cells having nonspecific suppressor function(34S-44). On the other hand, absorption with hybridoma without function(34S-281) removed the cytotoxic activity of anti-I-J^b sera against all hybrid cell lines. These results suggested that hybrid cell line 34S-281 has two different I-J determinants each of which was shared by either of two other hybridomas expressing different functional activities (34S-44 and 34S-704). This was confirmed by the results of the experiments that anti-I-J^b absorbed with both 34S-44 and 34S-704 could not react with 34S-281. These findings indicate that there are at least two genes within *I-J* subregion coding

Table IV. Heterogeneity of I-J Subregion Gene Products

Target cells	Suppressive activity	% Cytotoxicity by anti-I-J^b absorbed with					Determinants	
		no	34S-281	34S-704	34S-44	34S-704 34S-44		
34S-281	no	86	-	52	74	-	1	2
34S-704	specific	88	-	-	40	-		2
34S-44	non-specific	70	-	30	-	-	1	

for distinct products expressed on the functionally different subsets of T cells. Definitive answer should wait chemical analysis of the hybridoma-derived antigen-specific and non-specific suppressor molecules.

In any events, *I-J* determined molecules seem to be able to discriminate the fine polymorphism of *I*-region gene products expressed on other cell types to find out the proper partner to talk with.

ACKNOWLEDGMENT

We wish to thank Drs. M. Igarashi and M. Yamada for their help. We also wish to thank Dr. N. Shinohara for his generous discussion.

REFERENCES

1. Takemori, T., and Tada, T., *J. Exp. Med. 142,* 1241 (1975).
2. Taniguchi, M., Hayakawa, K., and Tada, T., *J. Immunol.116,* 542 (1976).
3. Tada, T., Taniguchi, M., and David, C.S., *J. Exp. Med.144,* 713 (1976).
4. Taniguchi, M., Tada, T., and Tokuhisa, T., *J. Exp. Med. 144,* 20 (1976).
5. Thèze, J., Kapp, J.A., and Benacerraf, B., *J. Exp. Med. 145,* 839 (1977).
6. Thèze, J., Waltenbaugh, C., Dorf, M.E.,and Benacerraf, B., *J. Exp. Med. 146,* 287 (1977).
7. Kontiainen, S., and Feldmann, M., *Eur. J. Immunol. 7,* 310 (1977).
8. Taniguchi, M., Saito, T., and Tada, T., *Nature. 278,* 555 (1979).
9. Taniguchi, M., and Miller, J.F.A.P., *J. Exp. Med. 146,*1450 (1978).
10. Tada, T., *In* "Immune System: Genetics and Regulation" (E. Sercarz, L.A. Herzenberg, and C.F. Fox, ed) p.354. Academic Press, New York (1977).

GENERAL DISCUSSION ON ANTIGEN-SPECIFIC SUPPRESSOR FACTORS

GOODMAN: Action across H-2 does not preclude molecular interaction at the cell surface involving I-region markers. A point of confusion with the factors is that some, such as Tada's are H-2 restricted whereas others, such as that of Kontiainen, seem not to be. It is not clear what the basis is for this; perhaps it involves the targets, which may be different.

KONTIAINEN: As antigen-specific suppressor factors act across H-2 (or species) barrier, the I-J coded determinants in factors acting on T-helper cells seem not to be essential for the suppressor function as such. However, they may well have other functions, e.g. act as a transport-piece or in "homing" of the suppressor factors *in vivo*.

FELDMANN: Since one can go across many H-2 barriers, it is not clear in every system that the Ia determinants are recognized. There are some recent reports that some helper factors also bear I-J; that could mean either that the I-J region is heterogeneous or that the I-J determinants are not implicit in a function.

TAUSSIG: We also wondered about the significance of the action of Ia-bearing helper factors across strain and species barriers. Most likely, the Ia chain is indeed involved in activity and the critical interaction sites are preserved in different strains and species; the polymorphic determinants are presumably not associated with those interaction sites.

TANIGUCHI: As mentioned in my report, there are two genes in the I-J subregion coding for determinants expressed on suppressor T-cells with different function. We have also published that I-J determined molecules are expressed on a subset of helper T-cells. These results suggest that there are at least three genes in the I-J subregion coding for different I-J determinants.

DIENER: It appeared some time ago that allogeneic restriction in specific (T) factor-B cell interaction relates to a factor obtained by extraction from carrier-educated T cells. Is there any consistancy as to the conditions which will yield allogeneically restricted factor?

ISBN 0-12-213950-X

TANIGUCHI: We have always obtained allogeneically restricted helper and suppressor factors by the physical extraction of educated T cells. I would like to make another comment about the H-2 restriction of T cell-derived factors. There are some discrepancies in the H-2 restrictions among antigen-specific factors. One of the alternative interpretations for this is as follows: T cells have two binding sites; one for antigen, the other for self- or allo-antigens. If conventional anti-Ia antisera contain anti-idiotypic antibody for self- or allo-antigen reactive receptors, the determinant on T cell or T cell-factor detected by anti-Ia antisera could be the receptor site for self- or allo-antigens. If this is the case, the receptor site for self- or allo-antigens may discriminate an H-2 barrier.

FELDMANN: The biochemical characterization of these factors is still incredibly primitive. However, certain advances have been made. In particular, the use of monoclonal cell lines and hybridomas to produce active material should now permit more effective analysis. The results of such studies suggest that there are at least two chains, as shown by Taussig. The effluent experiments of Taniguchi also suggest that there are at least two different chains. Of course this does not mean that there could not be even more components. The factor combining site certainly appears to be shared to some extent with antibody molecules and we have learned of two reports of idiotype markers on a helper and on a suppressor factor. There are also data indicating the presence of V_H markers on helper and suppressor factors. Would Goodman like to comment on the biochemical characterization of these factors?

GOODMAN: I cannot add much to the biochemical characterization of antigen-specific T cell molecules. We have an azobenzenearsonate (ABA) binding molecule from strain A/J T cells which looks, superficially, like Taussig's heavy chain. It has a nominal MW of 70 - 92,000, depending on the method, and is devoid of anti-Ig or anti-Ia reacitvity. We now have several T cell hybridomas which bind ABA and appear to express the major idiotype associated with this specificity, but as yet we have not characterized the products of their cells.

LEON: Since Taniguchi's material is obtained from extracted cells one can always raise the possibility that the apparent presence of I-J determinants and antigen-binding activity on two polypeptide chains (in contrast with Mozes' data) is due to a proteolytic cleavage. Similarly, differences in molecular weight values for these T cell molecules may also reflect differences in susceptibility to proteolytic cleavage, such as is found for IgD in relation to the other classes of immunoglobulin.

FELDMANN: For this group of molecules which have Ia determinants and combining sites related to Ig, there are a lot of questions which remain to be answered, besides the biochemical ones which seem to be foremost in many people's minds. Conceptually, some important points have remained untouched. How many different types of antigen-specific factors are there? Is the difference between factors which are genetically restricted in their action and those which are not, a technical artifact; or is it an indication that they are two different types of molecules? Is there a basic biological difference between suppressor factors with a MW of about 200,000 daltons from those with a MW of about 50,000? All we can say at the moment is that there is probably a *family* of helper and suppressor factors. Some of them may act not on antibody formation but on delayed hypersensitivity, a topic which we have not discussed at all. At this time, our questions probably resemble the state of discussion about immunoglobulins in the late 1940s when the typical question was: "Are the agglutinins different from the precipitins?" Some years from now, our questions will probably appear ludicrous to the protagonists at that time.

PATTERNS OF IN VIVO RELEASE OF LYMPHOKINES THEIR ENHANCEMENT AND INHIBITION

S. B. Salvin[1]
and
Ruth Neta

Department of Microbiology
University of Pittsburgh
School of Medicine[1]
and
University of Notre Dame[2]

Studies on the production of lymphokines in man and animals have been carried out in vitro by exposing lymphoid cells to a specific antigen or to a mitogen. Our research is concerned primarily with the formation and release of lymphokines in vivo in the intact animal. A phase of this work relating to the in vivo release of migration inhibitory factor (MIF) and type II interferon (IF II) with respect to other lymphokines and in different strains of mice is to be presented.

High titers of lymphokines released into the circulation in vivo were obtained in mice sensitized to components of the tubercle bacillus. Herein, mice were sensitized intravenously with 300 μg cell walls of Mycobacterium bovis strain BCG* in Drakeol-Tween 80 emulsion, and three weeks later were challenged intravenously with 50 mg old tuberculin (OT). The mice were exsanguinated at intervals after the intravenous challenge, and the resulting sera assayed for the presence of lymphokines. Appropriate controls of nonsensitized mice challenged with OT, sensitized mice not challenged with OT, and BCG-

**Obtained through the courtesy of Dr. Edgar Ribi, Rocky Mountain Laboratory, Hamilton, Montana.*

ISBN 0-12-213950-X

sensitized or normal mice challenged with lipopolysaccharide (LPS) yielded either non-detectable amounts of or low titers of MIF or IF II (1-3).

In the original studies using outbred Swiss white mice purchased from Taconic Farms, Germantown, New York, pools of 5 or more mice consistently yielded titers of MIF in the range of 1:128 to 1:512. The titer refers to that dilution of serum which inhibited migration of normal mouse peritoneal macrophages 20% or more (4). When other strains of mice were similarly assayed for their capacity to release MIF or IF II *in vivo* into the circulation, the amount of these lymphokines in the sera varied depending on the strain of mouse. Thus, C57Bl/KsJ, DBA/2, and BALB/cByJ all released MIF and IF II into the circulation in high titers. In contrast, AKR, CBA/Ca, and DBA/1 did not produce detectable quantities of these lymphokines. The three high-responders all belonged to the $H-2^d$ histocompatibility type, whereas the low-responders were either $H-2^k$ (AKR and CBA/Ca) or $H-2^q$ (DBA/1).

Studies were then initiated to determine whether this capacity of sensitized mice to respond to challenge with specific antigen could be altered by experimental manipulation. CFA has been shown to induce suppressor-cell activity (5). Accordingly, one group of mice was inoculated subcutaneously with complete Freund's adjuvant (CFA), containing 2 mg dead tubercle bacilli, two weeks before intravenous sensitization with BCG cell walls; a second group was inoculated subcutaneously one week after intravenous sensitization but two weeks before intravenous challenge with OT. Control mice were sensitized intravenously and three weeks later challenged with OT. The group of mice that had been treated with CFA before sensitization and challenge showed an enhanced release of IF II into the circulation; this result applied both to the high-responder and low-responder strains. In contrast, the group of mice that had been treated with CFA one week after sensitization but two weeks before challenge released less IF II into the circulation. Thus, the capacity to release MIF or IF II into the circulation seems to have a genetic basis, yet can be influenced somewhat by experimental conditions.

The strains of mice that had been studied for their capacity to produce MIF and IF II *in vivo* were also studied for their capacity to release other lymphokines into the circulation, such as lymphotoxin (LT), mitogenic factor (MF), and macrophage activating factor (MAF). Although strains of mice that released MIF also released quantities of IF II in parallel, the three other lymphokines did not follow this pattern, and appeared independently of the MIF and IF II, as well as of each other.

The possible relationship between the capacity to release MIF and the capacity to develop cell-mediated immunity was then investigated. DBA/2 mice, high responders of MIF and IF II, and DBA/1 mice, low-responders of MIF and IF II, were challenged intraoesophageally with 2 x 10^6 18-hour-old cells of Candida albicans, and the fecal pellets cultured quantitatively on Sabouraud's agar at daily intervals up to ten days after challenge. The DBA/2 mice completely eliminated the fungus from the stools in less than ten days, whereas the DBA/1 mice still had the fungus present in the stools on the tenth day after challenge. In addition, the highest counts in the fecal pellets of the DBA/2 mice were 10^1 to 10^2 fungal colonies per pellet on the third day after challenge, whereas the counts of the C. albicans in the fecal pellets of the DBA/1 mice were 10^3 to 10^5 on the tenth day after challenge (the last day of experimentation) and were apparently still rising. Thus, the strain of mouse (DBA/2) that could release high titers of MIF or IF II into the circulation was more resistant to intraoesophageal challenge with C. albicans than the strain (DBA/1) that did not release detectable quantities of the two lymphokines into the circulation.

In summary, the following observations have been made:

(1) in vivo release of serum-MIF and serum-IF II varies according to the genetic characteristics of the strain of mouse;

(2) subcutaneous treatment of the mouse with CFA either two weeks before or one week after intravenous sensitization with cell walls of BCG in Drakeol-Tween 80 emulsion may enhance or inhibit respectively the in vivo release of the two lymphokines;

(3) MIF and IF II seem to be released independently of three other serum-lymphokines, namely, mitogenic factor, lymphotoxin, and macrophage activating factor; and

(4) the capacity to release serum-MIF occurred in parallel with the capacity to resist intraoesophageal challenge with a sublethal dose of Candida albicans.

REFERENCES

1. Salvin, S. B., Youngner, J. S., and Lederer, W. H. "Migration inhibitory factor and interferon in the circulation of mice with delayed hypersensitivity". Infect. Immun. 7, 68 (1973).
2. Youngner, J. S. and Salvin, S. B. "Production and properties of migration inhibitory factor and inte-feron in the circulation of mice with delayed hypersensitivity". J. Immunol. 111, 1914 (1973).
3. Salvin, S. B., Ribi, E., Granger, D. L., and Youngner, J. S. "Migration inhibitory factor and Type II interferon in the circulation of mice sensitized with mycobacterial components". J. Immunol. 11e, 354 (1975).
4. Salvin, S. B. and Nishio, J. "In vitro cell reactions in delayed hypersensitivity". J. Immunol. 103, 138 (1969).
5. Neta, R. and Salvin, S. B. "Adjuvants in the induction of suppressor cells". Infect. Immun. 23, 360 (1979).

DISCUSSION

YOSHIDA: At what point after the i.v. OT (or CFA) challenge were the strain differences in lymphokine production in vivo compared?

SALVIN: The intravenous challenge was made with OT, never with complete Freund's adjuvant (CFA). Blood samples were taken 2 - 4 hours after this challenge and the sera assayed for lymphokines such as MIF and LT. The response of various strains of mice was explored in this way.

Our assay was based on the detection of enzymes in macrophages by the nitrobluetetrazolium test (NBT). Test sera were incubated with normal macrophages, NBT added, and the percentage of macrophages demonstrating blue granules determined.

PICK: Why did Salvin use oesophageal challenge to test for resistance to Candida? It seems rather unlikely that the gastrointestinal tract would be the best place to test for the role of CMI (and MIF) in resistance to infection.

SALVIN: Many Candida infections in man and mice start in the intestinal tract, where the fungus is usually present and becomes invasive under conditions of altered immunologic environment.

WAKSMAN: I might comment on Pick's question. Cell-mediated immunity is well expressed at the level of the mucosa. Sensitized lymphocytes which pass through the epithelium have been shown to respond to antigen with production of LK, including MIF, by a number of authors.

KIRCHNER: Interferon type I induction by viruses is under strict genetic control (de Maeyer). Has Salvin performed a genetic analysis in regard to type II interferon?

SALVIN: We are now carrying out such an analysis.

VILCEK: Has Salvin checked whether the interferon produced in animals has properties of type II interferon?

SALVIN: The interferon produced under our experimental conditions is type II in that it is heat stable.

VILCEK: Has Salvin tried to establish organ cultures from the animals after challenge, to determine the source of lymphokines?

SALVIN: This has not yet been done.

DAVID: Can Salvin transfer resistance to Candida by passive transfer of sera containing MIF and other lymphokines?

SALVIN: This has been done, and a limited degree of resistance was detected (by quantitative organ culture).

ZSCHIESCHE: Can Salvin tell us something about the kinetics of the four lymphokines studied. Are they similar or different?

SALVIN: In our studies thus far, MAF is produced at an earlier time (one hour) and persists longer (up to 24 hours after challenge) than MIF, LT or mitogenic factor, which produce maximum titers for only a brief period, i. e. about 2 - 4 hours post-challenge.

YOSHIDA: Does the appearance and/or disappearance of circulating interferon activity correlate in any way with the skin reactivity (or any other DTH expression) in the treated mice?

SALVIN: In reply to Yoshida we have carried out studies on the kinetics of lymphokine production and have determined at what times after OT intravenous challenge peak responses of several lymphokines have occurred. Since most of the lymphokines were released in maximum quantities 2 - 4 hours after challenge, this interval was utilized to compare strain differences rather than correlating any lymphokine presence or titer with DTH.

STUDIES ON DESENSITIZATION FACTORS: SUPPRESSIVE EFFECTS ON LYMPHOKINE PRODUCTION[1]

Takeshi Yoshida[2]
Toru Baba
Matsunobu Suko
Stanley Cohen

Department of Pathology
University of Connecticut Health Center
Farmington, Connecticut 06032
U.S.A.

Desensitization is defined as the suppression of a pre-existing delayed type hypersensitivity (DTH) state by the systemic administration of a large dose of homologous antigen. The unresponsiveness achieved by this treatment is usually antigen-nonspecific in contrast to the antigen-specific suppression observed in case of the immediate type hypersensitivity. In spite of potential importance of this phenomenon, for example as a experimental model for clinical anergy state, various biological reactions associated with the desensitization have never been fully investigated, and its underlying mechanism is still unclear (1-3). The present study has revealed that the desensitization of DTH manifests itself in at least three separable stages, each of which may be mediated by different soluble factors and/or cells.

Hartley guinea pigs were immunized with a combination of at least two unrelated antigens (100 μg each) in Freund's complete adjuvant(CFA). These antigens include egg albumin (EA), keyholelimpet hemocyanin (KLH), bovine gamma globulin (BGG), dinitrophenylated (DNP)-EA, DNP-KLH, DNP-BGG, and BGG-anti-BGG immune complex. The desensitization was achieved by an intravenous injection of one of immunizing antigen at the dose of

[1]*This study was supported by a NIH grant, AI-12225*
[2]*Recipient of PHS Research Career Development Award AI00082*

ISBN 0-12-213950-X

5 mg. Skin reactive factor (SRF) utilized in the present experiments was prepared as described previously (4). Briefly, the lymphocytes obtained from guinea pigs immunized with 100 μg of DNP-EA were cultured with 50 μg/ml of DNP-EA for 24 hrs. The culture supernatant was concentrated and fractionated by a Sephadex G-100 column chromatography. The active fraction was tested with the corresponding control fraction obtained similarly from the unstimulated culture supernatant. Skin reactions by SRF were observed at 4-6 hours after the intracutaneous injection. Skin reactions by antigens in immunized animals were examined by injecting 20 μg of them and recorded at 3 hours (for Arthus type) and 24 hours later.

During the first 24 to 36 hours (the first stage) after the systemic injection of an antigen into guinea pigs immunized with multiple antigens in CFA, a general suppression in various skin reactivities was observed. Thus, the reactions to SRF, histamine, compound 48/80, and passive cutaneous anaphylaxis, were all inhibited as well as the DTH skin reactions induced by antigens both specific and non-specific in relation to the desensitizing antigen. The strongest suppression was usually observed at 12 to 24 hours after the antigenic challenge. This time course is consistent with the appearance of the macrophage migration inhibitory factor (MIF) activity in the circulation as shown previously(5). In addition, the present study has revealed that macrophages and polymorphonuclear cells obtained from those animals are deficient in their ability to respond for chemotactic stimuli. Furthermore, this general suppression of skin reactivity was shown to be reversed by the intravenous injection of 1.0 ml of 1.0 M of α-L-fucose at the time of desensitization. This indicates that the suppression observed may be lymphokine-dependent. A more direct evidence was obtained by the systemic injection of MIF-rich supernatant into normal guinea pigs. As shown in Table I, vascular permeability increases induced by either SRF, PCA, or compound 48/80 were significantly reduced when 15 ml of MIF-rich supernatant was injected intraperitoneally in normal guinea pigs.

TABLE I. Suppression of Vascular Permeability by Intravenous Injection of Lymphokines

I.P. Injection	*SRF*	*PCA*	*Compound 48/80*
15 ml of MIF Sup.	*18.4± 3.0*[a]	*51.8± 13.2*	*34.8± 6.5*
15 ml of Control Sup.	*10.7± 2.1*	*22.9± 3.9*	*23.0± 6.2*

[a] *Mean ± S.D. of the amount of Pontamin sky blue (μg) recovered from the skin reaction sites according to the method by Nitta et al (6).*

These results clearly indicate the significance of the circulating lymphokines (e.g. MIF) during the first stage of the desensitization of the DTH.

In the second stage of the desensitization, occurring between 36 and 72 hours after the antigenic challenge, the delayed type skin reactions to both specific and non-specific antigens remained suppressed, while the other skin reactivities returned to normal. Since the reaction to SRF is normal while the DTH reactions are suppressed, it is most likely that a certain suppressive factor(s) is present in the circulation to inhibit the lymphokine production. In fact, the sera obtained from guinea pigs desensitized 1 to 4 days previously were found to contain a soluble factor which could block the production of MIF by immune lymphocytes stimulated with a specific antigen. Table II summarizes these results.

TABLE II. Effect of Serum from Desensitized Animals on the MIF Production In Vitro.

Serum Source[a]	*Days After Desensitization*[b]				
	1	*2*	*4*	*5*	*7*
Immunized	*55.7*[c]	*76.5*	*58.9*	*69.7*	*68.5*
Desensitized	*<u>99.5</u>*	*<u>88.8</u>*	*<u>81.5</u>*	*68.4*	*60.2*
Normal	*71.3*	*79.5*	*66.2*	*72.5*	*64.3*

[a] *Lymph node cells from animals immunized with DNP-EA in CFA were cultured with 50 μg/ml of DNP-EA in the presence of the testing serum.*

[b] *Immunized animals were desensitized on the 7th day of the immunization. Corresponding control or normal serum was obtained on the same day when the desensitized serum was collected. Therefore, control serum for the 1 day after the desensitization means the serum on the 8th day of the immunization.*

[c] *% migration index. Significantly suppressed reactions are underlined.*

These results seem to indicate a regulatory mechanism, where a lymphokine itself or the secondary products induced by the lymphokines may inhibit the further production of these soluble mediators. To test this hypothesis, the <u>in vitro</u> MIF production system was again utilized. First, we have produced MIF-rich and control supernatants by stimulating lymphocytes obtained from guinea pigs immunized with DNP-KLH in CFA. The lymphocytes obtained from the animals immunized with DNP-EA in CFA were incubated with these MIF-rich or control supernatant for 24 hours. After washing the cells, they were then cultured with 50μg/ml of DNP-EA for 24 hours. Control supernatant-treated as well as untreated lymphocytes could produce comparable amount of MIF(Migration Index or MI were 73.5 and 75.2). The MIF-treated lymphocytes, on the other hand, were not able to produce a significant amount of MIF (MI:90.9). As shown in our previous studies on monocyte disappearance phenomenon (5,7), monocytes and/or macrophages are definitely affected by the presence of the circulating MIF. This consideration has prompted us to examine if the macrophages treated by MIF can inhibit the production of MIF by stimulated lymphocytes. Macrophage monolayer cultures were established by removing non-adherent cells after 3 hours of incubation of peritoneal exudate cells in tissue culture dishes. They were then incubated with either MIF-rich or control supernatant obtained from DNP-KLH immune lymphocytes. The lymphocytes from DNP-EA-immune guinea pigs were added to these dishes and cultured with or without 50μg/ml of DNP-EA. As a result, the lymphocytes cultured with the MIF-treated macrophages could not produce MIF (MI: 88.7%), while the lymphocytes cultured with control macrophages, either untreated or control supernatant-treated, were able to generate significant amounts of MIF (MI: 63.5,& 60.3 respectively). The next obvious question is whether or not the suppression achieved by the MIF-treated macrophages is mediated by any soluble factor. To test this possibility, we have incubated macrophages with MIF-rich or control supernatant for 24 hours. The cells were washed by gently flushing them with fresh medium and cultured in fresh medium for another 24 hours. The cell-free supernatants were obtained from each culture and tested for their activity on lymphokine production. The immune lymphocytes when cultured in the supernatant obtained from MIF-treated macrophages were only able to generate significantly lower amount of MIF than the MIF activity found when the cells were cultured in the supernatant obtained from control-treated macrophages. This results clearly indicated that the MIF-treated macrophages are able to release a suppressive factor for MIF production by antigen-stimulated lymphocytes.

The data from these in vitro studies together with those from previous in vivo experiments may suggest strongly that the second stage of the desensitization in vivo of DTH may be mediated by a suppressive factor released from monocytes or macrophages activated by the circulating MIF.

After the 72 hours of the desensitization (the third stage), the only reaction that remains suppressed is the DTH to the specific antigen which is used for the desensitization. This suppression usually continues for at least 7 days. Mechanisms regulating this stage of the desensitization state are still unknown.

In summary, the data presented here suggest a new aspect of

the in vivo lymphokine activity, especially the significance of the systemic or circulating lymphokines. This is also the first report, as far as we know, describing that the production of lymphokines by immune T cells is regulated by a soluble factor(s). Together with MIFIF found as a regulator for B-cell MIF production (8), the suppressive factors described here may play important roles in the patho-physiological regulations of the efferent limb of the delayed type hypersensitivity.

REFERENCES

1. Dwyer,J.M. and Kantor,F.S. (1973). *J.Exp.Med. 137*,32.
2. Sonozaki,H., Papermaster,V.,Yoshida,T., and Cohen,S.(1975). *J.Immunol. 115*,1657.
3. Papermaster,V., Yoshida,T.,and Cohen,S.(1978). *Cell.Immunol. 35*, 378.
4. Yoshida,T.,Nagai,R.,and Hashimoto,T.(1973). *Lab.Invest. 29*, 329.
5. Yoshida,T.,and Cohen,S.(1974). *J.Immunol. 112*, 1540.
6. Nitta,R.,Hayashi,H., and Norimatsu,K. (1963). *Proc.Soc. Exptl.Biol.Med. 113*, 185.
7. Yoshida,T.,Benacerraf,B.,McCluskey,R.,and Vassalli,P.(1969). *J.Immunol. 102*, 804.
8. Cohen,S.and Yoshida,T. (1977). *J.Immunol. 119*, 719.

DISCUSSION

HADDEN: Many experiments indicate that prostaglandin production by macrophages is an important negative regulatory mechanism. I wonder what is the effect of indomethacin on the phenomena Yoshida described.

YOSHIDA: We have not tested that yet. By preliminary characterization studies, however, the substance generated from macrophages seems to be large in size (more than 20,000 daltons) and non-dialyzable, excluding the possibility of some compound of the prostaglandin series.

DE WECK: Do the animals sensitized also show anaphylaxis upon i.v. administration of antigen?

YOSHIDA: On the 7th day of immunization the animals were desensitized by 5 mg of one of the protein antigens mentioned. Under these conditions no anaphylaxis was observed, although a certain amount of circulating antibody was present. To minimize the participation of antibody, we immunized by injecting the antigen-antibody complex (e. g. BSA - anti-BSA complex made in antibody excess) with complete Freund's adjuvant into footpads or intramuscularly. When such guinea pigs were challenged i.v. with BSA, no anaphylaxis, rather desensitization of DTH was observed.

THE ARTIFICIAL GRANULOMA. II. INDUCTION OF PULMONARY GRANULOMA FORMATION BY EXOGENOUS, CIRCULATING AND LOCALIZED GRANULOMA-DERIVED LYMPHOKINES.[1]

Dov L. Boros
Lee Carrick, Jr.

Department of Immunology and Microbiology
Wayne State University School of Medicine
Detroit, Michigan

I. INTRODUCTION

There is a dearth of information on the *in vivo* role of inflammatory lymphokines in cell-mediated tissue reactions. Delayed skin reaction sites yielded chemotactic factors (1), explanted, chronically inflamed synovial tissue (2) and isolated schistosome egg granulomas (3) secreted *in vitro* MIF-active substances. Overt lymphokine production was also found in patients with sarcoidosis (4). Here, we present evidence that granuloma-produced lymphokines are involved in the initiation of the pulmonary granulomatous reaction.

II. MATERIALS AND METHODS

Female, CBA/J mice, 20–22 g were sensitized s.c. with 200 μg methylated bovine serum albumin (MeBSA) in complete adjuvant. Ten days later, state of delayed hypersensitivity was verified by positive footpad swelling. Mice were then challenged i.v. with 6000 Sepharose beads (50μ) covalently coupled with MeBSA. At 7 days the diameter of artificial granulomas, measured in stained lung sections, was: 154μ. Seven-day-old granulomas were isolated from the lungs of 40 mice by gentle homogenization. Lesions were cultured in RPMI-1640 without

[1]*Supported by NIH grants HL-19732 and HL-20104.*

ISBN 0-12-213950-X

serum, with 1 μg/ml of MeBSA. Supernatants were collected, concentrated, dialyzed and lyophilized. The antigen was removed by a QAE-Sephadex column, and the eluted samples were tested for MIF (capillary migration) and chemotactic activity (Boyden chamber). Supernatants were administered in untreated or heated (80°C, 60 min) form 1) intratracheally, 2) enclosed into osmotic minipumps (Alza, CA) and implanted i.p., 3) covalently bound to Sepharose beads. Mice given liquid lymphokines received i.v. beads, to provide a nidus for granuloma formation. At intervals after bead injections groups of 6-8 mice were sacrificed, their lungs fixed and processed. Granuloma diameters were measured in stained sections.

III. RESULTS

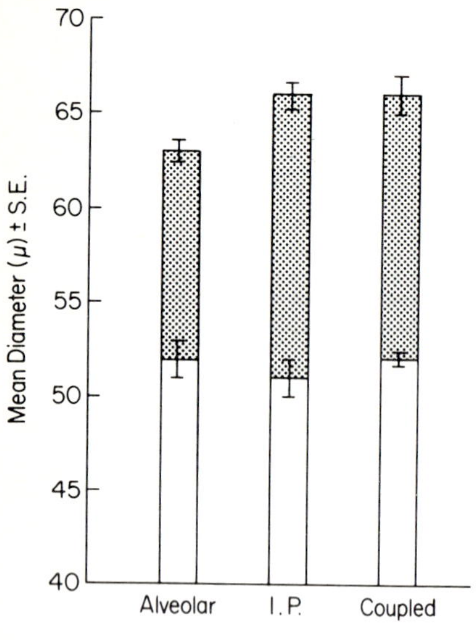

FIGURE 1. Granuloma induction by systemic or localized lymphokine.

Supernatants collected after 24 (24 sup) and 48 hr (48 sup) incubation were tested for lymphokine activity. At the range of 1-5 μg dry weight, 24hr sup showed strong macrophage migration inhibitory activity (48.7%) and chemotactic effect; 97.8% (compared with casein-induced control - 100%). In a similar range 48 hr sup showed an MMI of 43.4% but no chemotactic activity. Heat treatment abolished lymphokine activity. The 24 hr sup was administered to normal mice with i.v. injected beads which embolized the pulmonary microvasculature. Granuloma sizes measured at 96 hr are shown in Fig. 1. Deposited onto the alveoli in liquid or bead-bound form, or released at the rate of 1 μl/hr from the minipumps, lymphokine active sup (stippled bar) induced a significantly ($p<0.05$) larger mononuclear aggregation than the heated material (open bar). Histologically the beads were surrounded by layers of young mononuclear cells; many larger vessels showed cuffing. The kinetics of the granulomatous response is shown below. At 24 hr after bead injection and 40 hr after the start of lymphokine release, practically no reaction was seen around the beads.

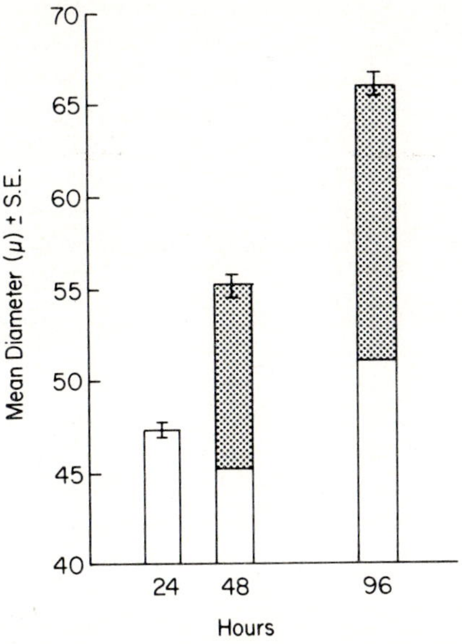

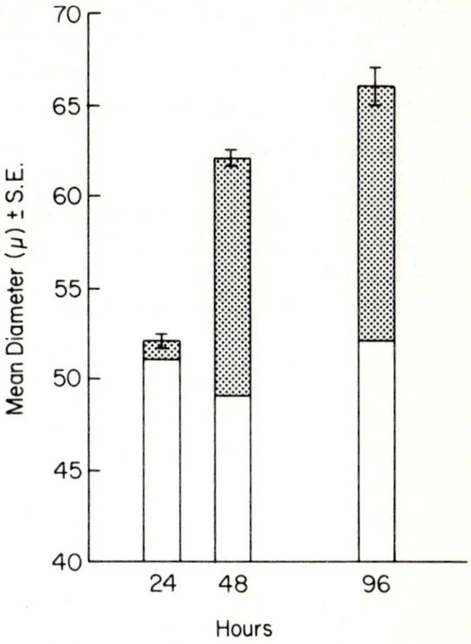

Kinetics of Granuloma Induction

FIGURE 2. Systemic lymphokine effect. (Minipump)

FIGURE 3. Localized lymphokine effect. (Coupled)

By 48 hr granulomas increased in size, and the reaction peaked at 96 hrs. Heated lymphokine induced sparse mononuclear infiltration (Fig. 2). Lymphokines administered in a bead-bound form induced a faster evolution of the lesions (Fig. 3). The 48 sup (bead-bound) induced a slower pace of granuloma development. Mean diameters (μ): 48 hr = 48 ± 2; 96 hr = 62 ± 3; 144 hr = 46 ± 3. Supernatant (24h) from bare bead-induced, foreign body lung granulomas had no MIF activity. In a bead-bound form it induced no reaction. (Mean diameter: 96 hr = 48 ± 1).

REFERENCES

1. Cohen, S., Ward, P.A., Yoshida, T., and Burek, C.L. (1973) *Cell. Immunol. 9*, 363.
2. Stastny, P., Rosenthal, M., Andreis, M., Cooke, D., and Ziff, M. (1975) *Ann. N.Y. Acad. Sci. 256*, 117.
3. Boros, D.L., Warren, K.S., and Pelley, R.P. (1973) *Nature 246*, 224.
4. Kataria, Y.P., LoBuglio, A.F., and Bromberg, P.A. (1976) *Amer. Rev. Resp. Dis. 113*, 315.

DISCUSSION

WAKSMAN: I compliment Boros on a significant simplification in a biologically important area. This is most elegant work. Is he looking also at the contributions to granuloma formation of the LK designated macrophage aggregation factor and macrophage fusion factor, discussed by Galindo a few years ago? It seems to me that he is under an obligation to study these, the more so as he began his presentation with a picture of a granuloma containing a giant cell, whose formation presumably depends on "MFF".

BOROS: I quite agree with Waksman. Though Galindo et al. described their macrophage fusion factor in the Mycobacterium model, it is more than likely that such a factor would also be produced by the artificial granuloma. Whereas presently we are preoccupied with the effects of chemotactic and MIF-active substances, we hope to move on to explore the presence and activity of additional lymphokines such as agglutination and fusion factors.

HADDEN: I would like to respond to Waksman's query about the macrophage fusion factor (MFF). We have confirmed the Galindo and Myrvik observations using more conventional protocols for MIF production with bovine gamma globulin. The factor produced in the rabbit elutes from sephadex G100 between 20 - 70,000 daltons and fuses both oil induced peritoneal and alveolar macrophages. In the guinea pig the phenomenon is variable and restricted to alveolar macrophages and to high concentration of lymphokine. Preliminary studies indicate that MFF, MIF and MMF/MGF are distinct.

WOOD: How does Boros explain the response of cells to the granule-bound lymphokine when the cell is physically separated from the bead surface? Is a granuloma formed at the mouth of the implanted micropump releasing lymphokines?

BOROS: There is no ready answer to Wood's question. Indeed we are baffled regarding the mode of action of the bead-bound lymphokine. Various possibilities include: (1) The lymphokine is slowly released from the bead, despite being covalently bound. (2) The lymphokine in its bound form interacts with blood and/or tissue components which release additional chemotactic etc. agents. (3) The recruited macrophages themselves may release additional chemotactic substances. The phenomenon is all the more noteworthy, since macrophages are visible in the alveolar spaces remote from the granulomatous foci.

In response to Wood's second question, the minipumps in the peritoneum are not surrounded either by granulomatous or fibrotic tissues.

PICK: Does Boros know which is the actual cell producing lymphokine in his lung granulomas? Obviously it could be a lymphocyte, but there are alternative possibilities.

BOROS: We have only circumstantial evidence for the origin of the lymphokine. First, the spleen cells of the granuloma-bearing mice *do* secrete MIF when specifically stimulated. Second, the foreign body granuloma which contains macrophages and fibroblasts does not secrete MIF. Hence the possibility that the lymphokine originates from fibroblasts as described by Feldman years ago, or less likely by macrophages. Obviously, final proof will require isolating the lymphocytes from dispersed granulomas and testing them for lymphokine activity. However, this poses a formidable technical difficulty because of the low yield of granuloma lymphocytes.

YOSHIDA: Masih and I have also found MIF and macrophage chemotactic factor (MCF) in the extracts of hypersensitivity lung granulomas (Masih and Yoshida, Am. J. Pathol. 95:381, 1979). In this guinea pig model, MIF was recovered mainly in the early phase of granuloma formation but not later on. MCF activity was only found sporadically.

BOROS: In our model, peak MIF activity from the lesions is detectable at 7 days, when the granuloma is at its full size. By the second week lymphokine production in the lesions has dropped significantly. These observations were made on MIF activity. We have no data on the presence of chemotactic lymphokine, beyond that of the first 7 days.

LOHMANN-MATTHES: Boros mentioned twice that the macrophages surrounding his beads were young macrophages. Was that statement derived from the literature or had he actually determined the age of these macrophages?

BOROS: We have not carried out any systematic delineation of the age and maturity of the macrophages surrounding the beads. There was a conspicuous absence of epithelioid cells and giant cells in such lesions. The staging of the lymphokine-induced granuloma macrophage was based on the description by Adams (Am. J. Pathol.) for the Mycobacterium-induced granuloma.

DAVID: Has Boros coupled lymphokines from other sources - say lymph node or spleen - to beads? This would allow him to do an important control, namely coupling the supernatant from *non*-stimulated sensitive lymphocytes free of MIF.

BOROS: Not yet. We were pleased to show at the first phase that substances obtained from the foreign-body granuloma, were incapable of generating a significant cellular reaction. David's suggestion is a most important control. The next phase will consist of experiments in which normal and antigen-stimulated spleen cell supernates will be examined in parallel for the elicitation of the granulomatous response.

COMMENT ON IN VIVO EFFECTS OF LYMPHOCYTE CULTURE SUPERNATES

PAPERMASTER: We have been studying the effects of crude lymphokine preparations injected intralesionally into tumors of patients and into skin sites of tumor-bearing animals to ascertain their therapeutic potential.

Our experimental model utilized the effect of intralesionally injected crude preparations from the human cell line RPMI 1788 in DBA mice growing subcutaneously inoculated tumors of the L 1210 type. The animals were challenged with 10^5 cells and inoculated on a ventral site. We followed the development of tumor size, morphology, metastasis and the survival curve. There is a highly significant difference between lymphokine-treated and control mice. At the beginning of the treatment (injection at 48 hour intervals) there is a slight increase in size of tumor followed by tumor shrinkage, eventual necrosis and sloughing of the lesions. Sometimes regrowth and even occasional metastasis occurs. In this particular tumor, metastasis can be followed at the single cell level, even in the spleen. Animals treated by local intra-tumor injection showed a highly significant increased survival with between 30 - 40 % of the animals surviving indefinitely. This is not viewed as a realistic tumor model, but rather an assay system of interest for evaluating the antitumor action of culture supernatants.

In patients, intracutaneous inoculation of the crude supernates causes a rather typical dermal lesion, showing a PMN and monocytic infiltrate, peak size at about 12 hours, and very similar to that described in the guinea pig years ago by Cohen and Yoshida. As candidates for local lymphokine therapy, patients with breast cancer and extensive local metastasis, resistant to Cytoxan, prednisone and 5-fluorouracil, have been used. Biopsies of locally injected lesions following the first inflammatory phase show centralized necrosis in healing lesions, remnants of inflammation, hemosiderin deposits and often a complete disappearance of tumor cells. In about 30 lesions treated, improvement or complete disappearance of tumor cells was observed by biopsy in about 50 % of the lesions treated, none of the non-treated control lesions showed these changes. In a subsequent study with Hersh on about 20 melanoma patients treated with similar preparations there was likewise a significant reduction in tumor size and in some cases complete disappearance of melanotic lesions within 48 hours.

ISBN 0-12-213950-X

SUMMING UP AND CONCLUDING REMARKS

COHEN S.: In seeking to look into the future by way of the past and present, it is appropriate to recall that one of the major themes of the First Lymphokine Workshop involved biologic generality. Lymphokines were recognized as having biologic activities similar to those of other mediator systems, such as the complement cascade, for example. Also, it was pointed out at that time that many different cell types could elaborate lymphokines. It was demonstrated that interferon had lymphokine-like properties and that lymphokines had interferon-like properties. Certain aspects of lymphokine-cell membrane interaction were found to be similar for several different factors. Many examples were given to show that the lymphocyte-derived mediators fit comfortably into the framework provided by the modern emphasis on the role of intercellular and intracellular signals in recognition, activation, and interaction phenomena.

One of the themes that seems to have emerged from the present meeting involves chemical generality. Here the magic words are *subunits* and *precursors*. There are hints from several laboratories as to subunit structure for at least MIF and LT, and perhaps other mediators as well. Some of the subunits may serve as precursors, or, alternatively, precursors may require cleavage for the expression of activity. We have heard that different pieces of the same lymphokine can have different properties, thus defining a kind of intramolecular heterogeneity. Examples of this can be found in some studies of MAF and TMIF. We have also heard that a given factor may have different biologic properties as a function of the assay system used to detect it (a kind of biological Heisenberg uncertainty principle). This appears to be the case for Type I interferon, and an even better defined synthetic tripeptide as well. Other themes of this meeting related to mechanisms of action of lymphokines and regulation and control of mediator activity. In these cases, also, there appear to be general principles and general physicochemical properties that hold for at least some of the mediators studied thus far.

It has also become apparent that the tools for future analysis of these various issues are either at hand or close to hand. Traditional physico-chemical procedures are yielding mediators of even greater purity. Several of us have provided, almost simultaneously, procedures for preparing antibody to and against LT. Hybridoma techniques give promise of ample quantities of better defined, monospecific antisera, useful not only

ISBN 0-12-213950-X

for purification and characterization studies, but also for studies of mechanism.

Thus, a number of interesting questions are now becoming answerable. I have listed some, not in any particular order, to point out some of the directions in which I sense lymphokine research will be directed.

1. What are the restrictions on the subpopulations of cell that can make lymphokines?
2. Is any given cell limited to the production of only a single lymphokine?
3. How many different lymphokines are there? There is already evidence that the actual number of distinct entities is far less than the 96 activities that have been cataloged. The concept of the "Mother Factors", a minimal set of lymphokine building blocks may prove to have some unifying value.
4. What is the nature of the initial interaction of mediator and target? Is there a finite period in which membrane binding can be demonstrated? Much of the data presently available is difficult to interpret because of sensitivity limitations. Is internalization of the mediator a requisite for the expression of activity? Is there a secondary signal inside the cell, and if so, what does it signal, and how?
5. How many molecules of mediator are necessary to activate a cell? We have heard that for interferon, the number may be one, a single molecule.

In this context, I consider it essential to emphasize that it *is* possible to do important and useful experiments with impure reagents, and it is moreover possible to comprehend mechanisms prior to an understanding of underlying chemistry. A little divine inspiration is all that is necessary.

A final set of questions that I think will be answered in the near future relate to regulation and control of lymphokine activity. Here it is important to distinguish between control at the level of lymphokine *production* and control at the level of *expression of activity.* As has been indicated, lymphokines can exert self-control, not only through feedback inhibition and suppressor mechanisms, but also by blocking the expression of their own activity. The latter can occur via pre-emption mechanisms as well as by the abolition of essential gradients.

Finally, I feel that we can confidently expect clinical applications, not only by the use of lymphokines for their phlogistic and cytotoxic effects, but especially by the use of well-defined anti-lymphokine antisera for more specific modes of immunosuppression than are currently available. New and improved assays will also facilitate lymphokine detection for prognostic and diagnostic purposes.

The past few years have convinced us that what we are studying is biologically relevant. The sense that emerges from the present meeting is that there is an underlying order to the whole field. The task ahead of us is to make that order visible and comprehensible.

PICK: These three days of extensive reporting, lively discussions, some controversy, and many private exchanges while strolling the garden paths of charming Schloss Wolfsberg have imprinted on my mind seven "messages" which not only accompany me on my return home but may well condition my own investigative outlook.

1. One of the most impressive messages is the fact that researchers working on interferon were so remarkably successful. I think the reasons for this are several, and classical lymphokinologists should note them well. In my opinion, the reasons for success were: a) persistence - as expressed by the belief that twenty years spent researching one subject is not too much; b) monomania - we would have been more successful had we expressed such "monomaniacal" behaviour; c) the belief that they were purifying a material which is not only interesting but also patently useful, and d) the fact that most of the work was done by people who were not immunologists by training (I am exempting from this stricture those few illustrious immunologists who did indeed contribute significantly to understanding interferon).

2. The second message is that the frequently heard apology that progress in investigating lymphokines is difficult because of poor assay techniques, does not stand up to criticism. The interferon assay is not that much better than many of the assays commonly used to quantitate lymphokines. Moreover, some thymic hormones have been isolated, sequenced and even synthesized despite rather poor assays.

3. A third message is that mediators are getting smaller and smaller. I think that this is a healthy trend since what we ultimately want are small peptides, (hopefully of few aminoacids) which constitute the active sites of lymphokines. To draw a parallel with immunoglobulins, we heard

too little about Fab and perhaps too much about Fc, at this meeting. An encouraging sign is the ever increasing use of separation under denaturing conditions. Urea, guanidine HCl, SDS, trichloracetic acid and high salt concentrations are proving friendlier than we had thought.

4. The fourth message is that even a very small mediator molecule, such as acetylcholine or histamine, can do more than one thing. Acetylcholine can activate a muscarinic or a nicotinic type of response depending on the existence of the corresponding receptors on the target cells and the same is true for histamine interacting with either H1 or H2 receptors. A similar multiplicity of biological effects is evident for complement components, some of which have been found to act as chemotactic attractants, histamine releasers and cytotoxic agents, depending on the nature of the target cell. We should also learn from complementologists that, as opposed to what is so frequently stated, the part can at times be as important as the whole.

5. The fifth message is that considerable information can be gained from the study of simple compounds mimicking lymphokine action. I refer not only to phorbol myristate acetate and the ionophore A23187, but mostly to the exciting studies performed with the chemotactic peptides of the formylmethionyl group and to those performed with tuftsin. I was surprised by the absence at this meeting of communications dealing with chemotactic lymphokines. I would like to remind the distinguished representatives of inflammatory lymphokines that a macrophage can be activated only if it has arrived on the scene.

6. There appears to be an unfortunate lack of concern, which became evident at this workshop, in the matter of bacterial and fungal contamination of culture supernatants, and especially with column eluates. I refer not only to the possibility of contamination with ubiquitous endotoxin but to other bacterial products as well. It is known, for instance, that staphylococcal toxins can act as both lymphokine inducers and lymphokine-mimicking agents. Too often the view prevails that these are simply and solely biochemical operations. Not so! It is essential to take appropriate precautions, to perform simple sterility tests on all lymphokine preparations and to include these in our written and oral reporting. It is unthinkable that the lymphokine community should work under conditions which would not be tolerated by the pharmaceutical industry in the production of eye drops.

7. The seventh and final message refers to the conspicuous lack of interest of macrophage activation enthusiasts in the actual mechanisms of target cell killing. This is somewhat similar to the dislike of meat-eaters to visit slaughterhouses. I do not think that such an issue will ever be resolved by electron microscopy.
   It has been reported somewhere in the Middle East, but not yet confirmed, that one day all of us will have to account for our deeds in front of someone who could best be described as an Unbiased Observer. That day, the macrophage activation expert will be asked: Why did you not investigate the reason for the heightened susceptibility of tumor cells to lymphokine-activated macrophages?

DIENER: Occasionally, philosophers on theories of scientific discovery have some useful comments for experimentalists; one that is brought to mind by this meeting is that because all horses have ears, not all animals having ears are horses. By analogy, 23 different investigators reporting the same molecular weight for a lymphokine which was assayed in 23 different ways are not necessarily dealing with the same molecule. While the biochemical and biophysical characterization of biologically active agents is a necessity, it must take its proper place within the hierarchy of experimental procedures, if confusion is to be avoided. I shall briefly outline what I mean by this. The first point to be considered when characterizing a putative lymphokine is its source of production and site of action. The difficulty of having to place a factor-mediated phenomenon within a conceptual framework is greatest when the source of factor is uncertain and its action is directed at more than one cell type. Such functional pleiotropy points to the presence of either a multifactorial system or an artifact. It is thus imperative to determine the physiological significance of the particular test system. Systems for which this has successfully been done include interferon, MIF and the T cell-derived helper factors that have all been shown to function in vivo. In vivo verification is still required for many of the systems that have nevertheless served as excellent tools in the ontogenic analysis of their target cells. The outstanding examples here are colony stimulating factors in the analysis of cell differentiation as well as lymphoproliferative factors derived from various sources of feeder layers.

The next consideration in the sequence of investigative steps is the necessity of associating functional markers with the lymphokine in question. In this respect, T cell-derived helper factors are particularly good examples. We know of three functional markers at present: antigen recognition, triggering specificity for a defined cell class and somewhat less certain, allogeneic restriction of the factor-target interaction.

The third point concerns serological markers. It became evident during the meeting that the availability of antibodies against a given factor offers an enormous advantage, notably when such antibody can be continuously obtained in large amounts. The monoclonal antibodies to osteoclast-activating factor serve here as an example. The strategy of factor-specific antibodies utilized in verifying the physiological action of a factor cannot be overemphasized. We need only to recall the demonstration that anti-MIF antibody blocks GVH.

My final criterion within the hierarchy of investigative procedures in factor analysis would be the biochemical markers. We have elaborated sufficiently on these markers in the course of our meeting to realize their advantages and shortcomings. Again, it has been demonstrated that antibody affinity chromatography is one of the most powerful tools for obtaining pure material from crude supernatants. Another necessity is to obtain large quantities of factor from factor-producing cells. Lymphokine-producing lymphoblastoid cell lines and feeder layers may help in such mass production as well as in the cloning of factor-producing cellular elements. For the future, we envision even more sophisticated technologies such as recombinant DNA techniques and cell-free synthesis of factors (such as interferon) or their biologically active fragments.

MAYER: I have been interested in kinetic methods of studying biological phenomena for a long time, so I could not resist the temptation to draw a kinetic curve of the interest and results obtained in the lymphokine field. There has been an appreciable increase in the slope of this curve during the 1970's, and I have a feeling that this increase in slope will continue and that we are entering into a logarithmic phase in this field.

As you know, much of my attention has been directed to the technical aspects of the subject since I feel that much can be gained by improving the technology. There has been a great deal of progress in assay methods and in physico-chemical characterization since the first Workshop at Bethesda. It is now quite clear that we have multiple molecular species with the same biological activity and, conversely, that in some cases the same molecular species may exhibit multiple activities. I would put emphasis on four items that will help us make progress. The first one is co-chromatography which will help resolve the question as to whether or not the same molecular species exhibits multiple activities. Secondly, the shape of the dose-response curve, which I have already mentioned several times, can teach us a great deal about the nature of the substances, besides being important in the presentation of the data. It can also give us indications about mode of action and requirements for cooperativity. There is need to pay more attention to the question of cooperativity, i. e., multiple factors cooperating with one another. That kind of information can also be obtained from careful accounting methods. By this I mean that when running a fractionation and putting in a certain number of biological units, it is very interesting to count up all the fractions and add up what one gets back. If only a very small part of the activity is recovered, a cooperative system should be suspected and, accordingly, fractions ought to be recombined and tested. Continuing the same line, I am sure all of us realize that the use of monoclonal antibodies from hybridomas will be a very powerful tool for assay purposes and for purification.

Let me now turn to the matter of functional purity. There has been much discussion about chemical purity; I would caution, however, that even highly sophisticated methods of assessing chemical purity, such as end group analysis, are sometimes not able to detect important contaminants present at low levels, e. g., 0.5 or 1 %. Even though that is very low, it can play a critical role. It has happened in the complement field: "classical" C3 (which we know now comprises C3, C5, C6, C7, C8 and C9) was prepared in highly purified form and shown to be homogenous by good physico-chemical methods and yet it contained all of those other proteins in sufficient quantities to function in a lytic sequence.

Finally, I would like to say a word about immunologic homeostasis. It is now clear that the alternative pathway of complement is a delicately poised homeostatic system. I think we will see more examples of immunologic homeostasis in studies of lymphokines. As we learn more about their mode of action and as we purify them, we will learn how to manipulate the immune system for the benefit of the host. This could be a useful approach to immunologic therapy. It will probably take a long time and may go well into the 21st century because it will require an enormous amount of biochemical work, a great deal of manpower, much faith and, of course, a lot of money. But I still draw this curve since I am convinced that it will indeed happen.

DE WECK: As the last in this small group of colleagues reflecting on the scientific record of our meeting here at Schloss Wolfsberg I would transmit some thoughts about the future rather than the immediate past, and identify some concrete steps we might take individually and jointly to improve the state of this, our chosen field. If nothing else, this conference will have made us once more acutely aware of the complexity of the subject, of a certain perhaps inevitable amount of confusion, but also of the considerable biological importance of the group of factors we have been considering.

The fact is that it has been puzzling to me to encounter, even now, immunologists who give little or no attention to lymphokines, monokines and other non antigen-specific mechanisms. For a good many immunologists, the foremost problem in immunology is the generation of a highly discriminating recognition mechanism by which differentiating lymphoid cell clones develop a highly effective memory system, similar to the grey cells of the brain. To use a medical comparison, there are a number of psychologists and psychiatrists in immunology to whom only the study of the brain seems of interest. However, as we know well, no organism functions without amplifying the brain signals, nor functions without nerves and muscles. Therefore, if someone wants to call this LK group the athletes of immunology, I have no objection. But in the course of this meeting you have shown that you are by no means "dumb" athletes.

In any case, it has become clear to most of us that the complexity and confusion we are presently experiencing in the lymphokine field has multiple origins:

1. The design of GOD (or its absent mindedness)
2. Low yields of purified materials
3. Complexity and variability of assay systems
4. A lack of standard reference preparations and monospecific antibodies with consequent precluding of the solution of our "identity problems"
5. Muddled nomenclature (more than need be!)

There are several concrete steps which can be taken to remedy this unhappy situation.

One way is to organize on a less haphazard scale cooperation between laboratories testing various activities on the same culture supernatants or fractions. Indeed such a cooperative arrangement is already under way as a common effort between several German laboratories and our group. Another positive step we could take is a more active approach to putting some order in LK nomenclature. A Nomenclature Subcommittee on Lymphokines of the IUIS does exist and has been reactivated and reorganized here at this meeting. The first aim of the Committee is to establish a list of all lymphokines and monokines described thus far and to investigate whether a consensus on nomenclature is to be achieved, at least on some of the factors which have been described. In order to do so, the Committee is ready to consider suggestions, which can be made by individuals or groups here at this meeting or colleagues elsewhere.

Another issue meriting serious consideration is an active exchange of reagents. It may be too early to organize this in an official manner. However, I cannot resist suggesting two new potentially helpful acronyms, namely ALHC (Anti-Lymphokine Hybridoma Club) and CLSES (Cell Line Supernatant Exchange System). If we succeed in increasing exchanges of this kind, it is almost certain that many of the noxious identity problems which have so provoked us during this meeting will be resolved by 1982, the date for the Third Lymphokine Workshop (which Stanley Cohen as chief organizer). It is to be hoped that by that time the expanding and proliferative phase in the number of factors and lymphokines to be considered will have given way to a shrinking process, in which some factors discussed here will have been shown by a combination of biological, biochemical, immunochemical and possibly structural criteria to be identical. This should not only facilitate our daily investigative life but also that of Stanley Cohen in organizing a somewhat less crowded program than the present one.

INDEX

V